Neuromuscular Disorder

DATE DUE

Demco, Inc. 38-293

NEUROLOGY IN PRACTICE:

SERIES EDITORS: ROBERT A. GROSS, DEPARTMENT OF NEUROLOGY, UNIVERSITY OF ROCHESTER MEDICAL CENTER, ROCHESTER, NY, USA

JONATHAN W. MINK, DEPARTMENT OF NEUROLOGY, UNIVERSITY OF ROCHESTER MEDICAL CENTER, ROCHESTER, NY, USA

Neuromuscular Disorders

EDITED BY

Rabi N. Tawil, MD
Professor of Neurology
University of Rochester Medical Center
Rochester, NY, USA

Shannon Venance, MD, PhD, FRCPCP
Associate Professor of Neurology
The University of Western Ontario
London, Ontario, Canada

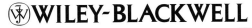

WILEY-BLACKWELL

A John Wiley & Sons, Ltd., Publication

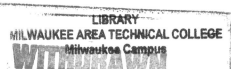

This edition first published 2011, ® 2011 by Blackwell Publishing Ltd

Blackwell Publishing was acquired by John Wiley & Sons in February 2007. Blackwell's publishing program has been merged with Wiley's global Scientific, Technical and Medical business to form Wiley-Blackwell.

Registered office: John Wiley & Sons Ltd, The Atrium, Southern Gate, Chichester, West Sussex, PO19 8SQ, UK

Editorial offices: 9600 Garsington Road, Oxford, OX4 2DQ, UK
The Atrium, Southern Gate, Chichester, West Sussex, PO19 8SQ, UK
111 River Street, Hoboken, NJ 07030-5774, USA

For details of our global editorial offices, for customer services and for information about how to apply for permission to reuse the copyright material in this book please see our website at www.wiley.com/wiley-blackwell

The right of the author to be identified as the author of this work has been asserted in accordance with the UK Copyright, Designs and Patents Act 1988.

Wiley also publishes its books in a variety of electronic formats. Some content that appears in print may not be available in electronic books.

Designations used by companies to distinguish their products are often claimed as trademarks. All brand names and product names used in this book are trade names, service marks, trademarks or registered trademarks of their respective owners. The publisher is not associated with any product or vendor mentioned in this book. This publication is designed to provide accurate and authoritative information in regard to the subject matter covered. It is sold on the understanding that the publisher is not engaged in rendering professional services. If professional advice or other expert assistance is required, the services of a competent professional should be sought.

The contents of this work are intended to further general scientific research, understanding, and discussion only and are not intended and should not be relied upon as recommending or promoting a specific method, diagnosis, or treatment by physicians for any particular patient. The publisher and the author make no representations or warranties with respect to the accuracy or completeness of the contents of this work and specifically disclaim all warranties, including without limitation any implied warranties of fitness for a particular purpose. In view of ongoing research, equipment modifications, changes in governmental regulations, and the constant flow of information relating to the use of medicines, equipment, and devices, the reader is urged to review and evaluate the information provided in the package insert or instructions for each medicine, equipment, or device for, among other things, any changes in the instructions or indication of usage and for added warnings and precautions. Readers should consult with a specialist where appropriate. The fact that an organization or Website is referred to in this work as a citation and/or a potential source of further information does not mean that the author or the publisher endorses the information the organization or Website may provide or recommendations it may make. Further, readers should be aware that Internet Websites listed in this work may have changed or disappeared between when this work was written and when it is read. No warranty may be created or extended by any promotional statements for this work. Neither the publisher nor the author shall be liable for any damages arising herefrom.

Library of Congress Cataloging-in-Publication Data
Neuromuscular disorders / edited by Rabi N. Tawil, Shannon Venance.
    p. ; cm. – (Neurology in practice)
  Includes bibliographical references and index.
  ISBN-13: 978-0-4706-5456-9 (pbk. : alk. paper)
  ISBN-10: 0-470-65456-2 (pbk. : alk. paper)
  ISBN-13: 978-1-119-97330-0 (ePDF)
  ISBN-13: 978-1-119-97333-1 (Wiley online library)
  [etc.]
  1. Neuromuscular diseases. I. Tawil, Rabi N. II. Venance, Shannon Lee,1959- III. Series: Neurology in practice.
  [DNLM: 1. Neuromuscular Diseases–diagnosis. 2. Neuromuscular Diseases–therapy. WE 550]
  RC925.5.N4733 2011
  616.7'44–dc23
                          2011014999

A catalogue record for this book is available from the British Library.

This book is published in the following electronic formats: ePDF 9781119973300; Wiley Online Library 9781119973331; ePub 9781119973317; mobi 9781119973324

Set in 8.75/11.75 pt Utopia by Toppan Best-set Premedia Limited
Printed and bound in Malaysia by Vivar Printing Sdn Bhd

1 2011

Contents

The colour plate section can be found facing page 228.

Contributor List

W. David Arnold, Department of Neurology, Division of Neuromuscular Medicine, The Ohio State University Medical Center, Columbus, OH, USA

Steven K. Baker, Department of Medicine, Physical Medicine and Neurology, Neuromuscular Disease Clinic, McMaster University Medical Center, McMaster University, Hamilton, Ontario, Canada

Nikhil Balakrishnan, Wake Forest University Baptist Medical Center, Winston Salem, NC, USA

Richard J. Barohn, Department of Neurology, University of Kansas Medical Center, Kansas City, KS, USA

James Burge, MRC Centre for Neuromuscular Diseases, and National Hospital for Neurology and Neurosurgery, UCLH FT, London, UK

Kate Bushby, Institute of Genetic Medicine, International Centre for Life, Newcastle upon Tyne, UK

Jean-Pierre Bouchard, Department of Neurological Sciences, Université Laval, CHA Hôpital Enfant-Jésus, Québec, Canada

Kristine Chapman, Division of Neurology, University of British Columbia, Vancouver, British Columbia, BC, Canada

Amy Chen, Department of Neurology, University of Rochester, Rochester, NY, USA

Emma Ciafaloni, Department of Neurology, University of Rochester, Rochester, NY, USA

Nigel Clarke, Institute for Neuroscience and Muscle Research, The Children's Hospital at Westmead, Sydney Medical School, University of Sydney, Sydney, NSW, Australia

James C. Cleland, Auckland City Hospital and University of Auckland School of Medicine, Auckland, New Zealand

Maxwell S. Damian, Cambridge University Hospitals Department of Neurology, Addenbrooke's Hospital Neurosciences Critical Care Unit, Cambridge, UK

Mazen M. Dimachkie, Neuromuscular Section, Department of Neurology, University of Kansas Medical Center, Kansas City, KS, USA

Annie Dionne, Department of Neurological Sciences, Université Laval, CHA Hôpital Enfant-Jésus, Québec, Canada

Valentina Emmanuele, Department of Neurology, Columbia University Medical Center, New York, NY, USA

Andrew G. Engel, Department of Neurology, Mayo Clinic, Rochester, MN, USA

Constantine Farmakidis, Columbia University Medical Center, Neurological Institute, New York, NY, USA

Steven A. Greenberg, Department of Neurology, Brigham and Women's Hospital and Harvard Medical School, Boston, MA, USA

Michela Guglieri, Institute of Genetic Medicine, International Centre for Life, Newcastle upon Tyne, UK

Michael G. Hanna, MRC Centre for Neuromuscular Diseases, and National Hospital for Neurology and Neurosurgery, UCLH FT, London, UK

Chad R. Heatwole, Department of Neurology, University of Rochester Medical Center, NY, USA

Michael K. Hehir, Department of Neurology, University of Rochester, Rochester, NY, USA

David N. Herrmann, Department of Neurology, University of Rochester Medical Center, Rochester, NY, USA

David Hilton-Jones, Department of Clinical Neurology, University of Oxford, and John Radcliffe Infirmary, Oxford, UK

Agnes Jani-Acsadi, Department of Neurology, Wayne State University, School of Medicine, Detroit, MI, USA

Nicholas Johnson, Department of Neurology, University of Rochester Medical Center, NY, USA

Petra Kaufmann, National Institute of Neurological Disorders and Stroke (NINDS), National Institutes of Health, Bethesda, MD, USA

Kurt Kimpinski, Department of Clinical Neurological Sciences, University Hospital and London Health Sciences Centre, University of Western Ontario, London, ON, Canada

John T. Kissel, Department of Neurology, Division of Neuromuscular Medicine, The Ohio State University Medical Center, Columbus, OH, USA

Richard A. Lewis, Department of Neurology, Wayne State University, School of Medicine, Detroit, MI, USA

Eric L. Logigian, University of Rochester Medical Center, Rochester, NY, USA

Matthew N. Meriggioli, Division of Neuromuscular Medicine, University of Illinois College of Medicine, Chicago, IL, USA

Hiroshi Mitsumoto, Eleanor and Lou Gehrig's MDA/ALS Research Center, Columbia University, New York, NY, USA

Jacqueline Montes, SMA Clinical Research Center, Department of Neurology, Columbia University, New York, NY, USA

Michael W. Nicolle, Department of Clinical Neurological Sciences, University of Western Ontario, and Myasthenia Gravis Clinic, University Hospital, London, ON, Canada

Kathryn North, Institute for Neuroscience and Muscle Research, The Children's Hospital at Westmead, Sydney Medical School, University of Sydney, Sydney, NSW, Australia

Araya Puwanant, Department of Neurology, University of Rochester Medical Center, Rochester, NY, USA

Catarina M. Quinzii, Department of Neurology, Columbia University Medical Center, New York, NY, USA

Donald B. Sanders, Duke University Medical Center, Durham, NC, USA

Amanda Sherwin, Vancouver Hospital, Vancouver, British Columbia, BC Canada

Christen Shoesmith, London Health Sciences Centre Motor Neuron Diseases Clinic, and University of Western Ontario, London, Ontario, Canada

Rabi Tawil, Neuromuscular Disease Unit, Fields Center for FSHD and Neuromuscular Research, University of Rochester Medical Center, Rochester, NY, USA

Ingrid Tein, Neurometabolic Clinic and Research Laboratory, Department of Pediatrics, Division of Neurology, and Genetics and Genome Biology Program, The Hospital for Sick Children, University of Toronto, Toronto, Ontario, Canada

Pariwat Thaisetthawatkul, Department of Neurological Sciences, University of Nebraska Medical Center, Omaha, NE, USA

Bjarne Udd, Neuromuscular Research Center, University of Tampere and Tampere University Hospital, Tampere; Folkhalsan Institute of Genetics, University of Helsinki, Helsinki; and Department of Neurology, Vasa Central Hospital, Vasa, Finland

Shannon L. Venance, Department of Clinical Neurological Sciences, University of Western Ontario, London, Canada

Matthew P. Wicklund, Department of Neurology, Penn State College of Medicine, Hershey, PA, USA

Douglas W. Zochodne, Department of Clinical Neurosciences, University of Calgary, Alberta, Canada

Acknowledgment

We wish to thank Karen Richards for her exceptional organizational skills and her tireless effort in keeping us, as well as all the authors, on task and on time.

Series Foreword

The genesis for this book series started with the proposition that, increasingly, physicians want direct, useful information to help them in clinical care. Textbooks, while comprehensive, are useful primarily as detailed reference works but pose challenges for uses at point of care. By contrast, more outline-type references often leave out the "how's and whys" – pathophysiology, pharmacology – that form the basis of management decisions. Our goal for this series is to present books, covering most areas of neurology, that provide enough background information for the reader to feel comfortable, but not so much to be overwhelming; and to combine that with practical advice from experts about care, combining the growing evidence base with best practices.

Our series will encompass various aspects of neurology, the topics and specific content chosen to be accessible and useful. *Neuromuscular Disorders* by R. Tawil and S. Vance, covers the commonly seen areas of acquired and inherited conditions of muscle, nerve, and the neuromuscular junction, which we hope will appeal to students, trainees, experts and practicing neurologists alike. The editors are expert in their field and have recruited superb contributors to share their views on best treatment and management options.

Chapters cover critical information that will inform the reader of the disease processes and mechanisms as a prelude to treatment planning. Algorithms and guidelines are presented, when appropriate. "Tips and Tricks" boxes provide expert suggestions. Other boxes present cautions and warnings to avoid pitfalls. Finally, we provide "Science Revisited" sections that review the most important and relevant science background material. Bibliographies guide the reader to additional material.

We welcome feedback. As additional volumes are added to the series, we hope to refine the content and format so that our readers will be best served.

Our thanks, appreciation and respect goes out to our editors and their contributors, who conceived and refined the content for each volume, assuring a high quality, practical approach to neurological conditions and their treatment.

And our thanks also go to our mentors and students (past, present, and future), who have challenged and delighted us; and to our book editors and their contributors, who were willing to take on additional work for an educational goal; and to our publisher, Martin Sugden, for his ideas and support, for wonderful discussions, and for commiseration over baseball and soccer teams that might not quite have lived up to expectations.

We would like to dedicate the series to Marsha, Jake and Dan; and to Janet, Laura and David.

And to Steven R. Schwid, MD, our friend and colleague, whose ideas helped shape this project and whose humor brightened our lives; but who could not complete this goal with us.

Robert A. Gross
Jonathan W. Mink
Rochester, July 2011

Preface

Neuromuscular diseases include acquired and inherited conditions of muscle, nerve, and the neuromuscular junction. As neuromuscular clinicians, we recognize that having a familiarity with and an approach to these disorders is important for all physicians for several reasons. First, many of the acquired neuromuscular disorders are eminently treatable and some can present as emergencies. Consequently, early recognition of these disorders is important. Second, and equally important, modern medical management has significantly improved the quality of life of many individuals living with inherited neuromuscular disorders. Therefore, most inherited neuromuscular disorders are now considered chronic illnesses and early recognition of complications specific for certain neuromuscular conditions may lead to lifesaving interventions. Finally, the manifestations of neuromuscular diseases span several medical specialties including cardiology, pulmonology, and gastroenterology, and an integrated, multidisciplinary approach to the management of these patients has become a standard of care.

The challenge in writing this introductory textbook is to provide accessible, useful information about an ever more complex field of study. Our understanding of the inherited neuromuscular disorders has grown exponentially since the discovery in 1987 of the Duchenne gene. This explosion of molecular information has both simplified the diagnosis and management of certain neuromuscular disorders and complicated that of others. From a clinically based classification of a handful of diseases, we now have dozens of neuromuscular diseases defined by specific gene defects. Molecular genetics has allowed exact clinical definition for some entities, while blurring the clinical boundaries of others as mutations in different genes sometimes result in clinically indistinguishable conditions. Complicating matters is the realization that identical clinical presentations may be seen with acquired and hereditary disorders.

Despite the increasing complexity of molecular classifications, the diagnosis of neuromuscular disorders remains a singularly clinical exercise. Ancillary testing, short of DNA testing, helps to narrow the differential but rarely results in specific diagnoses. Moreover, genetic testing is not always available to practitioners and, therefore, an accurate history and careful exam remain critical in providing the most useful clues to direct the diagnostic workup. Even where DNA testing is widely available, the history and exam are essential in determining the most efficient and cost-effective use of DNA diagnostics. In many instances today, DNA testing will be the first test ordered to confirm the clinical suspicion, sparing the patient other unnecessary diagnostic tests.

This textbook is meant as an introductory volume for trainees and generalists alike, providing a practical framework to approach patients presenting with problems that localize to the neuromuscular system. Four chapters describe the clinical approach to the major neuromuscular disease categories including diseases of the motor neuron, nerve, neuromuscular junction, and muscle. The textbook covers the spectrum of neuromuscular disorders from the common to the esoteric. Each chapter contains text boxes highlighting relevant information regarding the diagnosis and management of individual disorders. The short bibliography at the end of every chapter provides relevant references for those interested in a more in-depth understanding of specific disorders.

We hope that the authors' tips and tricks and cautions prove to be valuable in clinical practice. With the increasing complexity of the neuromuscular field, making a specific diagnosis may not be achievable in some cases except in specialized academic centers. More relevant, however, is that better understanding of the neuromuscular disorders and their associated complications, result in improved patient care.

Rabi N. Tawil, MD
Rochester
Shannon Venance, MD, PhD
London, Ontario

Neuromuscular Diseases: Approach to Clinical Diagnosis

Shannon Venance[1] and Rabi Tawil[2]

[1]Department of Clinical Neurological Sciences, University of Western Ontario, London, Ontario, Canada
[2]University of Rochester Medical Center, Neuromuscular Disease Unit, Rochester, NY, USA

Effective clinical diagnosis of neuromuscular disorders requires the thoughtful use of the physician's core clinical skills of history taking and examination. Hypotheses are generated based on the clinical presentation and history taking, and tested during the physical examination. Unique to neurosciences is the need for accurate localization within the nervous system, before arriving at the differential diagnosis and identifying the investigations needed to confirm the clinical diagnosis. Only then is confirmation of a clinical diagnosis possible. Once the determination is made that the history and exam are consistent with a disorder of the peripheral nervous system, the clinician has to decide if the presentation is a disorder of peripheral nerve, muscle, neuromuscular junction, or motor neuron. Complicating matters are neuromuscular disorders, such as amyotrophic lateral sclerosis (ALS) in which peripheral and central nervous system (CNS) signs and symptoms coexist. As a general rule, investigations are tailored to reflect the clinical reasoning process and the most likely diagnostic considerations. A diagnosis is important for different reasons in different circumstances and individuals. An accurate diagnosis directs treatment and management, permits a discussion of disease progression, potential complications, and, in certain cases, is required for peace of mind. The approach taken throughout this volume emphasizes a careful history and examination with an insightful approach to the use of newer imaging and molecular diagnostic techniques in arriving at a diagnosis.

History taking: generating hypotheses

The clinical presentations of neuromuscular disorders reflect dysfunction of the lower motor neuron and the peripheral aspects of the sensory and autonomic systems. Similar complaints may be non-neurological or seen with CNS disorders. The art of history taking, allowing the patient to tell his or her story, is a critical aspect in deciding if there is a neurological problem and, in particular, a neuromuscular disorder.

It is helpful to categorize symptoms as positive (e.g. cramping, twitching, stiffness, tingling, pins, needles, burning pain) or negative (e.g. weakness, loss of muscle, numbness, incoordination), recognizing that it is often negative symptoms that have ready correlates on examination. Conversely, examination may be entirely normal in a patient with only positive symptoms. Ask patients to clarify what a symptom means to

Neuromuscular Disorders, First Edition. Edited by Rabi N. Tawil, Shannon Venance.
© 2011 John Wiley & Sons, Ltd. Published 2011 by John Wiley & Sons, Ltd.

them (e.g. numbness may actually mean weakness or tingling or heaviness), and whether and how this affects their ability to function within their daily activities at work, school, or home. In general, someone with neurological weakness will state what activity they struggle with (e.g. a need for a hand rail on stairs) or a function no longer done (e.g. avoid steak and salads) rather than complain of weakness. Individuals with systemic illness such as cancer, congestive heart failure, or depression will often use the term "weakness" for fatigue or malaise. When appropriate, include a functional inquiry covering the autonomic nervous system.

Classify the onset as acute (hours to days), subacute (weeks to months), or chronic (months to years) and whether the temporal evolution of symptoms is static, progressive, episodic, or fluctuating. A patient presenting with rapidly progressive proximal and distal weakness with four extremity paraesthesiae and areflexia over 5 days is easily recognized as having Guillain–Barré syndrome or acute inflammatory demyelinating polyneuropathy. On the other hand, similar symptoms that relapse and remit over months to years would favor chronic inflammatory demyelinating polyneuropathy.

An organized methodical approach is emphasized in the following chapters to ensure that associated symptoms and any precipitating, aggravating, and alleviating factors are uncovered. The diagnostic possibilities in an adolescent presenting with exertional intolerance, myalgias, episodic myoglobinuria, and a normal examination will differ depending on the type of activity precipitating symptoms, e.g. high-intensity activity, of brief duration, associated with prolonged painful contractures suggests a glycogen storage disorder whereas endurance activities with symptomatic worsening during times of fasting and intercurrent viral illness suggest a disorder of lipid metabolism. A careful inquiry of function, review of systems, and social and occupational history, as well as attention to medication including herbal preparations and supplements, illicit drug use, alcohol, and other potential toxic exposures and hobbies may yield useful clues. A developmental history may be indicated and a three-generation detailed family tree, inquiring about ethnicity and consanguinity, is usually always appropriate if heritable conditions are in the differential diagnosis. It is not helpful simply to ask if anyone else in the family has a nerve or muscle problem.

Examination: testing your hypotheses

An initial assessment should consider all elements of the neurological examination to accurately localize within the nervous system and to determine whether the problem is isolated to the peripheral nervous system or also involves the CNS (e.g. ALS, mitochondrial cytopathies, congenital muscular dystrophies). A systemic examination should be part of the routine examination because many hereditary and acquired neuromuscular disorders will have associated systemic manifestations or are, in the case of acquired disorders, the result of a systemic illness. Most critical from a management point of view is the identification of cardiac and respiratory involvement.

☆ **TIPS AND TRICKS**

PRESENCE OF PROMINENT RESPIRATORY INVOLVEMENT
Think of:

- Acute/Subacute:
  - Guillian–Barré syndrome
  - myasthenia gravis
- Chronic:
  - amyotrophic lateral sclerosis
  - acid maltase deficiency
  - Duchenne dystrophy
  - myotonic dystrophy

☆ **TIPS AND TRICKS**

PROMINENT CARDIAC INVOLVEMENT
Think of:

- Cardiac conduction defects:
  - myotonic dystrophy
  - Emery–Dreyfuss syndrome
- Cardiomyopathy:
  - Duchenne dystrophy
  - limb–girdle muscular dystrophies
  - Pompe's disease (infantile onset)
  - mitochondrial myopathies
  - amyloidosis

A brief screening mental status may be indicated. Cognitive impairment is seen as a primary feature of some neuromuscular diseases (Duchenne muscular dystrophy, congenital myotonic dystrophy, mitochondrial cytopathies, frontotemporal dementia in ALS or secondary to the complications of the disease – confusion secondary to chronic respiratory failure and hypercapnia). A relevant cranial nerve examination might include assessment of fundi because pigmentary retinopathy can be a feature of some mitochondrial disorders, pupils (not involved in myasthenia gravis compared with fixed with botulism), eyelids, and extraocular movements. Trigeminal neuropathy may be seen with Sjögren's syndrome or other neuropathies. Facial weakness is prominent in a number of myopathies but may also be seen in some hereditary neuropathies. Subtle evidence of facial weakness may be an inability to bury the eyelashes. Sensorineural hearing loss may be evident in neuropathies and mitochondrial disorders. A high arched palate may be a clue to a longstanding, inherited disorder, and the quality of the voice, in addition to the elevation of the soft palate, highlights the involvement of nerves IX and X. In addition to tongue movement, the presence or absence of tongue atrophy (hypoglossal nerve involvement, ALS), hypertrophy (Duchenne muscular dystrophy, amyloidosis), and fasciculations should be noted. Neck flexion is often weaker than neck extension in many myopathies and myasthenia gravis, although there are exceptions.

✭ TIPS AND TRICKS

PRESENCE OF PTOSIS AND/OR OPHTHALMOPLEGIA
Think of:

- Acute/Subacute:
  - myasthenia gravis
  - Lambert–Eaton myasthenic syndrome
  - Miller-Fisher variant of Guillain–Barré syndrome
- Chronic:
  - myotonic muscular dystrophy
  - mitochondrial disorders
  - oculopharyngeal dystrophy
  - congenital myopathy

A vigilant motor examination at the first assessment yields useful clues because the patterns of weakness are informative. This should be preceded by careful inspection of the muscle for spontaneous movements such as fasciculations and myokymia, and assessment of muscle bulk. Attention to tone and reflexes can help differentiate neurogenic from myopathic conditions, as well as ruling out the presence of an upper motor neuron component. Direct percussion of the muscles with a reflex hammer can induce rippling, mounding, or myotonia which are important diagnostic clues. A systematic approach that includes all muscle groups about the shoulder, elbow, wrist, hand including the long finger and thumb flexors, hip, knee, and ankle may shorten the differential diagnosis. In inclusion body myositis for example, the quadriceps muscles and finger flexors are preferentially involved early in the disease. And, finally, observing the posture, stance, and gait, including a functional assessment by having the patient lift the arms above the head, walk on heels, toes, hop on either foot, rise from a squat, climb a few stairs, or rise from the floor, often yields important diagnostic information. An individual with a marked lumbar lordosis and Trendelenburg gait has a chronic problem, even if he or she dates symptom onset only back several months.

A careful sensory assessment of all modalities requires mapping out the territories on face, arm, leg, or trunk for perception of pinprick (± temperature) and vibration threshold (± joint perception). This assessment reveals patterns of individual nerve, multiple nerves, plexus, root, proximal, distal, or central involvement in individuals with sensory, balance, and coordination complaints, e.g. a subacute stocking-and-glove sensory loss to all modalities with absent reflexes and preserved strength points to a sensory neuronopathy and prompts a return to the history to make further inquiries about pyridoxine intake, dry eyes and mouth, etc. if not revealed initially. Coordination testing with attention to Romberg's sign and dysmetria are often abnormal in the face of marked large-fiber sensory deficits. Retained reflexes would be expected in the individual with painful, burning feet and a small-fiber neuropathy. The weal-and-flare "triple" skin response is often abnormal with small-fiber neuropathies affecting autonomic fibers. Attention to the skin, and any trophic (thinning, temperature, and color change) or sweating changes (absent or increased) in the feet may be early signs of the small thinly myelinated or unmyelinated fiber involvement.

Localization: defines your differential and investigations

Localization is most often apparent after a skilled history and physical exam are completed, although there are presentations that may still localize to several parts of the peripheral nervous system (e.g. proximal symmetrical weakness with absent reflexes may be nerve, neuromusculat junction, or muscle) and investigations will help to clarify.

Investigations: selection based on pre-test probability

Healthcare costs have risen dramatically in the past few years, and it is the responsibility of each physician to select the appropriate tests based on the most likely diagnosis, taking into consideration how management will be affected. A creatine kinase and thyroid-stimulating hormone (TSH) test in muscle disease, acetylcholine receptor antibodies and TSH in neuromuscular junction disorders and fasting glucose, and a glucose tolerance test and serum protein electrophoresis with immunofixation in neuropathy are first-line lab tests in the investigation of common presentations of neuromuscular disease. Additional tests will depend on the clinical scenario and what the likely yield will be. For example, uncovering a low-titer antinuclear antibody in a middle-aged woman with a subacute sensorimotor neuropathy and no symptoms or signs of connective tissue or autoimmune involvement is of little benefit and may prompt unnecessary investigation. With a high pre-test probability, specific antibodies, and immune and paraneoplastic markers have their place (e.g. positive, high-titer serum, voltage-gated, potassium channel antibodies confirm a clinical diagnosis of neuromyotonia).

Electrodiagnostic studies (nerve conduction studies, repetitive nerve stimulation, electromyography [EMG], somatosensory-evoked potentials, provocative testing) in skilled hands are generally always helpful in neuromuscular disorders. Electrodiagnostics will help confirm segmental lower motor neuron involvement in motor neuron disease, distinguish between axonal and demyelinating neuropathies, localize particular nerve roots or parts of the plexus, detect increment or decrement in neuromuscular junction disorders, and identify involved muscles in some myopathies to guide biopsy. It is important to note that electrodiagnostic studies are an extension of the history and physical exam, and rarely in and of themselves diagnostic. For example, the individual with the asymptomatic median neuropathy at the wrist on nerve conduction studies does not have carpal tunnel syndrome and the individual with small-amplitude, short-duration motor units with fibrillation potentials and positive sharp waves on EMG may have an inflammatory, toxic, or hereditary myopathy.

In many instances now, DNA analysis is clinically available for a number of disorders, in particular hereditary myopathies. It is appropriate, and less invasive, to confirm a clinical diagnosis with a genetic test in several hereditary myopathies including Duchenne/Becker muscular dystrophy, facioscapulohumeral muscular dystrophy (FSHD), myotonic dystrophy types 1 and 2, and oculopharyngeal muscular dystrophy. It is the responsibility of the ordering physician, however, to understand the sensitivity and specificity of tests ordered.

Muscle biopsy remains a critical investigation for diseases of muscle. However, the timing, site, and subsequent analysis and testing of the muscle, and the utility of a concomitant skin biopsy to generate fibroblast culture for enzymatic assays, are all decided based on the working diagnosis. Increasingly, in the literature, the use of magnetic resonance imaging to guide investigation of muscle disease is emerging; however, the benefits and costs over a careful history and examination in the clinical setting have yet to be determined. Nerve biopsies, on the other hand, are used infrequently in the investigation of neuropathies but remain critical in the diagnosis of vasculitic and amyloid neuropathies. A relatively new technique, punch skin biopsy for assessment of epidermal innervation, is helpful in the diagnosis of suspected small-fiber neuropathies that cannot be confirmed by electrodiagnostic testing.

Diagnosis: putting the story together

Ultimately, an accurate diagnosis is needed to facilitate management. The needs of individual patients will vary from simple to complex. Having a confirmed diagnosis, however, facilitates discussions with patients and their families. Communication is the cornerstone of effective therapeutic relationships, regardless of whether there are effective treatments for a condition (e.g. Guillain–Barré syndrome, myasthenia gravis) or whether management remains supportive around education, planning and problem-solving (FSHD, hereditary neuropathies, etc.). When possible, interprofessional healthcare teams should be used because they improve quality of life. Lifestyle and behavior adaptation are often required, in addition to medical and surgical approaches.

References

Amato AA, Russell JA. *Neuromuscular Disorders*. New York: McGraw Hill, 2008.

Dyck PJ, Thomas PK. *Peripheral Neuropathy*, 4th edn. New York: Elsevier Saunders, 2005.

Engel AG, Franzini-Armstrong C. *Myology*, 3rd edn. New York: McGraw Hill, 2004.

Washington University's Neuromuscular Homepage. http://neuromuscular.wustl.edu (a comprehensive, continually updated, reference for all neuromuscular disorders).

Part I

Myopathies

Approach to Diseases of Muscle

Matthew P. Wicklund

Department of Neurology, Penn State College of Medicine, Hershey, PA, USA

Muscle disorders nearly always present with weakness, much less often with myalgias, contractures or myoglobinuria, and rarely with chronic respiratory failure or cardiac dysfunction. The primary task is determining whether muscle, neuromuscular junction, nerve, or motor neuron accounts for the weakness. This task can generally be achieved through clinical, laboratory, and electrodiagnostic evaluation. Once the disorder has been localized to muscle, the goal is to delineate a syndromic or specific diagnosis. Finally, one should initiate treatment, if available, and, if not, optimize functional status.

History and examination offer the greatest clues in delineating the fundamental features of individual muscle disorders. Further studies such as blood and urine tests, electrodiagnostics, biopsy, and genetic testing then play only a confirmatory role. An orderly approach simplifies this quest, dissecting down to the most likely diagnoses.

Clinical history and examination

Start by asking *six questions* in the history.

1. What are the "negative" and/or "positive" symptoms?

Negative symptoms usually predominate and include weakness, atrophy, fatigue, and exercise intolerance. Patients with proximal leg weakness have difficulties squatting, negotiating stairways, and arising from toilets, chairs and car seats. Proximal arm weakness causes trouble lifting objects overhead, doing one's hair, and retrieving items from cupboards. With distal weakness, problems opening jars, turning keys, playing musical instruments, and tripping or scuffing toes are most prominent. Cranial muscle weakness may cause trouble with drinking through a straw, swallowing, whistling, blowing out candles, slurred speech, drooping eyelids and double vision.

Positive symptoms include myalgias, cramps, hypertrophy, contractures, stiffness, rippling and mounding of muscles, along with myoglobinuria. Although myalgias may complicate mitochondrial, inflammatory, toxic (statins), infectious (viral), endocrine (hypothyroid) and metabolic myopathies, pain without weakness most often implicates disorders of the bones, joints, or tendons. Muscle cramps are associated with dehydration, hyponatremia, azotemia, and myxedema, in addition to polyneuropathies and amyotrophic lateral sclerosis. They are not common in myopathies. Muscle contractures reflect the inability of muscle fibers to relax and are electrically silent on needle electromyography. Muscle contractures, along with myoglobinuria, occur in some metabolic myopathies. Muscle stiffness is generally associated with myotonic disorders such as the myotonic dystrophies, myotonia and paramyotonia congenita, the periodic paralyses, and hypothyroid myopathy. Rippling and mounding are uncommon, but

Neuromuscular Disorders, First Edition. Edited by Rabi N. Tawil, Shannon Venance.
© 2011 John Wiley & Sons, Ltd. Published 2011 by John Wiley & Sons, Ltd.

suggest muscle disease resulting from mutations in the gene for caveolin.

2. What is the temporal course?

It is important to note the timing of symptom onset: birth, childhood or adulthood. Most congenital myopathies have slow or static courses and their creatine kinase levels are normal or mildly elevated. Muscular dystrophies, glycogen storage diseases, mitochondrial cytopathies and inflammatory myopathies often arise during childhood or adolescence. Myotonic dystrophy, distal myopathies, inflammatory myopathies, and inclusion body myositis most often or always have onset in adults.

Rate of progression and duration of weakness also help categorize myopathies. Acquired disorders such as dermatomyositis and polymyositis progress over days, weeks, or months, whereas most genetic disorders advance over months or years. Weakness emerges intermittently in periodic paralyses and metabolic myopathies but advances relatively steadily in muscular dystrophies.

3. Is there a family history?

Patterns of inheritance include autosomal dominant, autosomal recessive, X-linked, and mitochondrial (exclusively maternal transmission). When inquiring about family history, do not just ask whether family members had a problem with their muscles. Query whether family members had trouble walking, climbing stairs or swallowing, or required an assistive device such as a cane, walker, or wheelchair.

4. Are there provocative factors?

Alcohol, steroids, statins and chemotherapeutic agents may cause weakness, whereas cocaine, alcohol, statins, and muscle-bulking agents sometimes provoke rhabdomyolysis. Episodic stiffness may be set off by cold temperatures (paramyotonia congenita), whereas a large carbohydrate meal (periodic paralysis) or fevers (carnitine palmitoyl transferase deficiency) may precipitate attacks of weakness.

5. Are other organ systems affected?

Delineating involvement in other organ systems not only helps narrow diagnostic possibilities, but assures referral to specialists for appropriate surveillance and treatment. Cardiac arrhythmias and congestive heart failure complicate Duchenne, Becker, Emery–Dreifuss, and limb–girdle muscular dystrophies, mitochondrial and nemaline myopathies, glycogenoses, polymyositis, and Andersen–Tawil syndrome. Early or prominent respiratory dysfunction may occur in acid maltase deficiency, mitochondrial myopathies, polymyositis, and several muscular dystrophies. Distinctive disorders are associated with particular organ system involvement such as gastrointestinal dysfunction (childhood dermatomyositis, mitochondrial disorders), hepatomegaly (glycogenoses), cataracts (myotonic dystrophy), skin rash (dermatomyositis), early joint contractures (Emery–Dreifuss muscular dystrophies), peripheral neuropathies (HIV, chemotherapeutic agents) and cancers (dermatomyositis, necrotizing myopathy).

> ### ☝ CAUTION!
>
> Although muscle disease itself leads to morbidity and even mortality, involvement of other organ systems is the usual ultimate cause of death in most patients. Consequently, when appropriate, involvement of other specialists, mostly cardiologists and pulmonologists, is critical in the care of patients with myopathies.

6. What is the pattern of weakness?

Depending on the myopathy, weakness initially manifests in particular muscle groups or regions of the body including ocular, pharyngeal, facial, respiratory, axial, and proximal or distal limb muscles. Commonly, more than one of these areas is affected. By determining the pattern of muscle involvement, the differential diagnosis can be narrowed considerably.

A careful examination places the patient into one of *six distinctive patterns* (Figure 2.1).

Proximal arms and legs

This "limb girdle" pattern is the one that most clinicians think of for myopathies. It is the most common and least specific pattern.

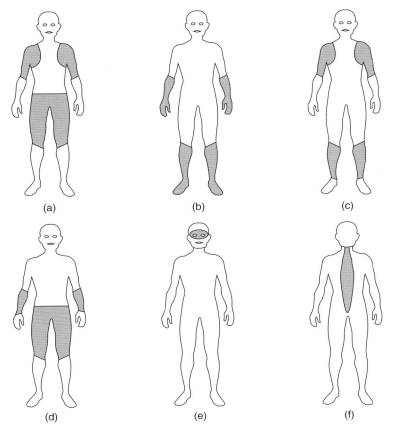

Figure 2.1. Patterns of muscle weakness: (a) proximal; (b) distal; (c) proximal arm with distal leg; (d) proximal leg with distal arm; (e) ptosis; and (f) axial muscles.

Dermatomyositis, polymyositis, and most dystrophies present with this pattern, as do congenital, mitochondrial, myofibrillar, endocrine, metabolic, and toxic myopathies. However, the history should have narrowed the possibilities. Inflammatory myopathies present acutely or subacutely. Weakness from birth suggests a congenital myopathy, whereas a 6-year-old boy with a Gower sign most likely has Duchenne dystrophy. A history of recently prescribed cholesterol-lowering drugs points toward a toxic myopathy.

Distal weakness

In these disorders, there is weakness of ankle dorsiflexion or plantar flexion, weakness of the wrists and fingers, or some combination thereof. Of the distal muscular dystrophies, Nonaka, Laing, and Miyoshi dystrophies have onset in children or young adults, whereas Markesbery–Griggs, Welander and Udd dystrophies present in middle age or older. The myofibrillar myopathies and myotonic dystrophy may also have primarily distal weakness.

Proximal arms and distal legs

In this "scapuloperoneal" pattern, the periscapular muscles, along with the anterior foreleg muscles, are most affected. The scapuloperoneal, Emory–Dreifuss and facioscapulohumeral muscular dystrophies fall into this category.

Proximal legs with distal arms

This is the classic pattern seen in most patients with sporadic inclusion body myositis. There is prominent weakness and wasting of the quadriceps (Figure 2.2) as well as wrist and finger flexors.

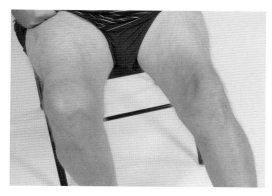

Figure 2.2. Marked atrophy of the quadriceps muscles in a patient with inclusion body myositis – note the asymmetry with greater atrophy on the left.

Ptosis and ophthalmoparesis

Ptosis with ophthalmoplegia is characteristic of a limited number of disorders, usually oculopharyngeal muscular dystrophy or mitochondrial myopathies. Even though patients have limited extraocular movements, they rarely complain of diplopia. Ptosis without ophthalmoplegia occurs in myotonic dystrophy along with the congenital and myofibrillar myopathies.

Axial musculature

The most prominent weakness in some patients may be of the neck (isolated neck extensor myopathy) or the paraspinous muscles (camptocormia). In isolation, these presentations may be due to muscle disease, but more often occur in disorders of the neuromuscular junction or motor neuron. Patients may also present with rigidity of the spine due not to weakness, but to contractures of the axial structures. This is commonly seen in congenital, Ullrich, and Emory–Dreifuss muscular dystrophies.

Finally, some patients remain relatively asymptomatic between attacks of weakness, stiffness, myoglobinuria, or pain, and thus do not fit into one of the above categories. Most of these patients have disorders in some way affecting components of the muscle membrane or energy pathways. Thus, the myotonias, periodic paralyses, metabolic myopathies, and drug ingestions fall into this category. However, over time, some of these may transform from episodic to progressive disorders.

Diagnostic tests

The six questions with six patterns help narrow the diagnosis considerably and determine what diagnostic tests should follow. Creatine kinase (CK) is the most valuable laboratory test and assists in narrowing the differential diagnosis. Markedly elevated CK levels occur in dystrophies with defects in the muscle membrane such as Duchenne dystrophy, some inflammatory myopathies, hypothyroid myopathy, and rhabdomyolysis. Inversely, CK levels may be disproportionately low in very weak patients with dermatomyositis or hyperthyroidism.

☆ TIPS AND TRICKS

Resting CK levels are influenced by muscle mass, gender, and race. Although, in most labs, the upper limit of normal (ULN) ranges from 160 international units per liter (IU/L) to 240 IU/L, studies show that race and gender have to be taken into account:

Group	Constituents	ULN (97.5%)
High	Black males	520 IU/L
Intermediate	Nonblack males and black females	345 IU/L
Low	Nonblack females	145 IU/L

☝ CAUTION!

Alanine aminotransferase (ALT) and aspartate aminotransferase (ALT) are present in both liver and muscle:

- ALT and AST rise commensurately with CK in myopathies and unless associated with elevation of γ-glutamyltransferase (GGT) do not indicate coexistent liver disease.
- Reciprocally, elevated ALT and AST without elevation of GGT should raise the consideration of a myopathy and trigger a check of serum CK.

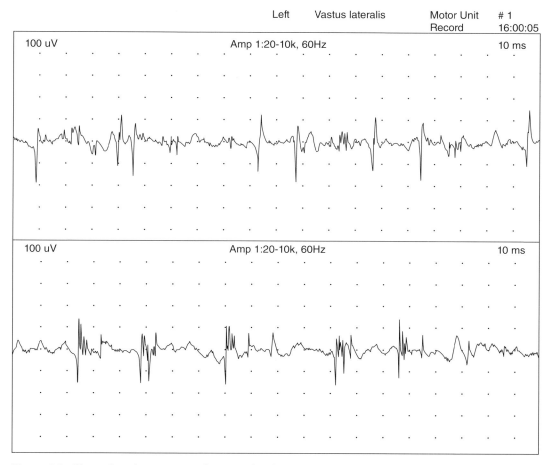

Figure 2.3. Short-duration (2–5 ms), low-amplitude (50–300 μV) motor units, some of which are polyphasic. EMG from a myopathy patient providing minimal contractile force, therefore demonstrating early recruitment.

Nerve conduction studies (NCS) and electromyography (EMG) help confirm a myopathic process and exclude other neuromuscular causes. Neuropathic disorders, neuromuscular junction disorders, and anterior horn cell disease may all mimic myopathies. NCS/EMG allows the examiner to distinguish between these possibilities. The presence of short-duration, low-amplitude motor units with early recruitment on EMG is useful in confirming a myopathy (Figure 2.3). EMG helps establish the extent and pattern of muscle involvement, the temporal course, and points the evaluator toward the most appropriate muscle group for biopsy. It is important to recognize that EMG can be normal in some of the indolent myopathies. EMG alone does not provide a specific diagnosis; results must be evaluated in the context of the patient's history, neurological exam, and other laboratory studies.

Imaging can be valuable in evaluation of muscle diseases. Computed tomography, muscle ultrasonography, and magnetic resonance imaging illuminate patterns of involvement, severity within and between muscles, stage of disease, and even clues to the underlying pathology. Imaging provides the advantages of being noninvasive and able to evaluate multiple muscles in one procedure. Imaging can also be used to guide selection of an appropriate muscle for biopsy.

If clinical and electrodiagnostic features suggest a myopathy, a muscle biopsy may be an appropriate test to confirm the diagnosis. However, if clinical features suggest a specific myopathy for which genetic testing is readily available, diagnostic DNA testing should precede a muscle biopsy. Selection of the appropriate muscle to biopsy is essential. Severely weak or normal strength muscles generally should not be biopsied. Light microscopy, electron microscopy, biochemical studies, and immune staining offer useful diagnostic clues. Typical myopathic features include central nuclei, both small and hypertrophic round fibers, split fibers, and degenerating and regenerating fibers (Plate 2.1). Chronic myopathies frequently have increased connective tissue and fat, whereas inflammatory myopathies show endomysial, perimysial, and/or perivascular mononuclear infiltrates. Electron microscopy is helpful in identifying ultrastructural changes in congenital, myofibrillar, and mitochondrial myopathies. Biochemical analysis of specific enzyme defects is essential in metabolic or mitochondrial myopathies.

Genetic testing is commercially available for many muscle diseases and should be guided by the clinical, laboratory, and electrodiagnostic features of the patient. Alternatively, distinctive muscle biopsy findings direct which individual DNA test or panel of tests is most appropriate for a definitive diagnosis. A definitive genetic diagnosis is important for a patient's peace of mind, an accurate prognosis, preemptive care for other organ system involvement, eligibility for research trials, and, importantly, for appropriate genetic counseling.

The approach described in this chapter offers a straightforward method to the diagnosis of muscle disease. Six questions about symptoms, temporal course, family history, triggers, other organ system involvement, and the distribution of weakness, combined with six patterns of weakness, allow the examiner to place patients into syndromes or distinct diagnoses. This guides laboratory testing, electrodiagnostic studies, imaging, biopsy, and genetic testing for a definitive diagnosis, which in turn directs appropriate therapy. The subsequent chapters fill in the details. Together with this framework, the reader will gain an ease in diagnosis of, and an expertise in, the diseases of muscle.

References

Black HR, Quallich H, Gareleck CB. Racial differences in serum creatine kinase levels. *Am J Med* 1986;**81**:479–87.

Carpenter S, Karpati G. *Pathology of Skeletal Muscle*, 2nd edn. Oxford: Oxford University Press, 2001.

Mercuri E, Pichiecchio A, Allsop J, et al. Muscle MRI in inherited neuromuscular disorders: past, present, and future. *J Magn Reson Imaging* 2007;**25**:433–40.

Preston DC, Shapiro BE. *Electromyography and Neuromuscular Disorders*, 2nd edn. Philadelphia: Elsevier, 2005.

Wong ET, Cobb C, Umahara MK. Heterogeneity of serum CK activity among racial and gender groups of the population. *Am J Clin Pathol* 1983;**79**:582–6.

Inflammatory Myopathies

Steven A. Greenberg

Department of Neurology, Brigham and Women's Hospital and Harvard Medical School, Boston, MA, USA

Classification and pathogenesis

The inflammatory myopathies are disorders in which muscle injury is in part mediated by the immune system. The three most frequently referred to subtypes are dermatomyositis (DM), inclusion body myositis (IBM), and polymyositis (PM); other categories are overlap syndromes (inflammatory myopathies occurring in patients with connective tissue diseases), necrotizing myopathy, eosinophilic myositis, and granulomatous myositis. Many patients with inflammatory myopathies cannot be assigned to any of these subtypes and may be classified as having nonspecific myositis.

Dermatomyositis

Dermatomyositis is a multisystem disease, predominantly affecting skin and muscle, but also affecting lung and other organs. Some patients have skin involvement only (amyopathic dermatomyositis). Dermatomyositis is not "polymyositis without rash"; its pathology and mechanism are entirely different.

Type I interferon-induced molecules are abundant in dermatomyositis muscle and skin biopsy specimens, and a recent autoantibody against one of these molecules (IFIH1) is highly specific for a subtype of dermatomyositis involving predominantly skin and lung.

> **⚙ SCIENCE REVISITED**
>
> Recent studies suggest that the type 1 interferon pathway is very active in dermatomyositis, providing opportunities for developing diagnostic biomarkers and therapeutic approaches.

Polymyositis

The term "polymyositis" encompasses a wide range of different diseases. Symmetric proximal weakness and certain muscle biopsy pathological features define this group, with considerable variation in how experts make this diagnosis. The alternative diagnosis of nonspecific myositis is appropriate for many patients. As a result of the marked heterogeneity of this category, unified mechanistic understanding is lacking. Many patients with "refractory polymyositis" have instead inclusion body myositis.

Inclusion body myositis

The term refers to an inflammatory myopathy that develops in mid or later life with a distinctive pattern of weakness involving asymmetric wrist flexor, finger flexor (Figure 3.1), and quadriceps weakness, and distinctive pathological features

Neuromuscular Disorders, First Edition. Edited by Rabi N. Tawil, Shannon Venance.
© 2011 John Wiley & Sons, Ltd. Published 2011 by John Wiley & Sons, Ltd.

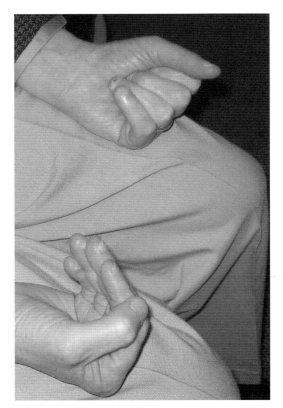

Figure 3.1. Asymmetric finger flexor weakness in inclusion body myositis. Patient is attempting to make a fist with both hands.

(inflammatory cells surrounding myofibers and rimmed vacuoles).

The mechanism of myofiber injury in IBM is poorly understood. Myonuclear abnormalities are present but have an unknown relationship with the mechanism of myofiber injury.

Clinical evaluation

General

The diagnosis of inflammatory myopathy and the specific subtype is based on a combination of clinical presentation, laboratory studies, and pathological findings in muscle biopsy samples. In general, symptoms of acute or subacute (weeks to months) muscle weakness (difficulty arising from a low chair, climbing up or down stairs, getting into a car, washing hair, brushing teeth,

or, in IBM, gripping objects) or skin rash (in dermatomyositis) are the presenting features. Patients presenting with prominent diffuse pain, often attributed to muscles, usually do not have an inflammatory myopathy. Pronounced lumbar lordosis and waddling gait, facial weakness, and scapular winging, signs of an indolent chronic myopathic process, should lead to considerations other than inflammatory myopathy.

Laboratory studies other than serum creatine kinase (CK) are of limited value to support or refute the diagnosis of inflammatory myopathy. The CK may be normal in active untreated DM. Serum "liver function tests" – aspartate aminotransferase (AST) and alanine aminotransferase (ALT) – may be elevated in inflammatory or other myopathies; these enzymes are present in muscle. Some patients with PM- or IBM-like clinical patterns of weakness may have associated HTLV-1 or HIV infection, so laboratory testing for these may be considered. Laboratory demonstration of autoantibodies, including antinuclear antibodies, anti-histidyl transfer RNA (anti-Jo-1) antibodies, anti-IFIH1 antibodies, and anti-Mi-2 antibodies may be helpful. The presence of anti-Jo-1 antibodies, associated with DM and PM, should raise suspicion for interstitial lung disease and prompt evaluation with pulmonary function tests, chest computed tomography (CT), and avoidance of methotrexate therapy because of the last's potential pulmonary toxicity. Chest CT is also useful for consideration of sarcoidosis and as part of a malignancy evaluation for adults with DM.

Muscle biopsy and the pathological examination of the specimen obtained are important diagnostic procedures for patients with suspected inflammatory myopathies. In general, a mild-to-moderately weak muscle is optimal for biopsy. Good choices often are the biceps and vastus lateralis, but specific cases need to be considered individually.

Dermatomyositis

Dermatomyositis affects children and adults. Adult DM generally presents as subacute progressive painless proximal weakness, a skin rash, or both. Juvenile DM may present similarly or as an acute or subacute febrile illness followed by skin, muscle, or sometimes multisystem involvement.

The skin involvement in DM may have diverse manifestations, including: a heliotrope rash (purplish discoloration) on the eyelids; an erythematous rash on the face, neck, and anterior chest ("V-sign"), upper back ("shawl sign"), elbows, or knees; a purplish scaly papular rash on the extensor surface of the hands (Gottron's papules); thickened and cracked skin on the dorsal and ventral surfaces of the hands ("mechanic's hands"); and other changes. Subcutaneous calcinosis is a significant problem in juvenile DM and uncommon in adult DM. Cutaneous symptoms in DM have a high impact on lowering quality of life in patients and include prominent pruritus.

The pattern of proximal limb weakness in DM is not distinctive and does not distinguish DM from many other myopathies. Significant muscle asymmetries or prominent distal (forearm or lower leg) weakness together with skin rash should prompt consideration of sarcoidosis, for which clinical involvement similar to DM has been recognized. Normal serum CK may be present in patients with progressive disease and does not exclude the diagnosis. When elevated serum CK is present in DM, reductions generally occur with treatment and elevation with relapse.

Additional evaluation of adult patients with DM should be performed because of its association with two other important clinical syndromes: interstitial lung disease and malignancy. Pulmonary function tests, chest CT, and laboratory testing for the presence of anti-histidyl-tRNA antibodies (anti-Jo-1 antibodies) should be considered in all patients with DM. Malignancy has been estimated to be associated with 6–45% of adult patients with DM, with age-associated increased risk particularly in women aged over 40. A malignancy evaluation, including physical examination (skin examination, breast and pelvic examinations in women, and testicular and prostate examination in men), blood studies (complete blood count, liver function tests, lactate dehydrogenase, prostate-specific antigen), stool for occult blood, CT (chest, abdomen, and pelvis), and colonoscopy should be considered in every adult patient with a new diagnosis of DM.

> ★ **TIPS AND TRICKS**
>
> - Malignancies are associated with 6–45% of patients with DM.
> - A malignancy evaluation is essential in patients diagnosed with DM.

Muscle biopsy is an important diagnostic procedure in DM. The most supportive diagnostic features of muscle biopsies for DM evident in routine clinical studies are the presence of perifascicular atrophy and the absence of multiple myofibers surrounded by inflammatory cells. Perifascicular atrophy refers to the presence of small myofibers that are slightly darker and bluish in color in hematoxylin and eosin sections, typically located at the edges of fascicles (Plate 3.1).

Inclusion body myositis

Inclusion body myositis affects adults in middle and later life. Onset before age 50 occurs in 18–20% of patients and then mostly after age 50. Diagnosis has historically been frequently delayed by a mean of 5–8 years from symptom onset.

The clinical presentation of IBM is distinct from that of other inflammatory myopathies. Atrophy and weakness of wrist and finger flexors and quadriceps are distinctive, and physical examination should focus on careful testing of these muscle groups. Comparison of wrist and finger extensors with corresponding flexors may demonstrate the greater involvement of the flexors and asymmetries (see Figure 3.1). Relative preservation of deltoids, in comparison to the forearm flexors, can be impressive, in marked contrast to the pattern of weakness seen in DM and PM. Involvement of tibialis anterior may also be distinctive in IBM. Dysphagia can be a significant problem with a prevalence estimated as high as 66%.

Serum CK is only modestly elevated; research criteria have proposed diagnostic criteria of an upper limit of 12 times the upper limit of normal, although patients with higher values, up to 16 times the upper limit of normal, have been reported.

On muscle biopsy, the presence of multiple myofibers surrounded by inflammatory cells and many myofibers with rimmed vacuoles is highly supportive of a pathological diagnosis of IBM. Both IBM and PM (see below) may have similar patterns with respect to the location of inflammatory cells as seen in routine studies. The pattern of inflammatory cells deep within fascicles surrounding and sometimes invading myofibers (Figure 3.2) is distinct from that of DM. What distinguishes IBM from PM in light microscopic examination is a sufficient number of rimmed vacuoles as well as the presence of signs of a chronic indolent process in IBM such as hypertrophied fibers and fibrosis. Difficulties with diagnosis occur in patients with typical clinical features but few inflammatory cells or with few rimmed vacuoles.

> ★ **TIPS AND TRICKS**
>
> - Unlike PM and DM, IBM presents with a distinct pattern of muscle weakness.
> - Finger flexors, wrist flexors, and quadriceps are selectively involved in IBM and associated with a "scooped-out" atrophic forearm flexor compartment and atrophy of quadriceps.

- In addition to the characteristic limb weakness, dysphagia occurs in most IBM patients.

Polymyositis

Patients with acquired myopathies, whose weakness improves with immunosuppressive therapies and relapses with taper of such therapy, but who lack the rash and pathological features of dermatomyositis, are challenging to classify. Depending on various criteria, such patients may be categorized as having polymyositis, nonspecific myositis, necrotizing myopathy, overlap syndromes, or other diagnoses. Patients with subacute progressive symmetric proximal arm and leg weakness, without skin rash and with muscle biopsy features of prominent inflammatory cells surrounding many muscle fibers, without perifascicular atrophy, are the patients who are most appropriately classified as having polymyositis or nonspecific myositis. Various research diagnostic criteria have been considered with regard to the challenges of PM diagnosis. The practical issues are avoiding misclassification of certain muscular dystrophies, particularly limb–girdle muscular dystrophy (LGMD), and

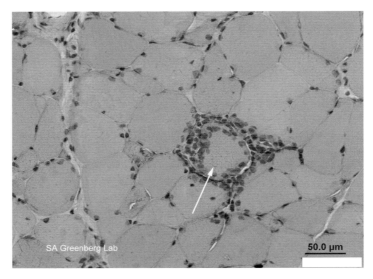

Figure 3.2. Inflammatory cells surrounding and invading a myofiber in inclusion body myositis (arrow).

IBM as PM. Most patients with LGMD and IBM meet widely used criteria for the diagnosis of PM.

As with DM, there is an association with interstitial lung disease, but no well-established association with malignancy. Serum CK is almost always elevated in patients with progressive PM. Connective tissue diseases should be considered through clinical evaluation and antinuclear antibody testing.

Treatment

Overall approach

IBM has no effective treatment and most experts choose not to treat with immunosuppressants because of lack of efficacy and the presence of side effects. Dermatomyositis, polymyositis, and necrotizing myopathy are usually treated with systemic immunosuppressive therapies.

Patients with cutaneous manifestations of dermatomyositis but without symptomatic weakness may be treated with systemic immuno-suppressivetherapies or topical glucocorticoids, topical tacrolimus, antipruritics, chloroquine, or other agents. The general approach is outlined in Figure 3.3.

Specific immunotherapies and their complications are discussed below. In general, high doses of corticosteroids are used initially to control disease and then tapered gradually. If relapse occurs on lower doses, 20 mg prednisone or less, the dose is increased and second agents, typically either methotrexate or azathioprine, are introduced for long-term control. Alternative approaches include use of therapies initially or early on to avoid prolonged use of corticosteroids. Some patients may be controlled with just monthly infusions of intravenous immunoglobulin (IVIG), or IVIG or methotrexate may

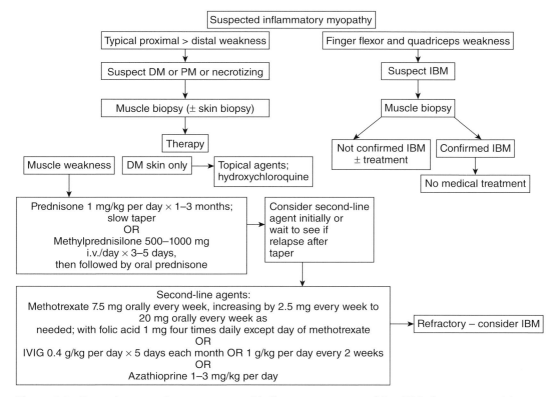

Figure 3.3. General approach to treatment of inflammatory myopathies. DM, dermatomyositis; IBM, inclusion body myositis.

be introduced early in the treatment course together with corticosteroids.

Prevention of osteoporosis

Corticosteroids are first-line agents for the treatment of DM and PM. Osteoporosis has been considered the single most debilitating effect of chronic steroid use, and significant bone loss occurs in the first 3–6 months of their use. Calcium (>1 g/day) and vitamin D (400 IU/day) have long been recommended. Increasingly, bisphosphonates are started the same day as initiation of glucocorticoid therapy. Bisphosphonate therapy should be avoided or used cautiously in premenopausal women given their potential teratogenicity. Alendronate (70 mg orally weekly) and risedronate (35 mg orally weekly) have both been shown in trials to prevent glucorticoid-induced osteoporosis. Patients need to take these medications with water fasting in the morning and remain sitting upright or standing for 30 minutes to prevent esophageal irritation. Other bisphosphonate approaches are available.

Risk of infection

Opportunistic infections with *Pneumocystis jiroveci*, *Leigonella*, *Candida*, *Aspergillus*, *Histoplasma*, and *Blastomyces* species, cytomegalovirus, and others occur in patients with DM and PM treated with immunosuppressants. In the largest reported series, 12% of 156 patients with DM or PM developed opportunistic infections, with a 28% mortality rate. Depressed lymphocyte counts may increase the risk. Prophylactic treatment with trimethoprim–sulfamethoxazole (Bactrim), given as one double strength tablet three times a week is effective prevention for *Pneumocystis jiroveci* pneumonia and should be considered in all patients receiving two or more immunomodulating therapies.

Before treatment, the history should be reviewed for tuberculosis (TB), a chest radiograph obtained, and, if suggestive of prior TB, TB skin testing performed. Patients with a history of TB or a positive purified protein derivative (PPD) should be treated with isoniazid together with immunosuppressive therapy.

Glucocorticoids

Glucocorticoids is used in a wide range of regimens, but one typical regimen for adults is prednisone 1 mg/kg per day dosing until definite and satisfactory improvement in strength occurs, usually with 1–3 months of treatment. Slow tapering by approximately 10 mg/month will then bring patients down to a dose of 20 mg/day after approximately 6 months of therapy. Treatment needs to be tailored to specific patients given a wide range of responses. Alternative approaches include initial high-dose intravenous treatment (methylprednisolone 1 g/day for 3–5 days) for patients with severe disease, weekly bolus intravenous therapies used particularly in aggressive approaches to juvenile DM, and alternate-day dosing of prednisone rather than daily dosing.

There is uncertainty with regard to alternate-day versus daily dosing of corticosteroids. One single uncontrolled study describing comparisons of these approaches in PM showed fewer side effects with alternate-day therapies, but this study did not compare patients with equivalent doses or control for severity of disease in patients for whom daily therapy might have been selected and maintained. In a controlled trial comparing alternate-day with daily therapy in a muscle disease (Duchenne muscular dystrophy), no difference in side effects was seen with equivalent dosing of these regimens. Studies in other diseases have shown no difference for bone loss for daily in comparison to alternate-day therapy.

Methotrexate

Methotrexate is commonly used for steroid-sparing effects. It has potential pulmonary toxicity, so it is important to exclude ILD in patients with DM or PM by chest CT scan, pulmonary function tests, and testing for anti-Jo-1 antibodies, and avoid its use if present. Methotrexate is given once a week in divided doses; a common approach starts with 7.5 mg/week (administered as 2.5 mg every 12 h three times). The dose may be increased by 2.5 mg/week, to as much as 20 mg/week orally. Higher doses are given parenterally by intramuscular injection, with doses higher than 40 mg/week uncommon. Folic acid 1 mg is given daily, except on the day of methotrexate dosing. The major side effects are alopecia, stomatitis, infection, anemia, and renal or liver toxicity.

In patients with inflammatory myopathies and interstitial lung disease, methotrexate should be avoided because of its potential pulmonary toxicity

Azathioprine

Azathioprine, similar to methotrexate, has a better long-term side-effect profile than corticosteroids. It has a very delayed onset and peak effect. As a result of the long delay in interpreting efficacy, the highest tolerated dose should be considered early, often 2.5–3 mg/kg per day, with attention to bone marrow suppression and hepatotoxicity. Monthly blood counts, liver function tests, and amylase levels are recommended, with mild lymphopenia being acceptable. Dosing can start at 50 mg/day and increase weekly by 50 mg, given once or twice a day. Abdominal pain and nausea, sometimes with frank pancreatitis, develop in a significant minority of patients, and require discontinuation and subsequent avoidance of this drug.

Intravenous immunoglobulin

Intravenous immunoglobulin can be used as initial treatment in severely affected patients with a goal of more rapid improvement, or occasionally as maintenance therapy in otherwise refractory patients or with a goal of reducing long-term corticosteroid use. Dosing is 2 g/kg total initially, divided over 2–5 days, and then repeat infusions every 2–4 weeks, with a total dosage of 1–2 g/kg per month.

Other immunomodulating therapies

As with other immune-mediated neurological diseases, many other immunomodulating therapies may be used for DM and PM, including cyclophosphamide, cyclosporine, tacrolimus, chlorambucil, and mycophenolate.

Bibliography

Amato AA, Barohn RJ. Evaluation and treatment of inflammatory myopathies. *J Neurol Neurosurg Psychiatry* 2009;**80**:1060–8.

de Padilla CM, Reed AM. Dendritic cells and the immunopathogenesis of idiopathic inflammatory myopathies. *Curr Opin Rheumatol* 2008; **20**:669–74.

Greenberg SA. Inflammatory myopathies: disease mechanisms. *Curr Opin Neurol* 2009; **22**:516–23.

Mastaglia FL. Inflammatory muscle diseases. *Neurol India* 2008;**56**:263–70.

Needham M, Mastaglia FL. Inclusion body myositis: current pathogenetic concepts and diagnostic and therapeutic approaches. *Lancet Neurol* 2007;**6**:620–31.

Salajegheh M, Pinkus JL, Taylor JP, et al. Sarcoplasmic redistribution of nuclear TDP-43 in inclusion body myositis. *Muscle Nerve* 2009; **40**:19–31.

Salajegheh M, Kong SW, Pinkus JL, et al. Interferon-stimulated gene 15 (ISG15) conjugates proteins in dermatomyositis muscle with perifascicular atrophy. *Ann Neurol* 2010;**67**: 53–63.

Sato S, Kuwana M. Clinically amyopathic dermatomyositis. *Curr Opin Rheumatol* 2010; **22**: 639–43.

Sato S, Hoshino K, Satoh T, et al. RNA helicase encoded by melanoma differentiation-associated gene 5 is a major autoantigen in patients with clinically amyopathic dermatomyositis: Association with rapidly progressive interstitial lung disease. *Arthritis Rheum* 2009; **60**:2193–200.

Tawil R, Griggs RC. Inclusion body myositis. *Curr Opin Rheumatol* 2002;**14**:653–7.

Toxic Myopathies

Steven K. Baker

Department of Medicine, Physical Medicine and Neurology, Neuromuscular Disease Clinic, McMaster University Medical Center, McMaster University, Hamilton, Ontario, Canada

Toxic myopathies are an important diagnostic consideration in neuromuscular clinics because the correct diagnosis and management often lead to clinical improvement in the absence of unnecessary treatment. The clinical presentations of toxic myopathies range from an indolent myopathy to acute rhabdomyolysis. Muscle damage can be caused by numerous drugs; in the classic case of toxic exposure, withdrawal of the offending agent usually leads to gradual improvement. Infrequently, however, an underlying myopathy may be triggered or unmasked by myotoxic medication. In these cases, drug withdrawal and occasionally a therapeutic intervention are required. A skeletal muscle biopsy is fundamental in the proper work-up of acquired muscle disease and can potentially support clinical suspicion of a toxic myopathy (Box 1). Pathological confirmation, when possible, is critical because patient exposure to a potentially myotoxic drug does not automatically inculpate the drug as pathogenic. Based on a combination of the pathological changes in muscle and/or the pharmacodynamics of the drug, a classification schema has been derived for the toxic myopathies (Box 4.1).

The actual incidence of toxic myopathies is unknown but it is estimated that less than 1% of all adverse drug reactions are ever reported, including inpatients admitted for severe drug reactions. Pathological changes have been detected in asymptomatic statin-treated patients, raising a question about whether all abnormalities in a muscle biopsy are pathological. This is particularly relevant in clinical practice when an individual with cardiovascular disease and dyslipidemia on a statin complains of leg fatigue, and has a biopsy revealing mild mitochondrial abnormalities and slight intramyocellular lipid accumulation, but there has been no attention paid to other diagnostic considerations (i.e. tight iliotibial bands, hip osteoarthritis, spinal stenosis, or radiculopathy) and the statin is inappropriately discontinued.

☝ CAUTION!

MUSCLE BIOPSY
Muscle biopsy evidence of reversible statin myopathy can occur without any overt clinical symptoms and with normal creatine kinase (CK) levels. Therefore, the decision to proceed with a muscle biopsy must be carefully considered and alternative explanations for the patient's symptoms should be explored. The treating physician should be fully aware of disorders that can predispose to cramping, leg heaviness/ fatigue, and myalgia.

Neuromuscular Disorders, First Edition. Edited by Rabi N. Tawil, Shannon Venance.

Box 4.1. Pathological categorization of toxic myopathies

Necrotizing: statins, fibrates
Inflammatory: statins, D-penicillamine, interferon-α, IM gene therapy
Myosinolysis: critical-illness myopathy
Type II fiber atrophy: steroids, cancer cachexia
Mitochondrial: azidothymidine (AZT), statins, germanium, fialuridine
Microtubular: colchicine, vincristine, podophyllin
Myofibrillar: emetine/ipecac intoxication
Curvilinear body: hydroxychloroquine
Vacuolar (hypokalemic): diuretics, laxatives, amphotericin, toluene, alcohol, black licorice

Box 4.2. Drugs interacting with statins

Amiodarone
Azole antifungals
Calcium channel blockers (diltiazem and verapamil)
Ciprofloxacin
Colchicine
Cyclosporine
Hypolipemics (cholestyramine, gemfibrozil and other fibrates, niacin, ezetimibe)
HIV protease inhibitors
Macrolide antibiotics (clarithromycin, erythromycin, azithromycin)
Nefazodone
Histamine H_2-receptor antagonists (cimetidine, ranitidine)
Sitagliptin (?)
Warfarin

Lipid-lowering medications

With virtually all the lipid-lowering drugs (statins, fibrates, bile acid-binding resins, and ezetimibe) implicated in muscle toxicity, many have theorized that cholesterol is critical to the skeletal muscle cell membrane and that lowering cholesterol may explain the class effect. This rationale seems to account for the potential myotoxicity of lipid-lowering drugs at a superficial level. However, direct evidence is lacking. In fact, human skeletal muscle cholesterol content increased after 8 weeks of simvastatin therapy (80 mg/day) and did not change in response to atorvastatin (40 mg/day). The role of cholesterol depletion in lipid-lowering myopathy remains uncertain at this point and alternative mechanisms may account for the toxic effect of this class of drugs.

Statins

At the pharmacodynamic level (i.e. their site of action) all statins act similarly by selectively binding to the active site of 3-hydroxy-3-methylglutaryl coenzyme A (HMG-CoA) reductase, inhibiting the enzyme competitively. However, at the pharmacokinetic level (i.e. absorption, distribution, metabolism, and excretion), the statins have metabolic differences related to their physiochemical properties, which in turn may translate into differences in myotoxic potential and the risks of interactions with other medications or toxins (Box 4.2). For example, medications that interact with the cytochrome P450 (CYP) CYP3A4 system may increase serum levels of some of the statins and must be used with caution. In addition to medications, there are number of comorbidities that predispose to statin myopathy.

> ✋ **CAUTION!**
>
> **DRUG INTERACTIONS WITH STATINS**
> The CYP3A4- and -2C9-dependent statins are subject to drug–drug interactions that could produce meaningful escalations in serum statin levels and cause myopathy. Therefore, ensuring normal liver and renal function and choosing non-interacting drugs will minimize the risk for myotoxicity. Indeed, a recent report, probing the adverse event reporting system of the Food and Drug Administration (FDA), demonstrated that the adverse event reporting rate ratio of simvastatin-induced rhabdomyolysis was 6.4 when comparing simvastatin-treated patients with and without a concomitant CYP3A4 inhibitor. Box 4.2 is a list of the various drugs known to interact with statins.

Adding another layer of complexity is the discovery that individual variation in the gene encoding human organic anion-transporting polypeptide C (*SLCO1B1*) may influence serum statin levels and be associated with statin myopathies, e.g. a single risk allele (Val174Ala) in *SLCO1B1* accounts for 60% of the myopathic reactions to simvastatin.

The mechanisms responsible for statin-induced muscle breakdown are not known. Numerous risk factors have been identified. Much interest has focused on the role of coenzyme Q_{10} (CoQ_{10}), also referred to as ubiquinone. CoQ_{10} is a fat-soluble compound that transfers electrons in the electron transport chain of the mitochondria. Statins lower CoQ_{10} levels in the blood and are thought to reflect an effect on low-density lipoprotein (LDL)-cholesterol. Statins, by blocking HMG-CoA-reductase, impair isoprenoid synthesis and this in turn should lower CoQ_{10} levels, but definitive evidence for this mechanism is lacking. Nevertheless, case reports have documented lactic acidosis in response to statin therapy, implying a primary mitochondrial pathogenesis.

★ **TIPS AND TRICKS**

RISK FACTORS FOR STATIN MYOPATHY

- Advanced age
- Diabetes
- Drug–drug interactions (i.e. amiodarone, cyclosporine, colchicine)
- Female sex
- Hypothyroidism
- Liver failure
- Pre-existing muscle disorder
- Renal failure

Impaired metabolic activity involving the breakdown of fatty acids and carbohydrates represents alternative mechanisms supported by class III evidence, e.g. statins have been reported to exacerbate or trigger muscle complaints and hyperCKemia in patients who harbor single heterozygous mutations in genes known to cause metabolic myopathies (i.e. *PYGM*, *CPTII*).

Calcium dysregulation is another hypothesis regarding the pathogenesis of statin myopathy. Capacchione et al. reported a case of a 30-year-old physically fit African–American man who was started on simvastatin (20 mg daily) 1 month before developing exertional rhabdomyolysis (CK > 10 000 IU) from a benign 2.5 mile walk. Genetic screening revealed multiple polymorphic variations in calcium-handling proteins. This highlights the potential myopathic triggering effect of statins in individuals who possess a latent genetic diathesis. Patients with a history of exertional rhabdomyolysis should not be started on statins until a thorough neuromuscular work-up has been completed. Patients with a history of malignant hyperthermia and rippling muscle disease should be monitored closely for adverse effects.

Immune factors have also been postulated to play a role in the development of statin myopathy/myositis in a subset of patients. There are reports of cases with inflammatory infiltrates on muscle biopsy consistent with dermatomyositis and polymyositis; however, there are also patients who develop a myopathy in which the biopsy reveals MHC-1 upregulation but with no evidence of inflammatory infiltration – referred to as a necrotizing myopathy (NM). NMs can be idiopathic, paraneoplastic, or secondary to a connective-tissue disorder. The observation that a NM can develop after statin discontinuation suggests that previously restricted epitopes may be exposed by statin therapy through a toxic mechanism, and this may trigger a subsequent autoimmune myopathy manifesting either necrotizing or inflammatory changes.

Given that numerous mechanisms may account for statin myopathy it is not surprising that a variety of neuromuscular diseases can potentially be triggered or "unmasked" by statin treatment. In certain circumstances it may be advisable to avoid statin therapy in patients with pre-existing muscle disorders and choose a bile-acid resin or low-dose fibrate as the safest alternative. An approach to inform clinical decision-making around patients suspected of statin myopathy is suggested below (Figure 4.1).

Fibrates

Fibrates are also myotoxic in some individuals. They decrease plasma triglycerides by decreasing

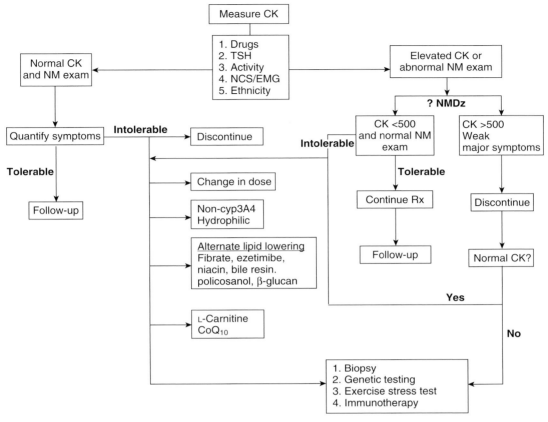

Figure 4.1. Management algorithm for statin-induced muscle disease. The box under "Measure CK" highlights five immediate considerations when assessing a patient with suspected statin myopathy. Drug interactions, hypothyroidism, exertional hyperCKemia, active denervating radiculopathy or neuropathy, and ethnic-specific CK references should be ruled out as the preliminary steps in the work-up process. CK, creatine kinase; CoQ_{10}, coenzyme Q_{10}; CYP, cytochrome P450; EMG, electromyography; NCS, nerve conduction studies; NM, neuromuscular; NMDz, neuromuscular disease; Rx, therapy; TSH, thyroid-stimulating hormone. (Reproduced from Baker SK, Samjoo IA. A neuromuscular approach to statin-related myotoxicity. *Can J Neurol Sci* 2008;**35**:8–21,with permission from *Canadian Journal of Neurological Sciences*.)

hepatic production and increasing their breakdown. They decrease the triglyceride very-low-density lipoprotein synthesis by increasing β-oxidation of fatty acids in the liver. Gemfibrozil inhibits the oxidative capacity of the CYP3A4 isoenzyme and is more myotoxic than fenofibrate, particularly when combined with statins that are CYP3A4 dependent (i.e. atorvastatin, simvastatin, and lovastatin). Acute NMs and rhabdomyolysis are seen with the fibrates, and may be more prominent with combination therapy of statins and gemfibrozil.

Ezetimibe
Ezetimibe is a novel cholesterol-lowering drug that binds to the Niemann–Pick C1-like 1 (NPC1L1) transporter, which regulates intestinal cholesterol absorption at the brush-border surface and whole-body cholesterol homeostasis. Ezetimibe alone or in combination with a statin may trigger a myopathy. Phillips et al. noted that most statin-intolerant patients also failed to tolerate ezetimibe because of recurrence of myopathic symptoms. Careful follow-up and monitoring are required for any statin-intolerant

patient on initiation of alternative lipid-lowering therapies.

Amphiphilic drugs

Cationic amphiphilic drugs contain both a hydrophilic and a hydrophobic region. It is the hydrophobic, or lipid-soluble, region that interacts with acidic/anionic phospholipids of membranes, leading to myeloid debris imbibed within lysosomes appearing as autophagic vacuoles.

Choloroquine and hydroxychloroquine

The antimalarial drugs chloroquine and hydroxychloroquine are commonly used in the treatment of connective tissue diseases. Ocular side effects include corneal deposits and, rarely, a retinopathy, or in certain cases, a "bull's eye" maculopathy. Sensory peripheral neuropathy

and cardiac toxicity can develop in addition to the myopathy. The myopathy is insidious and painless. Respiratory failure was reported in three patients with multiple comorbidities. Electrodiagnostics findings may include fibrillations, positive sharp waves, and action potentials of small amplitude, short duration, early recruitment, and polyphasic motor units. Muscle biopsy shows vacuolar degeneration and the distinct presence of curvilinear bodies, a finding that is diagnostic of hydroxychloroquine myopathy (Figure 4.2). An acute myopathy triggered by the addition of colchicine or atorvastatin (personal observation) in the setting of a chronic indolent hydroxychloroquine myopathy may occur. Thus, patients should be carefully questioned about the presence of myopathic symptoms before starting a second potentially myotoxic drug.

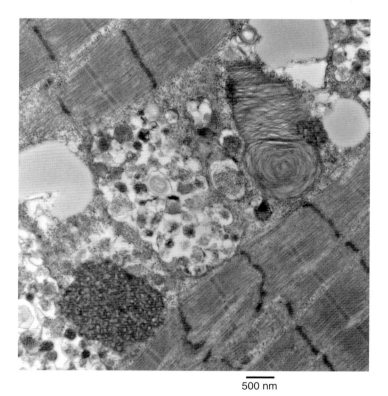

500 nm

Figure 4.2. Electron microscopic study of hydroxychloroquine myopathy. Note, the widespread and striking number of pleomorphic intracytoplasmic lysosomal inclusions. There are characteristic accumulations of concentric membranous myelinoid figures. Almost all inclusions contained characteristic curvilinear bodies. Capillaries showed thickening and multiplication of the basal lamina. Direct magnification; ×25 000.

Amiodarone

Amiodarone is a class 3 antiarrhythmic drug that prolongs phase 3 of the cardiac action potential. Amiodarone is fat soluble and therefore widely distributed in fat, muscle, skin, liver, and lungs. It is extensively metabolized by CYP3A4 and so must be used with caution when combined with CYP3A4-dependent statins. Thyrotoxicosis, hypothyroidism, cerebellar ataxia, sensorimotor mixed axonal/demyelinating polyneuroathy, pulmonary fibrosis, bone marrow suppression, dermatological reactions, and myopathy are among the reported toxicities attributed to amiodarone. Given the potential for thyrotoxicity, a dysthyroid myopathy should be considered in the differential diagnosis. The combination of nerve and muscle toxicity resulting in a neuromyopathy will produce both proximal and distal weakness. Drug withdrawal leads to an unpredictable recovery but most experience considerable improvement.

> ### ✋ CAUTION!
>
> **PHARMACOVIGILANCE**
> **Amiodarone** should not be prescribed to patients taking simvastatin at doses greater than 20 mg/day. Investigators found that the baseline use of amiodarone was associated with an 8.8 relative risk for myopathy [definite (CK >10 times upper limit of normal or ULN) and incipient myopathy (CK more than three times the ULN + five times the baseline level)] in those patients assigned to 80 mg simvastatin after 1 year of follow-up. If amiodarone is to be prescribed with a statin, **pravastatin** is preferred because there is less of a drug–drug interaction.

Antimicrotubular drugs

Colchicine

Colchicine, used for the treatment of gout, is a known tubulotoxin and disrupts microtubule assembly by binding to the α and β monomers of tubulin. Membranous organelles such as lysosomes and autophagic vacuoles are transported along the microtubule-dependent cytoskeletal lattice. HyperCKemia is typically present with proximal weakness which can develop rapidly, particularly in patients with impaired kidney function and additional myotoxic drug exposure. A distal sensory or sensorimotor neuropathy can also be present as in hydroxychloroquine and amiodarone. Pathological changes on biopsy reveal a lysosomal vacuolar myopathy. Type I fibers appear to be preferentially affected in colchicine myopathy.

> ### ✋ CAUTION!
>
> **PHARMACOVIGILANCE**
> **Colchicine** should not be administered in a dose >0.6 mg/day if renal dysfunction exists. Renal clearance accounts for approximately 10–20% of colchicine's total body clearance. Therefore, eligible patients should have a creatinine clearance above 50 mL/min.
> Colchicine is also metabolized through hepatic demethylation via CYP3A4. Therefore, the lipophilic/CYP3A4-dependent statins (i.e. atorvastatin, simvastatin, and lovastatin) may cause muscle damage through dual mechanisms of pharmacokinetic interactions and direct myotoxicity. The non-CYP3A4-dependent statins (i.e. pravastatin, rosuvastatin, and fluvastatin [2C9]) must also be used with caution in combination with colchicine.

Antimitochondrial drugs

HIV related: zidovudine (azidothymidine)

Zidovudine (3′-azido-3′-deoxythymidine, AZT), a nucleoside analog reverse transcriptase inhibitor (NRTI), was the first antiretroviral drug for treatment of acquired immune deficiency syndrome (AIDS). The toxic effect of AZT on skeletal muscle is due to an inhibitory effect on DNA polymerase γ, a nuclear-encoded mitochondrial enzyme involved in mitochondrial DNA replication. Mitochondrial toxicity can occur with both short-term and long-term therapy. AZT myopathy presents with slowly progressive proximal weakness, myalgias, and fatigue. The CK may be elevated but cannot be relied on to gauge severity. Muscle biopsy may reveal ragged-red fibers, cytochrome oxidase-negative fibers, paracrystalline inclusions, and an absence of inflammatory infiltrate.

In addition to AZT-induced mitochondrial myopathy, HIV infection can be associated with inflammatory myopathies (i.e. polymyositis, inclusion body myositis), NM, type 2 atrophy secondary to HIV-wasting syndrome, and a skeletal muscle microvasculitis. If the CK is markedly elevated, an AZT-induced myositis or rhabdomyolysis is more likely the cause. Due to frequent diagnostic uncertainty, a muscle biopsy is necessary to delineate the underlying pathology and guide clinical management. For example, AZT myopathy calls for drug withdrawal whereas a patient with an inflammatory myopathy would be treated with steroids and/or intravenous immunoglobulins. The newer NRTIs such as lamiduvine (3TC), zalcitabine (ddC), and didanosine (ddI) are considered somewhat safer than AZT, as are the other highly active antiretroviral therapies (HAART) – tenofir, lopinavir/ritonavir. However, as ritonavir is a pharmacoenhancer of lopinavir, and other protease inhibitors, through its inhibition of CYP3A, caution must be used when co-prescribing other CYP3A(4)-dependent drugs.

Drug-induced myosis

D-Penicillamine

D-Penicillamine is the prototypic drug implicated in induction of immune-mediated disorders including systemic lupus erythematosus, morphea, pemphigus, glomerulonephritis, myasthenia gravis, polymyositis, and dermatomyositis. The incidence of poly- and dermatomyositis caused by D-penicillamine is approximately 0.6%. Drug withdrawal may permit clinical recovery but immunosuppressive therapy is occasionally required.

Phenytoin

Phenytoin blocks voltage-gated neuronal sodium channels in a use-dependent fashion and therefore inhibits repetitive firing. Rarely, myotoxicity can occur in the form of hypersensitivity myositis, dermatomyositis, or rhabdomyolysis. Hepatitis, rash, myalgia, and fever may also be present. A biopsy from one patient whose CK peaked at 242 000 U/L revealed early necrosis and

sarcoplasmic dissolution with no signs of inflammatory infiltrate or vasculitis. The myopathy generally improves with drug withdrawal.

Procainamide

Procainamide, a class IA antiarrythmic, exerts its effect through sodium channel blockade. It is estimated that 20–30% of patients treated with long-term procainamide develop a lupus-like syndrome and 83% possess antinuclear antibodies. Vasculitis, pure red cell aplasia, agranulocytosis, and thrombocytopenia may also occur. A toxic myopathy is less common than the lupus-like syndrome but perivascular inflammatory infiltrates consisting of mononuclear cells and macrophages were demonstrated in a biopsy and this suggested a low-grade polymyositis. Drug withdrawal should prompt a recovery within a few weeks but immunotherapy may be necessary.

Miscellaneous drugs

Steroids

Chronic steroid excess of both endogenous (i.e. Cushing's syndrome) and exogenous origin can produce a slowly evolving proximal myopathy that is characterized by type II muscle fiber atrophy (particularly IIB), although type I fibers may also be slightly atrophic. Glucocorticoids shift skeletal muscle protein metabolism into a catabolic state. This effect is mediated by several key genes. Steroid therapy induces glutamine synthetase, atrogin-1 (plus other genes that cause muscle atrophy, i.e. atrogenes), and myostatin. Glutamine, testosterone, selective androgen receptor modulation, insulin-like growth factor-1, and growth hormone have been shown to offset the atrophying effects of glucocorticoids on muscle.

Bibliography

Abdel-Hamid H, Oddis CV, Lacomis D. Severe hydroxychloroquine myopathy. *Muscle Nerve* 2008;**38**:1206–10.

Baker SK, Samjoo IA. A neuromuscular approach to statin-related myotoxicity. *Can J Neurol Sci* 2008;**35**:8–21.

Barclay CL, McLean M, Hagen N, Brownell AK, MacRae ME. Severe phenytoin hypersensitivity with myopathy: a case report. *Neurology* 1992; **42**:230–3.

Bradley WG, Lassman LP, Pearce GW, Walton JN. The neuromyopathy of vincristine in man. Clinical, electrophysiological and pathological studies. *J Neurol Sci* 1970;**10**:107–31.

Capacchione JF, Sambuughin N, Bina S, Mulligan LP, Lawson TD, Muldoon SM. Exertional rhabdomyolysis and malignant hyperthermia in a patient with ryanodine receptor type 1 gene, L-type calcium channel alpha-1 subunit gene, and calsequestrin-1 gene polymorphisms. *Anesthesiology* **112**:239–44.

Chariot P, Abadia R, Agnus D, Danan C, Charpentier C, Gherardi RK. Simvastatin-induced rhabdomyolysis followed by a MELAS syndrome. *Am J Med* 1993;**94**:109–10.

Christopher-Stine L, Casciola-Rosen LA, Hong G, Chung T, Corse AM, Mammen AL. A novel autoantibody recognizing 200-kd and 100-kd proteins is associated with an immune-mediated necrotizing myopathy. *Arthritis Rheum* **62**:2757–66.

Dalakas MC. Toxic and drug-induced myopathies. *J Neurol Neurosurg Psychiatry* 2009;**80**: 832–8.

Engel JN, Mellul VG, Goodman DB. Phenytoin hypersensitivity: a case of severe acute rhabdomyolysis. *Am J Med* 1986;**81**:928–30.

Fontiveros ES, Cumming WJ, Hudgson P. Procainamide-induced myositis. *J Neurol Sci* 1980;**45**:143–7.

Grable-Esposito P, Katzberg HD, Greenberg SA, Srinivasan J, Katz J, Amato AA. Immune-mediated necrotizing myopathy associated with statins. *Muscle Nerve* **41**:185–90.

Link E, Parish S, Armitage J, et al. SLCO1B1 variants and statin-induced myopathy – a genomewide study. *N Engl J Med* 2008;**359**:789–99.

Magarian GJ, Lucas LM, Colley C. Gemfibrozil-induced myopathy. *Arch Intern Med* 1991;**151**: 1873–4.

Meier C, Kauer B, Muller U, Ludin HP. Neuromyopathy during chronic amiodarone treatment. A case report. *J Neurol* 1979;**220**: 231–9.

Niemi M, Schaeffeler E, Lang T, et al. High plasma pravastatin concentrations are associated with single nucleotide polymorphisms and haplotypes of organic anion transporting polypeptide-C (OATP-C, SLCO1B1). *Pharmacogenetics* 2004;**14**:429–40.

Metabolic Myopathies

Ingrid Tein

Neurometabolic Clinic and Research Laboratory, Dept. of Pediatrics, Division of Neurology, and Genetics and Genome Biology Program, The Hospital for Sick Children, University of Toronto, Toronto, Ontario, Canada

Utilization of bioenergetic substrates in exercise

Symptoms in muscle energy defects are directly related to a mismatch between the rate of ATP utilization (energy demand) and the capacity of the muscle metabolic pathways to regenerate ATP (energy supply). This energy supply/demand mismatch impairs energy-dependent processes that power muscle contraction (weakness, exertional fatigue), mediate muscle relaxation (muscle cramping, tightness), and/or maintain membrane ion gradients necessary for normal membrane excitability (fatigue, weakness) and muscle cell integrity (muscle pain, injury, myoglobinuria). In metabolic myopathies, the specific metabolic mediators of premature fatigue, cramping, pain, and muscle injury are complex and vary among the different metabolic disorders.

bioenergetic pathway in working muscle depends on the type, intensity, and duration of exercise and also on diet and physical conditioning. In the first 5–10 min of moderate exercise, high-energy phosphates are used to first regenerate adenosine triphosphate (ATP). This is followed by muscle glycogen breakdown, which is indicated by a sharp rise in lactate during the first 10 min. Blood lactate levels then drop as muscle triglycerides and blood-borne fuels are used. After 90 min, the major fuels are glucose and free fatty acids (FFAs). During 1–4 h of mild-to-moderate prolonged exercise, muscle uptake of FFAs increases approximately 70% and, after 4 h, FFAs are used twice as much as carbohydrates.

⚘ SCIENCE REVISITED

The primary source of energy for resting muscle is derived from fatty acid oxidation (FAO). At rest, glucose utilization accounts for 10–15% of total oxygen consumption and both slow- and fast-twitch fibers have similar levels of glycogen content. The choice of

Disorders of glycogen, lipid, or mitochondrial metabolism may cause two main clinical syndromes in muscle: (1) acute, recurrent, reversible muscle dysfunction with exercise intolerance and acute muscle breakdown or myoglobinuria (with or without cramps) and (2) progressive weakness. Progressive weakness and recurrent myoglobinuria can also occur together in a given disorder.

Neuromuscular Disorders, First Edition. Edited by Rabi N. Tawil, Shannon Venance.
© 2011 John Wiley & Sons, Ltd. Published 2011 by John Wiley & Sons, Ltd.

Clinical syndrome of myoglobinuria and mechanisms

A common presentation for metabolic myopathies is recurrent myoglobinuria. Myoglobinuria is a clinical syndrome, not just a biochemical state.

an attack of myoglobinuria, which require careful monitoring, are potentially life-threatening respiratory failure, renal failure, and cardiac arrhythmias.

Etiologies of myoglobinuria can be divided into hereditary and sporadic forms. The sporadic etiologies that may precipitate an attack in an otherwise normal individual can be divided into those related to exertion, crush injury, ischemia, toxins and drugs, metabolic depression, abnormalities of body temperature, infections, progressive muscle disease, and those that appear to be idiopathic. A comparison of myoglobinuria related to exertion, heat stroke, neuroleptic malignant syndrome and malignant hyperthermia is given in Table 5.1.

The hereditary forms (Box 5.1) are particularly important because they are recurrent and suggest underlying pathogenic mechanisms. This may have implications for treatment strategies, preventive measures and genetic counseling. These forms may be divided into three groups based on whether the biochemical abnormality is known, incompletely characterized, or unknown. In the first group, there are at least 25 recognized disorders. All are autosomal recessive in inheritance with the exception of three X-linked disorders. The mitochondrial defects may be autosomal

Table 5.1. Heat, fever, and myoglobinuria

	Exercise induced Myoglobinuria	Malignant Hyperthermia	Malignant Neuroleptic syndrome	Heat Exhaustion/Heat stroke
Myoglobinuria	+	+	+	+
Provoking factor	Exercise	Halothane	Neuroleptics	Exercise/Exposure
Tachycardia	+	+	+	+
Acidosis	+	+	+	+
DIC	+	+	+	+
Muscle rigidity	0	+	+	0
Onset duration	Minutes	Minutes	Days	Minutes
Familial attacks	Rare[a]	Rare	None	None

[a]Hereditable biochemical abnormality may be identified.
DIC, disseminated intravascular coagulation.
Reproduced from Rowland LP. Myoglobinuria. *Can J Neurol Sci* 1984;**11**:1–13 with permission from Canadian Journal Of Neurological Science.

Box 5.1. Heritable causes of exercise intolerance and recurrent myoglobinuria

Biochemical abnormality known

1. **Glycolysis/Glycogenolysis**
   Phosphorylase[a]
   Phosphofructokinase
   Phosphoglycerate kinase[a]
   Phosphoglycerate mutase[a]
   Lactate dehydrogenase[a]
   Phosphorylase "b" kinase
   Debrancher
   Aldolase A[a]
2. **Fatty acid oxidation**
   Carnitine palmitoyltransferase II[a]
   Long-chain acyl-CoA dehydrogenase
   Very-long-chain acyl-CoA dehydrogenase
   Medium-chain acyl-CoA dehydrogenase
   Short-chain L-3-hydroxyacyl-CoA
      dehydrogenase[a]
   Trifunctional protein/long-chain
      L-3-hydroxyacyl-CoA dehydrogenase[a]
   Medium-chain 3-ketoacyl-CoA thiolase[a]
   Acyl-CoA dehydrogenase 9 (ACAD9)[a]
3. **Pentose phosphate pathway**
   Glucose-6-phosphate dehydrogenase[a]
4. **Purine nucleotide cycle**
   Myoadenylate deaminase
5. **Respiratory chain**
   Complex II[a] and aconitase
   Coenzyme Q
   Multiple mitochondrial DNA deletions [a]
   Complex I[a]
   Complex III (cytochrome *b*)
   Complex IV (cytochrome oxidase)[a]
6. **Triglyceride and membrane phospholipid biosynthesis**
   LPIN1 – muscle-specific phosphatidic
      acid phosphatase[a]

Biochemical abnormality incompletely characterized
Impaired long-chain fatty acid oxidation[a]
Impaired function of the sarcoplasmic
   reticulum in familial malignant
   hyperthermia (predisposition in central
   core disease)[a]

Abnormal composition of the sarcolemma
   in, for example, Duchenne and Becker
   muscular dystrophy[a]

Biochemical abnormality unknown
Familial recurrent myoglobinuira[a]
Repeated attacks in sporadic cases[a]

[a]Etiologies that have been documented to cause recurrent myoglobinuria beginning in childhood.
Modified from Tein I, DiMauro S, Rowland LP. Myoglobinuria. In: Rowland LP, DiMauro S (eds), *Handbook of Clinical Neurology*, vol 18. *Myopathies*. Amsterdam: Elsevier Science Publishers BV, 1992.

recessive, autosomal dominant, X-linked, sporadic, or inherited by maternal mitochondrial transmission.

In FAO disorders, attacks of myoglobinuria are precipitated after mild-to-moderate prolonged exercise when fatty acids are the key energy source in exercising muscle. These attacks may be further exacerbated by inadequate caloric intake as in fasting or infection with vomiting, which further limit blood glucose. Other risk factors include infection, during which metabolic processes preferentially favor FAO; this persists despite glucose administration, thereby increasing the dependence on FAO. There may also be fever with shivering thermogenesis and vomiting with fasting, making this a common trigger. Cold exposure may be detrimental as shivering depends upon involuntary muscle activity which primarily depends upon long-chain fatty acids (LCFAs). Emotional stress has also been a recognized precipitant. Other possible mechanisms relate to the toxicity of elevated FFAs arising proximal to the block, especially LCFAs which may be membranotoxic.

Myoadenylate deaminase and glucose-6-phosphate dehydrogenase (G6PD) deficiencies have not been conclusively linked to causation because both enzymes may be absent in asymptomatic people.

There appear to be differences in the distribution of etiologies of heritable myoglobinuria in adults versus children. In a study of 100 cases of recurrent childhood-onset myoglobinuria, only

24% of children were diagnosed biochemically – 16 with carnitine palmitoyltransferase (CPT) II deficiency and 7 with various glycolytic/glycogenolytic defects. These children were divided into two groups: a type I exertional group with exertion as the primary precipitating factor and a type II toxic group with infection and/or fever and leukocytosis as the primary precipitants. The type II toxic childhood group was distinguished from the type I exertional childhood- and adult-onset groups by its etiologies, which were limited to FAO defects and slight female predominance in contrast to the marked male predominance in the latter two groups. The type II toxic group was further distinguished by its earlier age at onset of attacks of myoglobinuria, the presence of more generalized disease (e.g. ictal bulbar signs, encephalopathy, seizures, developmental delay), and a higher mortality rate. In a study of 77 adult patients, Tonin et al. identified the enzyme abnormality in 36 patients: CPT II deficiency in 17 patients; glycolytic/glycogenolytic defects in 15 patients; and combined CPT II and myoadenylate deaminase in one individual. The most common etiology overall for recurrent myoglobinuria in children, boys and girls, is CPT II deficiency and in adults is phosphorylase deficiency followed by CPT II deficiency. Differentiation of classic CPT II from phosphorylase deficiency is given in Table 5.2.

Glycolytic/glycogenolytic disorders

The clinical features, affected tissues, and enzyme defects of the muscle glycogenoses are shown in Table 5.3. Glycogen accumulation in muscle may or may not be present. Phosphorylase deficiency or McArdle's disease is the most common glycogenosis resulting in recurrent myoglobinuria. Certain defects such as phosphorylase (PPL) and phosphofructokinase (PFK) deficiencies can be detected on muscle histochemical staining.

Individuals with defective glycolysis/glycogenolysis are most vulnerable during the initial stages of intense exercise, and they must rest soon after starting exercise because of muscle cramps. However, if they continue to exercise at low intensity for 10–12 min, they are then able to continue for a longer time. This is known as the *second-wind phenomenon* and has been attributed to a metabolic switch from carbohydrate to fatty acid utilization and to increased circulation, with increased availability of blood glucose from hepatic glycogenolysis.

The forearm ischemic exercise test is a useful test for the detection of enzymatic defects in the non-lysosomal glycogenolytic and glycolytic pathways.

> ### ★ TIPS AND TRICKS FOR PERFORMING FOREARM ISCHEMIC EXERCISE TEST
>
> After 1 min of repetitive maximal grip exercise under ischemic conditions, blood samples from the antecubital vein are sequentially obtained at 1, 3, 5, 7, 10, and 15 min. In healthy individuals there is a four- to sixfold increase of lactate over baseline, with the peak occurring at 1–2 min after exercise, which declines to baseline values by 15 min. This is paralleled by a similar fivefold or more increase in ammonia, with levels generally peaking at 2–5 min after exercise in individuals with normal myoadenylate deaminase activity. In individuals with a defect in glycolysis/glycogenolysis, there is an insufficient rise in lactate (less than twofold), with a compensatory and exaggerated increase in ammonia, which also indicates sufficient effort on the part of the individual. An insufficient lactate rise has been demonstrated in PPL, debrancher, PFK, phosphoglycerate kinase (PGK), phosphoglycerate mutase (PGAM), and lactate dehydrogenase (LDH) deficiencies but not in acid maltase or phosphorylase b kinase deficiency. The major limitation of this test is that the rise of venous lactate in individuals who do not have a defect in this pathway is highly dependent on the patient's ability and willingness to exercise. Therefore patients in whom lactate levels are low due to poor effort, or to placement of the venous line in other than the median cubital vein, show proportionally blunted ammonia responses. The test should be immediately truncated if the patient develops an acute cramp, because myonecrosis may occur in an individual with a glycolytic disorder.

Table 5.2. Differentiation between disorders of glycogen versus lipid metabolism resulting in exercise intolerance and/or myoglobinuria

	Glycolytic/Glycogenolytic	Fatty acid oxidation
	Phosphorylase deficiency	Carnitine palmitoyltransferase II deficiency "adult type"
Symptom onset in exercise	Early (first few minutes)	Late (particularly after 1 hour)
Second wind	+	−
Myalgia	Cramps	Stiffness
Fixed weakness	More common	Less common
Elevated interictal creatine kinase	+	−
Abnormal forearm ischemic lactate test	+	−
Delayed ketogenesis	−	+
Muscle biopsy	± glycogen storage	± lipid storage

Taken with permission from Tein I. Approach to muscle cramps, exercise intolerance and recurrent myoglobinuria. Proceedings of the 38th Annual Meeting of the Canadian Congress of Neurosciences. Muscle Diseases Course, Quebec City, Canada, 2003: 1–29 (CME course).

Treatment in PPL deficiency includes the administration of glucose or sucrose and Vitamin B6. However glucose is ineffective in PFK and more distal glycolytic disorders. Acid maltase deficiency (AMD) may present with three very different clinical presentations including: (1) severe generalized disease of infancy described by Pompe, which is fatal before age 2 years and involves diffuse infantile hypotonia, macroglossia, respiratory weakness, cardiomyopathy, myopathy, hepatomegaly, and anterior horn cell disease; (2) a juvenile variant affecting exclusively muscle with onset in childhood and death by the second or third decade; and (3) a milder, adult-onset variant simulating limb–girdle myopathy. Enzyme replacement therapy appears promising in childhood and late-onset AMD. A high protein diet has been advocated for PPL, phosphorylase b kinase, and PFK deficiencies.

Fatty acid oxidation disorders

Defects in FAO are an important group of disorders because they are potentially rapidly fatal and a source of major morbidity encompassing a spectrum of clinical disorders, including recurrent myoglobinuria, progressive lipid storage myopathy, neuropathy, pigmentary retinopathy, progressive cardiomyopathy, recurrent hypoglycemic hypoketotic encephalopathy or Reye-like syndrome, seizures, and cognitive delays (**Table 5.4**). There is frequently a family history of sudden unexpected death syndrome (SIDS) in siblings as these are all autosomal recessive disorders. Early recognition and prompt institution of therapy and appropriate preventive measures, and in certain cases specific therapy, may be life saving and significantly decrease long-term morbidity, particularly with respect to central nervous system sequelae. There are at least 21 recognized enzyme defects in FAO. Newborn screening of blood spot acylcarnitines has been instituted in a number of countries and has contributed to the early detection of these disorders. The most common defect is medium-chain acyl-CoA dehydrogenase (MCAD) deficiency with an incidence as high as 1 in 8930 live births in the Pennsylvania newborn screening program. There are differentiating biochemical profiles of the FAO disorders. The clinical picture, in combination with an analysis of serum acylcarnitines, urinary organic acid profiles, and urinary acylglycines, may suggest a specific site of defect and the chain-length specificity of the defect (e.g. short, medium, or long chain), after which

Table 5.3. Clinical presentation of muscle glycogenoses

Type	Enzyme defect	Affected tissues	Clinical presentation
II Infancy	Acid maltase	Generalized	Cardiomegaly, weakness, hypotonia, death age <1 year
II Childhood	Acid maltase	Generalized	Myopathy simulating Duchenne dystrophy, respiratory insufficiency
II Adult	Acid maltase	Generalized	Myopathy simulating limb girdle dystrophy or polymyositis, respiratory insufficiency
III	Debrancher	Generalized	Hepatomegaly, fasting hypoglycemia, progressive weakness
IV	Brancher	Generalized	Hepatosplenomegaly, cirrhosis of liver, hepatic failure, myopathy, cardiomyopathy, APBD
V	Muscle phosphorylase	Skeletal muscle	Intolerance to intense exercise, cramps, myoglobinuria
VII	Muscle phosphofructokinase	Skeletal muscle RBCs	Intolerance to intense exercise, cramps, myoglobinuria
VIII	Phosphorylase kinase	Liver	Asymptomatic hepatomegaly
VIII	Phosphorylase kinase	Liver and muscle	Hepatomegaly, growth retardation, hypotonia
VIII	Phosphorylase kinase	Skeletal muscle	Exercise intolerance, myoglobinuria
VIII	Phosphorylase kinase	Heart	Fatal infantile cardiomyopathy
IX	Phosphoglycerate kinase	Generalized	Hemolytic anemia, seizures, learning disability, intolerance to intense exercise, myoglobinuria
X	Muscle phosphoglycerate mutase	Skeletal muscle	Intolerance to intense exercise, myoglobinuria
XI	Muscle lactate dehydrogenase	Skeletal muscle	Intolerance to intense exercise, myoglobinuria
XII	Aldolase A	Skeletal muscle RBCs	Nonspherocytic hemolytic anemia, exercise intolerance, weakness
XIII	β-Enolase	Skeletal muscle	Exercise intolerance

Modified from DiMauro S, Lamperti C. Muscle glycogenoses. *Muscle Nerve* 2001;**24**:985.
APBD, adult polyglucosan body disease; RBCs, red blood cells.

Table 5.4. Clinical features associated with specific genetic defects of fatty acid oxidation

Deficiency	Fasting disorder	Tissue involved	Hypoketotic hypoglycemia	Altered carnitine	Dicarboxylic acids	Reye-like syndrome	SIDS
LCFAUD	+	L	+	+	NR	NR	NR
OCTN2	+	H, M	+	+	NR	+	NR
CPT I	+	K	+	+	NR	+	NR
TRANS	+	H, M, (Mg)	+	+	NR	+	+
CPT II (mild)	±	M, Mg, P	NR	+	NR	NR	NR
CPT II (severe)	+	H, M, Mg, L	+	+	NR	+	+
VLCAD/LCAD	+	H, M, Mg, L	+	+	+	+	+
ACAD9	+	B, H, L, M, Mg	+	+	+	+	NR
Trifunctional/LCHAD	+	H, M, Mg, L, N, P, R	+	+	+	+	+
Dienoyl-CoA reductase	NR	M, D, B, (H)	NR	+	NR	NR	NR
MCAD	+	(Mg)	+	+	+	+	+
SCAD	+	M, B, D, H	±	+	+	NR	+
SCHAD	+	H, M, Mg, L	+	+	+	NR	+
ETF and ETF/Qo	+	M, H, K, B, D	+	+	+	NR	+
HMG-CoA lyase	+	B, P	+	+	+	+	+?

Modified from Tein I. Fatty acid oxidation and associated defects. *American Academy of Neurology Proceedings.* Seattle. Madison, WI: Omnipress, 1995.

ACAD9, acyl-CoA dehydrogenase 9; B, brain; CPT, carnitine palmitoyltransferase; D, dysmorphic features; ETF, electron transfer flavoprotein; H, heart; HMG, β-hydroxy-β-methylglutaryl; K, kidney; L, liver; LCAD, long-chain acyl-CoA dehydrogenase; LCFAUD, long-chain fatty acid uptake defect; M, muscle; MCAD, medium-chain acyl-CoA dehydrogenase; Mg, myoglobinuria; N, neuropathy; NR, no case yet reported; OCTN2, plasmalemmal high-affinity carnitine transporter; P, pancreatitis; Qo, coenzyme Q oxidoreductase; R, retinopathy; SCAD, short-chain acyl-CoA dehydrogenase; SCHAD, short-chain L-3-hydroxyacyl-CoA dehydrogenase; TRANS, carnitine acylcarnitine translocase; trifunctional, long-chain enoyl-CoA hydratase + long-chain L-3-hydroxyacyl-CoA dehydrogenase + long-chain 3-ketoacyl-CoA thiolase; VLCAD, very-long-chain acyl-CoA dehydrogenase.

specific enzyme assays in fibroblasts and molecular mutation analysis may be done to confirm the specific gene defect and screen family members.

General treatment approaches include the strict avoidance of precipitating factors such as prolonged fasting, prolonged aerobic exercise (>30 min), and cold exposure leading to shivering thermogenesis. A high carbohydrate load before exercise is advisable with a rest period and repeat carbohydrate load at 15 min. In the event of progressive lethargy, obtundation, or poor oral intake because of vomiting, urgent intravenous glucose therapy is indicated (8–10 mg/kg per min glucose infusion). In general, it is advisable to institute a high-carbohydrate, low-fat diet with frequent feedings throughout the day, particularly a bedtime snack, commensurate with the nutritional needs of the child given his or her age with the aid of a metabolic dietician. Augmentation of the diet with essential fatty acids (at 1–2% of total energy intake) is often used to reduce the risk of essential fatty acid deficiency. Flaxseed, canola, walnut, or safflower oils can be used for this purpose. To delay the onset of fasting overnight in children who manifest symptoms of early morning hypoglycemia, the nightly institution of uncooked cornstarch will prolong the postabsorptive state and delay fasting. Cornstarch provides a sustained-release source of glucose, thereby preventing hypoglycemia and lipolysis, but may result in undesirable weight gain.

Specific measures include riboflavin substitution in certain cases of multiple acyl-CoA dehydrogenase deficiencies, medium-chain triglyceride (MCT) oil in long-chain FAO disorders, and oral prednisone and docosahexaenoic acid (essential polyunsaturated fatty acid or PUFA) in myoneuropathic long-chain 3-hydroxyacyl-coenzyme A dehydrogenase (LCHAD) deficiency. Bezafibrate, a peroxisome proliferator-activated receptor (PPAR) agonist, increases long-chain FAO in deficient fibroblasts and is being considered as a future mode of therapy, although individuals should be monitored for possible drug-induced increase in serum CK because there have been rare reports of myoglobinuria in patients with renal insufficiency who tend to accumulate the drug. Carnitine therapy is absolutely essential in the high-affinity plasmalemmal carnitine transporter (OCTN2) defect, of questionable value in short- and medium-chain FAO defects, and potentially deleterious in long-chain FAO disorders.

Mitochondrial disorders

The prevalence of mtDNA point mutations that cause disease is estimated as 1/5000 to 1/10 000 and the frequency of mtDNA mutations among healthy individuals as 1/200. This suggests that mitochondrial diseases are among the most common metabolic disorders. *POLG* mutations are a major cause of human disease, possibly accounting for up to 25% of all patients with mitochondrial disease, with a variety of clinical syndromes, in which the autosomal recessive mutations tend to cause mtDNA depletion and present in childhood, whereas the dominant mutations tend to cause adult-onset disease with multiple secondary deletions of mtDNA.

Mitochondrial diseases are clinically heterogeneous. There may be variation in the age at onset, course, and distribution of weakness in pure myopathies. On average, the age of onset reflects the level of mutation and the severity of the biochemical defect; however, other factors including nuclear genetic and/or environmental factors can also affect the expression of disease. Additional features may include exercise intolerance and premature fatigue. The most common presenting clinical features include short stature, sensorineural hearing loss, migraine headaches, ophthalmoparesis, myopathy, axonal neuropathy, diabetes mellitus, hypertrophic cardiomyopathy, and renal tubular acidosis. Additional features may include stroke-like episodes, seizures, myoclonus, retinitis pigmentosa, optic atrophy, ataxia, gastrointestinal pseudo-obstruction, and hypoparathyroidism. Inheritance may be autosomal recessive which accounts for most cases, autosomal dominant, X-linked, or maternal mtDNA transmission (Box 5.2). In the case of mtDNA mutations, the expression of the phenotype depends upon the ratio of mutant to wild-type mtDNA in a given tissue and the tissues involved.

The diagnosis of mtDNA-related disorders requires a careful *synthesis* of the clinical history, signs, mode of inheritance with detailed family pedigree, laboratory data (serum lactate and

Box 5.2. Genetic classification of mitochondrial respiratory chain diseases

Defects of mitochondrial DNA

1. **Mutations in mitochondrial protein synthesis**
   A. mtDNA rearrangements:
      a. Single-deletions (usually sporadic)
      b. Duplications or duplications/ deletions (maternal transmission)
   B. mtDNA point mutations (maternal transmission):
      a. tRNA genes
      b. rRNA genes
2. **Mutations in protein-coding genes**
   a. Complex I (ND) genes
   b. Complex III – cytochrome *b*
   c. Complex IV (COX I, II, III)
   d. Complex V (ATPase 6) genes

Defects of nuclear DNA (mendelian transmission)

1. **Defects of the respiratory chain subunit genes – complex I, II, III**
2. **Defects in respiratory chain assembly ancillary proteins – complex I e.g. *NDUFA12L*; complex III, e.g. *BCS1L*; complex IV, e.g. *SURF1*, *SCO2*, *LRPPRC*; complex V, e.g. *ATPAF2***
3. **Defects in coenzyme Q10 biosynthesis, e.g. *CABC1*, *COQ2*, *COQ8*, *ADCK3*, *PDSS1*, *PDSS2***
4. **Defects of intergenomic signaling required for mtDNA integrity and replication**
   Multiple deletions of mtDNA – *POLG1*, *ANT1*, *PEO1*, *ECGF1*, *POLG2*, *TYMP*
   Depletion of mtDNA – *TK2*, *DGUOK*, *POLG1*, *SUCLA2*, *SUCLG1*, *MPV17*, *RRM2B*, *PEO1*, *TYMP*
5. **Defects of mitochondrial transport machinery – *TIMM8A*, *SLC25A3*, *ABCB7***
6. **Defects in mtDNA translation – *GFM1*, *MRPS16*, *TSFM*, *TUFM*, *PUS1*, *DARS2***
7. **Alterations mitochondrial membrane lipids in which RC is embedded – *TAZ***

8. **Alterations in mitochondrial fission and fusion – *MFN2*, *OPA1*, *DLP1***
9. **Defects in mitochondrial apoptosis – *FASTKD2***

Modified from Vu TH, Hirano M, DiMauro S. Mitochondrial diseases. *Neurol Clin N Am* 2002;**20**:809–39; DiMauro S. Mitochondrial diseases. *Biochim Biophys Acta* 2004;**1658**: 80–8; DiMauro S, Schon EA. Mitochondrial disorders in the nervous system. *Annu Rev Neurosci* 2008;**31**:91-–123; Rahman S, Hanna MG. Diagnosis and therapy in neuromuscular disorders: diagnosis and new treatments in mitochondrial diseases. *J Neurol Neurosurg Psychiatry* 2009;**80**:943–95; Finsterer J, Harbo HF, Baets J, et al. EFNS guidelines on the molecular diagnosis of mitochondrial disorders. *Eur J Neurol* 2009;**16**:1255–64.

alanine, glucose, hematological, liver and renal function studies, calcium metabolism, etc.), neuroophthalmological examination (including possibly an electroretinogram or ERG), evoked potentials, particularly auditory brain-stem responses (ABRs), neuroradiological findings (including magnetic resonance spectroscopy for lactate elevation), exercise physiology studies, muscle histology, electron microscopy and bio-chemistry, echocardiography and EKG, and molecular genetic studies.

⭐ **TIPS AND TRICKS FOR MUSCLE BIOPSY ANALYSIS**

Muscle histology may be helpful if there are ragged red fibers (RRFs) on Gomori's trichrome stain, signifying a proliferation of subsarcolemmal mitochondria, although RRFs are not specific for mitochondrial disorders and a number of mitochondrial disorders do not have RRFs. Proper handling and processing of the muscle biopsy are key for the biochemical assay of respiratory chain enzymes, especially complex I which is highly labile, and for the analysis of mtDNA depletion and deletions.

Approach to investigation of recurrent myoglobinuria

Based on the clinical features and screening biochemical tests, a practical approach can be derived for the prioritized investigation of recurrent myoglobinuria (Figure 5.1). If there is a history of true muscle cramps within the first minutes of high-intensity exercise or of a "second-wind" phenomenon, this would suggest a glycolytic or glycogenolytic disorder. If there is a history of muscle stiffness after mild-to-moderate prolonged exercise (e.g. >1 h) or of myoglobinuria precipitated by fasting or cold exposure,

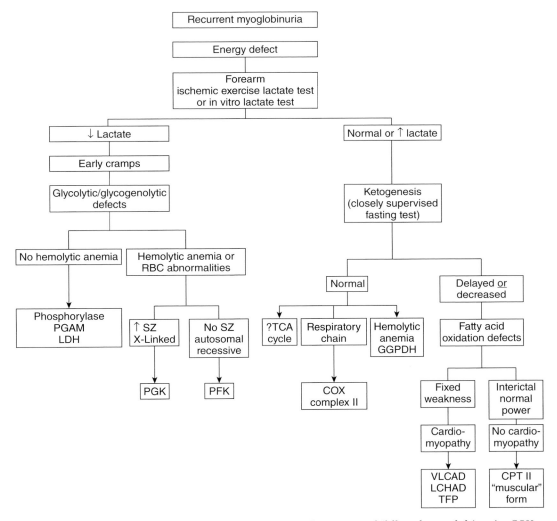

Figure 5.1. Algorithmic approach to the investigation of recurrent childhood myoglobinuria. COX, cytochrome oxidase; CPT, carnitine palmitoyltransferase; G6PDH, glucose-6-phosphate dehydrogenase; LCHAD, long-chain L-3-hydroxyacyl-CoA dehydrogenase; LDH, lactate dehydrogenase; PFK, phosphofructokinase; PGAM phosphoglycerate mutase; PGK, phosphoglycerate kinase; RBC, red blood cell; SZ, seizures; TCA, tricarboxylic acid cycle; TFP, trifunctional protein; VLCAD, very-long-chain acyl-CoA dehydrogenase. (Modified from Fejerman N, Chamoles NA (eds), *New Trends in Pediatric Neurology.* International Congress Series 1033. Amsterdam: Elsevier Science Publishers BV, 1993, with permission from Elsevier. pp 185-194)

this would suggest a defect in FAO. The first clinical test would be the forearm ischemic exercise test. In the young child in whom this is not possible, an in vitro lactate test may be performed on the muscle biopsy to test the integrity of the glycolytic pathway. If lactate production is insufficient (less than a three- to fourfold rise) and there is an exaggerated rise in ammonia, this would suggest a block in the glycogenolytic/glycolytic pathway. The defects in glycolysis/glycogenolysis can be divided into two groups: those in which there is an associated hemolytic anemia and those without hemolytic anemia. The forearm ischemic exercise test can also be used to assess whether there is an appropriate rise (three- to fourfold) in ammonia. If ammonia production is insufficient and there is an exaggerated rise in lactate, this would suggest a defect in the purine nucleotide cycle such as myoadenylate deaminase deficiency.

If there is adequate lactate production, the next important question relates to whether there is any evidence for deficient ketogenesis. If ketogenesis appears normal, the considerations include a defect in the pentose phosphate pathway (G6PD deficiency), which may be distinguished by the presence of hemolytic anemia. Other considerations would include the mitochondrial encephalomyopathies secondary to defects in the respiratory chain or mtDNA, which may be suspected if there are marked elevations of serum lactate (more than twofold) and certain characteristic clinical features such as failure to thrive, short stature, and sensorineural hearing loss, or perhaps a maternal pattern of inheritance.

If there is evidence of delayed or deficient ketogenesis, a defect in FAO should be suspected. Of the possibilities, the most common defect is that of the classic "adult" myopathic form of CPT II deficiency, in which there is typically adolescent-onset recurrent myoglobinuria, with normal power between episodes, and no associated cardiomyopathy or overt liver disease. This contrasts with the fixed lipid storage myopathy and cardiomyopathy seen in LCAD/very long-chain acyl-coenzyme A dehydrogenase (VLCAD), long-chain 3-hydroxyacyl-CoA dehydrogenase (LCHAD)/trifunctional protein deficiency (TFP), and short-chain 3-hydroxyacyl-CoA dehydrogenase (SCHAD) deficiencies. The common "adult" myopathic form of CPT II deficiency contrasts with the rare "infantile" hepatic form of CPT I deficiency, which presents with recurrent hypoglycemic/hypoketotic encephalopathy and seizures, precipitated by fasting or infection, and in which there are no significant muscular manifestations. Thus, the careful consideration of the history, and physical exam, followed by a series of selected, prioritized screening investigations, should allow the clinician to reach a presumptive diagnosis, to be confirmed by more specific and intensive investigations.

Bibliography

DiMauro S, Lamperti C. Muscle glycogenoses. *Muscle Nerve* 2001;**24**:984.

DiMauro S. Mitochondrial diseases. *Biochim Biophys Acta* 2004;**1658**:80–8.

DiMauro S, Mancuso M. Mitochondrial diseases: therapeutic approaches. *Biosci Rep* 2007;**27**: 125–37.

Elliott HR, Samuels DC, Eden JA, Relton CL, Chinnery PF. Pathogenic mitochondrial DNA mutations are common in the general population. *Am J Hum Genet* 2008;**83**:254–60.

Quinzii CM, DiMauro S, Hirano M. Human coenzyme Q10 deficiency. *Neurochem Res* 2007;**32**: 723–7.

Rowland LP. Myoglobinuria. *Can J Neurol Sci* 1984;**11**:1–13.

Spiekerkoetter U, Lindner M, Santer R, et al. Treatment recommendations in long-chain fatty acid oxidation defects: consensus from a workshop. *J Inherit Metab Dis* 2009;**32**: 498–505.

Taivassalo T, Dysgaard Jensen T, Kennaway N, et al. The spectrum of exercise tolerance in mitochondrial myopathies: a study of 40 patients. *Brain* 2003;**126**:413–23.

Taivassalo T, Gardner JL, Taylor RW, et al. Endurance training and detraining in mitochondrial myopathies due to single large-scale mtDNA deletions. *Brain* 2006;**129**: 3391–401.

Tein I. Recurrent childhood myoglobinuria. In: Fejerman N, Chamoles NA (eds), *New Trends in Pediatric Neurology*. International Congress Series 1033. Amsterdam: Elsevier Science Publishers BV, 1993: 185–94.

Tein I. Metabolic myopathies. In: Swaiman KF, Ashwal S, Ferriero D (eds), *Pediatric Neurology*, 4th edn. St Louis, MO: Mosby-Yearbook Inc., 2006: 2023–73.

Tein I, DiMauro S, De Vivo DC. Recurrent childhood myoglobinuria. *Adv Pediatr* 1990; **37**:77–117.

Tein I, DiMauro S, Rowland LP. Myoglobinuria. In: Rowland LP, DiMauro S (eds), *Handbook of Clinical Neurology*, vol 18. *Myopathies.* Amsterdam: Elsevier Science Publishers BV, 1992.

Tonin P, Lewis P, Servidei S, et al. Metabolic causes of myoglobinuria. *Ann Neurol* 1990;**27**:181–5.

Vu TH, Hirano M, DiMauro S. Mitochondrial diseases. *Neurol Clin N Am* 2002;**20**:809.

Zeharia A, Shaag A, Houtkooper RH, et al. Mutations in LPIN1 cause recurrent acute myoglobinuria in childhood. *Am J Hum Genet* 2008;**83**:489–94.

Mitochondrial Myopathies

Michio Hirano, **Valentina Emmanuele**, and **Catarina M. Quinzii**

Department of Neurology, Columbia University Medical Center, New York, NY, USA

Mitochondrial diseases encompass a large and expanding number of clinically and etiologically heterogeneous disorders. The unusual diversity of mitochondrial myopathies mainly results from the dual genetic origin of the organelle (Figure 6.1). This chapter focuses on mitochondrial diseases that predominantly affect muscle, which is frequently affected due to its high energy requirements.

⚙ SCIENCE REVISITED

Mitochondria are essential for the production of adenosine triphosphate (ATP), the energy currency of the cell. Reducing equivalents (electrons), mainly derived from the catabolism of fatty acids and carbohydrates, are shuttled through the four multisubunit complexes (I–IV) of the respiratory chain, embedded in the mitochondrial inner membrane, and generate a proton gradient that is utilized by complex V to generate ATP, a process known as oxidative phosphorylation (OXPHOS).

Mitochondria are the products of mitochondrial DNA (mtDNA) and nuclear DNA (nDNA); mutations in either genome can cause human disease. More than 200 point mutations and hundreds of deletion mutations of mtDNA have been reported. The mitochondrial genome is *maternally inherited*; therefore, mtDNA defects are typically transmitted from mothers to all progeny. Phenotypic expression of mtDNA defects depends upon *heteroplasmy* (amount) and *tissue distribution* of the mutation. The level of heteroplasmy must exceed a critical level (threshold) to produce biochemical and clinical effects. Mutations of mtDNA are designated by "m." followed by the nucleotide position and change (e.g. m.3243A>G).

As mtDNA maintenance depends on numerous factors encoded by nDNA, there is a variety of defects of intergenomic communication, primary nuclear gene disorders that cause mtDNA instability. The instability of the mitochondrial genome primarily manifests as mtDNA depletion, multiple deletions, or both.

General clinical features

Virtually every organ system can be affected by mitochondrial dysfunction and as a consequence, mitochondrial disorders often present as complex multisystemic diseases. Despite their protean clinical presentations, mitochondrial diseases manifest specific clinical symptoms and signs that should alert clinicians to suspect a mitochondrial disease (Box 6.1).

Neuromuscular Disorders, First Edition. Edited by Rabi N. Tawil, Shannon Venance.
© 2011 John Wiley & Sons, Ltd. Published 2011 by John Wiley & Sons, Ltd.

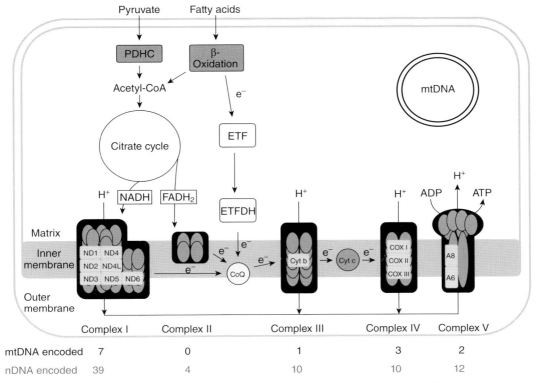

Figure 6.1. Schematic representation of mitochondrial metabolism. Respiratory chain components or complexes encoded by nuclear DNA are grey ovals; subunits encoded by mitochondrial DNA are white rectangles. CoQ, coenzyme Q; Cyt *c*, cytochrome *c*; ETF, electron-transferring flavoprotein; ETFDH, electron-transferring flavoprotein dehydrogenase; $FADH_2$, flavin adenine dinucleotide (reduced form); NADH, nicotinamide adenine dinucleotide (reduced form); ND, NADH dehydrogenase; PDHC, pyruvate dehydrogenase complex.

Furthermore, particular combinations of clinical manifestations define distinct disorders such as: Kearns–Sayre syndrome (KSS), mitochondrial encephalomyopathy with stroke-like episodes (MELAS), myoclonus epilepsy with ragged-red fibers (MERRF), and mitochondrial neurogastrointestinal encephalomyopathy (MNGIE).

Among the pure or predominantly myopathic forms of mitochondrial diseases, ptosis, progressive external ophthalmoplegia (PEO), or both are particularly common. Extraocular muscles contain abundant quantities of mitochondria and are vulnerable to defects of the mitochondrial respiratory chain. The onset of ptosis and PEO is usually insidious and symmetric, so diplopia and blurred vision are often mild or absent.

Skeletal myopathy is also common. As with most myopathies, neck flexor and proximal limb muscles are disproportionately weaker than other muscles. Serum creatine kinase (CK) levels may be normal or elevated. Many patients complain of premature fatigue out of proportion to the weakness. This exercise intolerance is intuitively compatible with a defect of oxidative phosphorylation (OXPHOS), but challenging to diagnose due to its subjective nature. In such cases, formal exercise testing can be helpful.

Along with muscle, the nervous system is also frequently affected, and consequently, mitochondrial diseases often present as encephalomyopathies. Common central nervous system manifestations include: epilepsy, myoclonus, migraine headaches, stroke-like episodes at a

Box 6.1. Clinical features of mitochondrial encephalomyopathies

Muscle
Exercise intolerance
External ophthalmoplegia
Ptosis
Oropharyngeal weakness
Limb weakness
Decreased muscle bulk
Elevated creatine kinase[a]
Myoglobinuria
Respiratory muscle weakness

Central nervous system
Leigh syndrome
Epilepsy (partial, generalized, or myoclonus)
Myoclonus
Migraine-like headaches
Stroke-like episodes at a young age
Ataxia
Optic neuropathy
Pigmentary retinopathy
Dementia
Learning disability
Leukodystrophy
Extrapyramidal signs
Motor neuron disease

Peripheral nervous system
Sensorimotor neuropathy

Endocrine systems
Diabetes mellitus
Hypothyroidism
Growth hormone deficiency with short stature
Hypoparathyroidism
Delayed puberty
Infertility
Irregular menses
Hirsutism

Heart
Cardiac conduction block
Hypertrophic cardiomyopathy
Pre-excitation syndrome

Renal
Tubular acidosis (de Toni–Fanconi–Debré syndrome)
Bartter-like syndrome

Pancreas
Exocrine deficiency

Liver
Elevated transaminases
Steatosis
Hepatic failure

Hematological
Pancytopenia
Sideroblastic anemia

Gastrointestinal tract
Dysmotility
Intestinal pseudoobstruction

Psychiatric
Depression
Schizophrenia-like episodes

Dermatological
Purpuric lesions
Hirsutism

Other
Cataracts
Lipomas

[a]Usually mild except in mtDNA depletion syndrome.

young age, ataxia, optic neuropathy, pigmentary retinopathy, dementia, and psychomotor regression. Peripheral neuropathies are frequent, but often overlooked, in mitochondrial disease patients. The neuropathy is typically axonal, but is mainly demyelinating in MNGIE. Sensorineural hearing loss is commonly associated with mitochondrial encephalomyopathies.

Visceral organ systems affected in mitochondrial diseases include the gastrointestinal system and liver manifesting as gastrointestinal dysmotility and hepatic steatosis. Heart involvement includes cardiomyopathy (often starting as hypertrophic cardiomyopathy), cardiac conduction block, or pre-excitation (Wolff–Parkinson–White) syndrome. Among mitochondrial endocrinopathies, diabetes mellitus is particularly common, but hypothyroidism, growth hormone deficiency, and hypoparathyroidism also occur. Box 6.2 defines the mitochondrial encephalopathies.

Box 6.2. Clinical definitions of mitochondrial encephalomyopathies

Progressive external ophthalmoplegia (PEO)
Ptosis and PEO generally beginning in childhood or young adulthood
Mitochondrial myopathy (ragged-red and COX-deficient fibers)
Oropharyngeal, facial, and limb myopathy may be present

Kearns–Sayre syndrome
Onset before age 20
Ophthalmoparesis
Pigmentary retinopathy
Plus, at least one of the following:
CSF protein >100 mg/dL
Cardiac conduction block
Cerebellar syndrome

Sensory ataxic neuropathy, dysarthria, ophthalmoplegia (SANDO)
Sensory ataxia
Peripheral neuropathy
Dysarthria
PEO

Mitochondrial encephalopathy, lactic acidosis, and stroke-like episodes (MELAS) syndrome
Stroke at a young age (typically before age 40 years)
Encephalopathy (seizures, dementia, or both)
Ragged-red fibers, lactic acidosis at rest, or both

Myoclonus epilepsy ragged-red fibers (MERRF) syndrome
Myoclonus
Epilepsy
Cerebellar syndrome
Myopathy with ragged-red fibers

Mitochondrial neurogastrointestinal encephalomyopathy (MNGIE) syndrome
Ophthalmoparesis, ptosis or both
Peripheral neuropathy
Gastrointestinal dysmotility
Cachexia
Leukoencephalopathy on brain imaging
Mitochondrial abnormalities: lactic acidosis or muscle biopsy showing ragged-red fibers, cytochrome *c* oxidase (COX)-deficient fibers, or multiple deletions or depletion of mtDNA

Leigh syndrome
Onset typically in infancy or childhood
Neurodevelopmental regression or delay
Clinical manifestations of disease in the brain stem, basal ganglia, or both.
Bilateral lesions of the basal ganglia and midbrain brain stem by brain CT, brain MRI (T_2-weighted hyperintense lesions), or by autopsy analysis of the patient or similarly affected sibling.
Elevated lactate or pyruvate in blood, CSF, or both
The following features are often present: hypotonia, feeding difficulty, respiratory abnormalities, vision loss, optic atrophy, pigmentary retinopathy, oculomotor palsies, nystagmus, dystonia, and ataxia.

Myopathic form of mtDNA depletion syndrome
Infantile or childhood onset myopathy
Serum CK is typically elevated
Mitochondrial myopathy (ragged-red and COX-deficient fibers, severe depletion of mtDNA)

Reversible infantile myopathy with COX deficiency
Diffuse weakness, hypotonia, and respiratory insufficiency due to myopathy
Spontaneous improvement by age 2–3 years
COX deficiency in muscle

Progressive external ophthalmoplegia

Ptosis and PEO typically present in childhood or adolescence in a symmetric fashion and are one of the most common myopathic presentations of mitochondrial disease. As the onset and progression are usually gradual, the term "chronic progressive external ophthalmoplegia" (CPEO) has been used. Weakness of oropharyngeal, facial, neck flexor, and limb muscles is frequently associated with extraocular mitochondrial myopathy. Respiratory muscle weakness may occur in some patients. About half the patients with PEO harbor a pathogenic mtDNA single deletion that is typically sporadic, but women harboring this type of mutation have a 4–11% risk of transmitting the mtDNA deletion to progeny. In addition, maternally inherited mtDNA point mutations, as well as autosomal dominant or recessive nDNA mutations, can cause PEO. Among the mtDNA mutations, the m.3243A>G transition, which is the most common cause of MELAS, is a frequent cause of maternally inherited PEO. Mutations in the *POLG* gene, encoding the mitochondrial polymerase γ, are the most common causes of autosomal dominant or recessive PEO.

The differential diagnosis of mitochondrial PEO includes other causes of ophthalmoplegia including congenital and autoimmune myasthenia gravis and congenital myopathies. Typically, in mitochondrial diseases, ptosis and PEO are noted in childhood or adolescence, in contrast to the infantile onset of most cases of congenital myasthenia gravis and congenital myopathies. Oculopharyngeal muscular dystrophy (OPMD), similar to mitochondrial PEO, manifests prominent ptosis, ophthalmoparesis, and weakness of pharyngeal, facial, and limb muscles. In OPMD, however, ptosis is more severe than ophthalmoparesis whereas in PEO both are usually severe. The diseases can also be distinguished based on age at onset with OPMD occurring in the fourth to sixth decades, whereas PEO typically begins before age 20.

Diagnostic testing for mitochondrial PEO is guided by family history. Maternally inherited PEO suggests an mtDNA point mutation, which can be detected in blood. In contrast, sporadic mitochondrial PEO is most often due to a single large-scale mtDNA deletion, which is typically undetectable in blood; therefore, muscle biopsy is often necessary to screen for ragged-red and cytochrome *c* oxidase (COX)-deficient fibers and to identify the pathogenic mutation by Southern blot analysis. In addition, Southern blot analysis may reveal mtDNA multiple deletions, which are characteristic of autosomal dominant or recessive forms mitochondrial PEO. *POLG* mutations are the most frequent causes of mendelian inherited PEO with multiple deletions of mtDNA, and can be identified in blood. Other causes of autosomal dominant PEO with mtDNA multiple deletions include mutations in *C10orf2* (encoding a mitochondrial helicase called "Twinkle"), *ANT1*, and *POLG2* (encoding the accessory subunit of polymerase γ).

✭ TIPS AND TRICKS

The diversity of mitochondrial myopathies provides diagnostic challenges even for experienced physicians. Clinicians should inquire about the following clinical features: exercise intolerance, migraine headaches, diabetes mellitus, short stature, and hearing loss.

Detailed family history is important because evidence of maternal inheritance may be subtle when dealing with an mtDNA point mutation.

☟ CAUTION

Although hallmarks of mitochondrial myopathies, ragged-red fibers (RRFs) and cytochrome *c* oxidase (COX)-deficient fibers in muscle, they are not seen in all mitochondrial diseases and are present at low levels (<2%) in normal aged individuals. Thus, quantification of abnormal muscle fibers and correlation with the age of the patient is critical.

Activities of mitochondrial respiratory chain enzymes can be measured in muscle. In mitochondrial myopathies, there may be defects of single or multiple respiratory chain enzymes, or even normal enzyme activities. Thus, biochemical tests alone are not sufficient to exclude mitochondrial diseases.

Low levels of multiple deletions of mtDNA are also detectable in muscle by polymerase chain reaction (PCR) in normal aged individuals, so estimating amounts of the deletions by Southern blot or quantitative PCR is often useful.

As PEO may evolve into PEO-plus or KSS, it is important to perform yearly electrocardiograms and echocardiograms to screen for cardiac conduction defects and cardiomyopathy, basic metabolic and liver function panels to detect renal or liver dysfunction, fasting glucose to detect diabetes mellitus, and audiometry to identify hearing loss.

Treatment of PEO is symptomatic. Ptosis that obscures vision may be treated with eyelid crutches or surgery to place eyelid slings, which are preferable to blepharoplasty, which can impair eyelid closure and lead to exposure keratitis. Cocktails of nutritional supplements and vitamins are often administered to patient and typically include: coenzyme Q_{10} (CoQ_{10}) (50–100 mg three times a day), L-carnitine (300 mg three times a day), thiamine (50–200 mg daily), riboflavin (50–600 mg daily), vitamin K_3 (5–80 mg daily), vitamin C (1000–4000 mg daily), and α-lipoic acid (up to 400 mg three times a day). As sensorineural hearing loss in mitochondrial diseases is typically due to cochlear dysfunction, severe hearing loss (i.e. inability to conduct telephone calls) often responds to cochlear implants.

Kearns–Sayre syndrome

PEO is a prominent feature of KSS, originally described as the triad of external ophthalmoplegia, retinitis pigmentosa, and onset before age 20 years plus at least one of the following features: heart block, cerebellar ataxia, or cerebrospinal fluid (CSF) protein >100 mg/dL. The cardiac conduction block may progress to lethal complete heart block. Additional features include hearing loss, oropharyngeal, facial, and limb muscle weakness, cognitive impairment, growth hormone deficiency, and diabetes mellitus. Secondary folate deficiency in CSF is observed in KSS. Cardiomyopathy and renal tubular acidosis occasionally occur in KSS and may be severe. KSS is usually sporadic and about 90% of cases are caused by a single deletion of mtDNA, but, as noted in the description of PEO, symptomatic women can transmit the mutation to their children.

As progressive external ophthalmoplegia with ptosis is the most prominent early feature of this syndrome, the differential diagnoses include disorders that cause PEO as described above. Niemann–Pick type C disease (NPC) can be misdiagnosed as KSS in children; however, the ophthalmoparesis of NPC is due to supranuclear palsy rather than ocular myopathy.

The diagnostic evaluation of KSS begins with routine blood tests, including complete blood count, serum electrolytes, liver function tests, blood urea nitrogen, creatinine, lactate, and pyruvate. These tests may reveal kidney or liver dysfunction. Elevated lactate and pyruvate at rest are common, and these values may increase dramatically after moderate exercise. Electrocardiogram and echocardiogram must be performed to screen for heart block and cardiomyopathy. Finally, muscle biopsy is performed to confirm the diagnosis. RRFs on modified Gomori's trichrome stain and other features of mitochondrial dysfunction may be found. Mitochondrial enzyme activities can be measured in whole muscle homogenate or isolated mitochondria. Muscle mtDNA should be screened by Southern blot analysis for the presence of single deletion of mtDNA.

Treatment of KSS is as described for PEO. In addition, folate deficiency in the CSF of KSS patients has prompted some clinicians to give folate or folinic acid.

PEO-plus

In addition to myopathic PEO and multisystemic KSS, there are other syndromes with prominent PEO plus other clinical manifestations, e.g. sensory ataxic neuropathy dysarthria ophthalmoplegia (SANDO) is a clinically recognizable condition associated with RRFs and COX-negative fibers, and multiple deletions of mtDNA in muscle usually due to autosomal recessive *POLG* mutations. The triad of PEO, hearing loss, and optic atrophy is also associated with mtDNA multiple deletions and is due to autosomal dominant mutations in the *OPA1* gene. In addition to the triad, patients may develop skeletal myopathy, ataxia, and peripheral neuropathy.

Mitochondrial neurogastrointestinal encephalomyopathy

This autosomal recessive multisystem mitochondrial disorder is clinically recognizable by the unusual combination of six features:

1. Progressive external ophthalmoplegia
2. Severe gastrointestinal dysmotility
3. Cachexia
4. Peripheral neuropathy
5. Diffuse leukoencephalopathy on magnetic resonance imaging (MRI) of the brain
6. Evidence of mitochondrial dysfunction (histological, biochemical, or genetic abnormalities of the mitochondria).

The patients are typically thin throughout life, but become strikingly emaciated as the disorder progresses. The average age at onset is 18 years, but varies from early childhood to the fifth decade. The mean age at death is 38 years.

Brain MRI reveals diffusely increased T_2-weighted signal in the white matter. Most MNGIE patients have lactic acidosis at rest. Nerve conduction and electromyographic studies usually reveal abnormalities consistent with a demyelinating neuropathy. Muscle biopsy may reveal RRFs that are COX negative as well as neurogenic changes. The disorder is due to mutations in the *TYMP* gene encoding thymidine phosphorylase (TP). The prominent gastrointestinal manifestations can be misattributed to celiac disease, inflammatory bowel disease, superior mesenteric artery syndrome, and anorexia nervosa. MNGIE patients presenting with neuropathy can be misdiagnosed as having chronic inflammatory demyelinating polyneuropathy or Charcot–Marie–Tooth disease. MNGIE-like phenotypes have also been associated with mutations in *POLG, RRM2B*, and the m.3243A>G "MELAS" mutation.

Despite significant morbidity and mortality, allogeneic hemopoietic stem cell transplantation has shown anecdotal success in correcting the biochemical defects of thymidine and deoxyuridine metabolism and ameliorating clinical manifestations.

Exercise intolerance due to mtDNA mutations

A small group of patients manifesting severe exercise intolerance, sometimes associated with myoglobinuria, fixed proximal limb weakness, or both, are associated with mutations in mtDNA. Unlike patients with defects of glycogen metabolism who present with intense exercise-induced muscle stiffness or cramps, or patients with lipid metabolism defects who develop symptoms after prolonged exertion, fasting, or both, this group of patients experiences premature muscle fatigue, which, in some cases, has been labeled chronic fatigue syndrome or fibromyalgia. Clues to the diagnosis of mtDNA mutation include elevated resting lactic acid and RRFs or pre-RRFs. This condition does not obey the typical rules of mitochondrial genetics because all patients are sporadic and the mutations and clinical manifestations were restricted to skeletal muscle. Most cases of mtDNA mutation-associated exercise intolerance are due to defects in the *CYTB* gene encoding cytochrome *b*. In addition, mtDNA mutations in *ND* genes encoding subunits of complex I, *CO* genes encoding complex IV subunits, and tRNA genes have been associated with exercise intolerance.

Coenzyme Q_{10} deficiencies

A vital component of the mitochondrial respiratory chain, CoQ_{10} (or ubiquinone) shuttles electrons from mitochondrial complexes I and II, as well as electron-transferring flavoprotein dehydrogenase (ETFDH), to complex III (see Figure 6.1). Deficiencies of CoQ_{10} can be primary, due to autosomal recessive mutations in the gene required for ubiquinone biosynthesis, or secondary, due to mutations in genes not directly related to CoQ_{10} production. Phenotypes associated with CoQ_{10} deficiency include: encephalomyopathy, cerebellar ataxia with marked cerebellar atrophy, infantile multisystemic disease (mainly encephalopathy with steroid-resistant nephrotic syndrome), isolated nephrotic syndrome, and isolated myopathy. The myopathic CoQ_{10} phenotype manifests lipid storage in muscle biopsy and some cases are secondary CoQ_{10} deficiencies due to *ETFDH* mutations. It is important to diagnose CoQ_{10} deficiencies because patients can respond dramatically to CoQ_{10} supplementation (initial doses of 30 mg/kg per day in children and up to 2400 mg/day in adults divided into three daily doses). Of great importance, blood levels of CoQ_{10} can be influenced by dietary intake, so CoQ_{10} deficiency cannot be diagnosed by serum measurements but rather by assessment in muscle or cultured fibroblasts.

Mitochondrial DNA depletion syndrome

The clinical presentations of mtDNA depletion syndrome (MDS) are variable, even within a single family. Onset may be congenital or soon after birth, generally leading to death within the first year of life. However, onset can also be in infancy or childhood with survival beyond the second decade. A variety of clinical phenotypes is reported of which two involve muscle:

1. Congenital myopathy, with neonatal weakness and hypotonia requiring assisted ventilation, and death before age 1 year. Renal dysfunction may also be present.
2. Encephalomyopathy with psychomotor retardation, muscle hypotonia, and weakness, and sometimes lesions on a brain MRI of the basal ganglia and brain stem indicative of Leigh syndrome.

Lactic acidosis is severe in infants with congenital forms of MDS, but lactate can be normal or only mildly elevated in children with infantile myopathy. Serum CK is markedly elevated in children with myopathy.

MDS is an autosomal recessive condition and has been linked to mutations in nine genes. Mutations in the *TK2* gene, which encodes thymidine kinase 2, cause the myopathic form of MDS.

The differential diagnosis of the myopathic form of MDS includes congenital myopathies, muscular dystrophies, and acquired myopathies. Treatment is limited to symptomatic and supportive care.

Infantile myopathies with COX deficiency

There are two forms of infantile myopathies with COX deficiency: fatal infantile myopathy (FIM) and reversible infantile myopathy (RIM), which is also known as benign infantile myopathy (BIM). The fatal form presents as generalized muscle weakness during infancy, respiratory muscle insufficiency, lactic acidosis, and death before age 1 year due to COX deficiency. In contrast to the patients with the fatal syndrome, some infants present with severe myopathy and lactic acidosis soon after birth, but improve dramatically and are virtually normal by age 2–3 years. Lactic acidosis and muscle histological abnormalities also resolve. As a result of the remarkable spontaneous improvement, the syndrome has been called reversible infantile myopathy or benign infantile myopathy. The latter term is misleading because the disorder can be fatal if patients are not properly managed in the critical first few months of life. This condition is due to a homoplasmic m.14674T>C mt-tRNA^{Glu} mutation.

Acknowledgments

Dr Hirano is supported by grants from the NIH (R01 HD056103, R01 HD057543, RC1 NS070232), Muscular Dystrophy Association (MDA), Santhera Pharmaceutical, and by the Marriott Mitochondrial Disorder Clinical Research Fund (MMDCRF).

Bibliography

DiMauro S, Hirano M, Schon EA. *Mitochondrial Medicine*. Oxon: Informa Healthcare, 2006.

DiMauro S, Hirano M. Mitochondrial DNA deletion syndromes. GeneReviews (online) April 19, 2007. Available at: www.ncbi.nlm.nih.gov/bookshelf/br.fcgi?book=gene&part=kss (accessed August 30, 2010).

Hirano M. Kearns Sayre syndrome. *Medlink Neurol* 2010. Available at: www.medlink.com (accessed August 30, 2010).

Hirano M, Nishigaki Y, Marti R. Mitochondrial neurogastrointestinal encephalomyopathy (MNGIE): a disease of two genomes. *Neurologist* 2004;**10**:8–17.

Horvath R, Kemp JP, Tuppen HA, et al. Molecular basis of infantile reversible cytochrome *c* oxidase deficiency myopathy. *Brain* 2009;**132** (Pt 11):3165–74.

Milone M, Massie R. Polymerase gamma 1 mutations: clinical correlations. *Neurologist* 2010;**16**:84–91.

Quinzii CM, Hirano M. Coenzyme Q and mitochondrial disease. *Dev Disabil Res Rev* 2010;**16**: 183–8.

Zeviani M, Lamperti C, DiMauro S. Disorders of nuclear–mitochondrial intergenomic signaling. In: Gilman S (eds), *Medlink Neurology*. San Diego, CA: Medlink Corp., 2010.

Dystrophinopathies

Shannon L. Venance

Department of Clinical Neurological Sciences, University of Western Ontario, London, Canada

Duchenne muscular dystrophy (DMD) and Becker (BMD) muscular dystrophy are allelic, X-linked recessive disorders of progressive muscle wasting and weakness caused by mutations in the dystrophin gene, *DMD*. DMD remains the most common muscular dystrophy, whereas BMD is a milder variant with a later onset and a more variable clinical course. Dystrophin deficiency is also an under-appreciated diagnostic consideration in females of any age with muscle complaints. The clinical spectrum in men and women, however, ranges from an asymptomatic elevated creatine kinase (CK) to a severely affected DMD phenotype, with onset in both males and females ranging from childhood to late adulthood. Genetic confirmation of a clinical diagnosis provides diagnostic certainty, facilitates appropriate management, permits genetic counseling, and is essential for future therapeutic trials.

Epidemiology

Dystrophinopathies are the most common of the inherited muscle diseases. The incidence of DMD is 1 in 3500 live male births and BMD approximately one-tenth of the incidence of DMD. The new mutation rate in the dystrophin gene is high, and a third of patients will not have a family history. Despite the absence of accurate incidence and prevalence data in females, the mothers and sisters of all affected individuals should be considered at risk. Similarly, all daughters of men affected by BMD will be obligate carriers.

> ### ★ TIPS AND TRICKS
>
> - Keep dystrophin deficiency in the differential diagnosis for both muscle and cognitive complaints.
> - Think of a dystrophinopathy in any male or female at any age presenting with an elevated CK or unexplained transaminases, exertional myalgias, myoglobinuria, or proximal weakness with or without diaphragm weakness or cardiomyopathy.
> - Dystrophin deficiency is also a consideration in children and adults presenting with cognitive dysfunction (e.g. delayed language development, autism, learning disorders, attention-deficit hyperactivity disorder and impaired intelligence).

Clinical presentations

Duchenne muscular dystrophy

The classic presentation of DMD includes delayed gross motor milestones, difficulty running, and increasing falls in young boys. Examination

Neuromuscular Disorders, First Edition. Edited by Rabi N. Tawil, Shannon Venance.
© 2011 John Wiley & Sons, Ltd. Published 2011 by John Wiley & Sons, Ltd.

shows calf pseudohypertrophy, and proximal hip girdle weakness manifested by a waddling gait and use of a Gower maneuver to get up from a supine position. Serum CK is markedly elevated (20–200 times normal). Many affected boys will also have cognitive dysfunction. Diagnosis is made between 3 and 5 years of age.

Progression is relentless, with loss of ambulation occurring by 12 years of age. Weakness of the diaphragm begins while boys are ambulatory and annual pulmonary function testing should be initiated early. With transition to a wheelchair, progressive kyphoscoliosis significantly worsens respiratory function. Monitoring for progressive scoliosis is essential in nonambulatory patients because some individuals may need spinal fusion to help maintain their respiratory function. Ultimately, it is the chronic respiratory failure that is the primary cause of death in DMD, typically in the late 20s or early 30s. Early involvement of pulmonologists is essential. The introduction of noninvasive ventilation (NIV) has altered the natural history and has extended the survival of boys with DMD well into adulthood. Nocturnal ventilation is useful for symptoms of ineffective ventilation such as morning headaches, reduced energy and appetite, nocturnal anxiety, and nightmares. Cough assist devices can help patients with poor cough to clear secretions and prevent infections. Tracheostomy and assisted mechanical ventilation may be pursued by some patients and families late in the disease course.

All boys with DMD develop signs of cardiac involvement, usually with asymptomatic tachycardia. An electrocardiogram (EKG) commonly shows sinus tachycardia, prominent Q waves, right ventricular hypertrophy, and a short P–R interval. Echocardiography with cardiology evaluation is recommended annually from age 10. Management may include angiotensin-converting enzyme (ACE) inhibitors and β blockers.

However, less than 40% of individuals with DMD will be symptomatic from a cardiac standpoint, likely related to the decreased demand on the heart after the transition to a wheelchair.

Optimal care for DMD requires a well-coordinated multidisciplinary healthcare team that anticipates and manages the multisystemic manifestations and complications of DMD. Glucocorticoids (prednisone 0.75 mg/kg per day and deflazacort 0.9 mg/kg per day) slow the decline of muscle strength and function in boys with DMD. Observational cohort data suggest that ambulation is prolonged in boys treated with glucocorticoids and benefit is maintained once nonambulatory, with a reduced risk of scoliosis, a slower deterioration in pulmonary function, and potential benefits to the heart. Despite this, there is marked variability in clinical practice with regard to dosing regimens and time to initiate treatment. Recent recommendations suggest individualized treatment based on consideration of functional status (start once no longer gaining in motor skills), age (>2 years but <8 years of age), and after assessment of risk factors for the many side effects of steroids. Similarly, there are no stopping rules; dosing may be adjusted to minimize side effects such as weight gain, mood and behavior changes, cataracts, and long bone and vertebral compression fractures. It remains common for young men with advanced DMD to continue their steroid regimen indefinitely. Seasonal flu shots are recommended in all boys and they should be supplemented with vitamin D if the serum 25-hydroxy-vitamin D is low.

Initiation of nocturnal ventilation requires coordination and provision of resources in the home and community, along with education of patients and families. Advanced care planning is critical for facilitating shared decision-making, and should be introduced early and revisited regularly in a systematic manner.

Becker dystrophy

In contrast to the fairly stereotypical presentation in DMD, there is a highly variable presentation with BMD. Any male at any age presenting with a symmetric limb–girdle pattern weakness should be tested for a dystrophinopathy, even in the absence of a positive family history. Although many affected males present in adolescence, onset of muscle weakness in the fourth and fifth decades and beyond is well described. Early involvement of the quadriceps in men aged over 40 may erroneously suggest the diagnosis of inclusion body myositis if a dystrophinopathy is not considered. In general, the older the age of symptomatic onset is, the milder the disease.

There may also be learning difficulties, and attention and behavioral problems in adolescents and men with BMD.

By clinical consensus, patients with a dystrophinopathy who remain ambulatory past the age of 16 years are said to have BMD. Adolescent boys who lose the ability to walk independently between 12 and 16 years of age were historically classified as having an intermediate phenotype between DMD and BMD. However the use of glucocorticoids has blurred this distinction.

Similar to DMD, all affected individuals should be screened with pulmonary function tests (seated and repeated supine) and cardiac investigations biannually. Symptomatic cardiac involvement secondary to dilated cardiomyopathy and/or arrhythmia is much more likely in men with BMD. EKG findings are similar to those seen in DMD. Referral to cardiology is indicated in all symptomatic individuals and management may require the use of ACE inhibitors and β blockers. Relatively preserved limb muscle strength likely permits more dynamic activity and increased cardiac demand. Importantly, cardiac failure may be the initial manifestation in some patients. Chronic respiratory failure secondary to diaphragm involvement and ineffective nighttime ventilation may also lead to right heart failure and management involves initiation of nocturnal assisted ventilation. Life expectancy is reduced for men with significant involvement of the heart or diaphragm.

☆ TIPS AND TRICKS

Pulmonary function tests should be done seated and repeated supine. A drop in lung volumes of more than 15–20% indicates diaphragm weakness and the need for closer monitoring. Maximal expiratory pressures and peak cough flow values are useful to follow expiratory force that is necessary to clear airways.

Asymptomatic/minimally symptomatic

It is reasonable to keep mild dystrophin deficiency in mind when assessing any individual presenting with exertional intolerance, myalgias, myoglobinuria, or a persistent elevation of CK (or unexplained elevation of transaminases). This is true regardless of age or gender. However, the diagnostic yield increases in the presence of subtle clues on history (e.g. clumsiness as a child or being at the "back of the pack" when running in gym class; toe walking; affected family members), exam (presence of calf or tongue hypertrophy), and electrophysiology (small-amplitude, short-duration motor units with or without fibrillation potentials and positive sharp waves). All affected individuals, regardless of symptoms, should have a baseline pulmonary and cardiac assessment with periodic follow-up.

X-linked dilated cardiomyopathy

X-linked dilated cardiomyopathy (XLDCM) is a rare manifestation of dystrophin deficiency restricted to cardiac muscle resulting from mutations affecting the cardiac isoform of dystrophin. The age of onset ranges from childhood to late adulthood, with most patients presenting in the second and third decades of life. Clinical presentations include asymptomatic EKG and echocardiogram changes, reduced exercise tolerance, exertional dyspnea, leg swelling, and frank heart failure. Diagnosis is based on X-linked inheritance, endocardial biopsy with dystrophin immunostaining, and DNA analysis. The clinical course is rapidly progressive with approximately a 50% mortality rate over 5 years without cardiac transplantation.

Dystrophin deficiency in females

First-degree female relatives of any male with a dystrophinopathy are at risk and should receive genetic counseling and DNA analysis. The majority of female carriers will be asymptomatic, although approximately 10% will manifest symptoms. Carriers may be minimally symptomatic with exertional muscle pain, cramps or even isolated calf hypertrophy. Mild ECG and echocardiogram abnormalities have been detected in asymptomatic carriers. Serum CK values are helpful when elevated, but it is important to note that 30% of carriers will have normal CK values. If the family history is documented and a specific mutation identified, targeted DNA analysis is the first step in confirming diagnosis.

Any asymptomatic woman with an affected male child should have DNA analysis on leukocytes to establish whether she is a carrier. This is essential both for genetic counseling and for monitoring women who are carriers. If DNA analysis does not reveal a mutation, the possibilities include a new mutation in the son or a germline mutation in the mother (dystrophin mutation in the oocytes only). Prenatal screening is available for families with an affected son if the genetic diagnosis was confirmed.

⚠ CAUTION!

- A normal CK value in a woman does not rule out carrier status because 30% of carriers will not have an elevated CK.
- DNA analysis or dystrophin immunostaining on muscle biopsy will confirm dystrophin deficiency if the mutation is not restricted to the germline.

The clinical presentations of manifesting carriers include myalgias, proximal muscle weakness, and/or cardiomyopathy. Muscle weakness often presents asymmetrically. Cognitive dysfunction may also be a feature. Rarely, a young girl will present with a severe DMD-like phenotype presumed to be on the basis of an XO karyotype (Turner syndrome) or nonrandom (skewed) X-chromosome inactivation. However, there is some evidence that specific mutations may result in manifestations in females even in the presence of random, nonskewed, X inactivation. Management of manifesting carriers is similar to DMD and BMD in males, and is focused on surveillance of cardiorespiratory status to anticipate and prevent complications while maintaining functional status. Similar to BMD, there are no clinical trials of glucocorticoids in manifesting females.

Differential diagnosis of dystrophinopathy

Although muscle diseases are uncommon, the probability of an acquired or hereditary myopathy is similar. It is therefore important to consider treatable etiologies in the workup (although unlikely in young boys with a classic DMD presentation). In adults with a subacute or chronic presentation, consider inflammatory myopathies, thyroid and other endocrine myopathies, as well as myotoxic insults (e.g. statin- and other drug-induced myopathies). Dystrophin deficiency should always be considered in individuals with partially steroid responsive or refractory "polymyositis." And, although dystrophinopathy is the most common hereditary muscle disease, other limb–girdle muscular dystrophies may present identically, in particular LGMD 2C-F and 2I (see Chapter 8). Clinicians should consider alternative diagnoses in any patient in whom dystrophin gene sequencing is negative.

Approach to diagnosis

Dystrophinopathy should be suspected in any child or adult with progressive limb girdle weakness, elevated serum CK values, myalgias, or evidence of cardiomyopathy. Intellectual impairment may also be a presenting feature. Patients may present with any combination of these features, or have minimal symptoms. A detailed family pedigree is important.

In DMD, the presentation is stereotypical. Onset between age 3 and 5 years with enlarged calves, a waddling gait, and a Gower maneuver to get up from a supine position in the setting of marked elevation in serum CK is highly suggestive. In most patients with DMD, the earliest and most involved muscles are glutei, thigh abductors, and triceps initially, followed by progressive weakness in quadriceps, deltoids, tibialis anterior, and biceps. Neck flexors are usually involved early in DMD and subtle weakness is best detected when supine. The pattern of muscle involvement in BMD is similar to DMD, although the severity and age at onset are highly variable. There may be enlargement of muscles such as the calves and tongue. Mild-to-moderate elevation in serum CK values at rest is characteristic in BMD, although some patients will only manifest with elevation of CK after exertion. EKG features are similar in both DMD and BMD and include findings consistent with ventricular hypertrophy; the echocardiogram may reveal reduced left ventricular ejection fraction.

Genetic testing

Confirmation of diagnosis requires DNA analysis of the dystrophin gene. Targeted mutation analysis is done if there is a positive family history and the mutation is known. Otherwise, a number of techniques may be used to screen for deletions and duplication in the dystrophin gene (multiplex polymerase chain reaction [PCR] and multiplex ligation-dependent probe amplification being two of the more common). These methods, targeting mutation hotspots, typically pick up about 70% of DMD mutations. If the initial screening is negative, direct sequencing, where available, is undertaken and provides near 100% sensitivity in the diagnosis of DMD. Alternatively, pathological confirmation is required by demonstrating the lack of dystrophin immunostaining in a muscle biopsy.

SCIENCE REVISITED

The dystrophin gene is large, consisting of 79 coding exons with a high new mutation rate. Mutations disrupting the reading frame of the dystrophin gene (out of frame), lead to a truncated, rapidly degraded message and virtual absence of dystrophin expression in muscle, and a DMD phenotype. Conversely, in-frame mutations result in a truncated but partially functional protein or reduced quantity of full-length dystrophin associated with the milder BMD and other dystrophinopathy phenotypes. This "reading-frame rule" holds true for approximately 90% of the mutations in dystrophinopathies. Most mutations are deletions and duplications, although the remaining mutations are small deletions, insertions, and nonsense and splice site mutations

Muscle biopsy

If genetic testing is unrevealing or if dystrophin deficiency is only one of several diagnostic considerations, a muscle biopsy of a mildly affected muscle is indicated. Pathological features are typically those of a chronic active myopathic process with foci of active muscle fiber necrosis and regeneration surrounded by mononuclear inflammatory infiltrates. Immunostaining of dystrophin is absent in DMD, variably reduced in males with BMD, and may show a mosaic pattern in affected females. Immunoblotting identifies the presence of abnormal quality or quantity of the dystrophin protein. Genetic confirmation is indicated if participation in clinical trials in being considered.

Electromyography

There is no role for electromyography (EMG) in young boys with clinically suspected DMD. However, in patients with mild BMD or in the workup of proximal weakness or other muscle presentations, EMG may be helpful in confirming an underlying myopathic process and in selecting an appropriate muscle for biopsy. A normal EMG study does not, however, exclude a myopathic process and, similarly, EMG features of an active necrotizing myopathy with muscle membrane irritability (i.e. fibrillation potentials and positive sharp waves) must not be misinterpreted summarily as "an inflammatory myopathy."

Conclusions

Dystrophinopathies are a diagnostic consideration in males and females of all ages presenting with weakness, myalgias, and elevated CK. On one hand, DMD with its classic presentation is readily diagnosed. On the other hand, a high index of suspicion results in accurate and genetically confirmed diagnoses in males with BMD and female carriers. Management remains supportive with comprehensive healthcare teams until such time as disease-modifying therapies become available.

SCIENCE REVISITED

Genetic therapies in the dystrophinopathies are directed at gene replacement (viral vectors or plasmid delivery of dystrophin gene constructs, stem cell or myoblast transplantation) or gene modification (using small molecules or antisense oligonucleotides to target specific mutations). The latter approach has the potential for personalized gene therapy directed at modifying point mutations or frameshift deletions, to restore the reading frame and convert a DMD phenotype to a milder BMD phenotype. A number of proof-of-principle and early phase clinical trials in DMD are under way or have been completed.

Bibliography

Aartsma-Rus A, Van Deutekom JC, Fokkema IF et al. Entries in the Leiden Duchenne muscular dystrophy mutation database: An overview of mutation types and paradoxical cases that confirm the reading frame rule. *Muscle Nerve* 2006;**34**:135–44.

Bushby K, Finkel R, Birnkrant DJ, et al. Diagnosis and management of Duchenne muscular dystrophy, part 1: diagnosis, and pharmacological and psychosocial management. *Lancet Neurol* 2010;**9**:77–93.

Bushby K, Finkel R, Birnkrant DJ, et al. Diagnosis and management of Duchenne muscular dystrophy, part 2: implementation of multidisciplinary care. *Lancet Neurol* 2010;**9**:177–89.

Cyrulnik SE, Fee RJ, Batchelder A, et al Cognitive and adaptive deficits in young children with Duchenne muscular dystrophy (DMD). *J Int Neuropsychol Soc* 2008;**14**:853–61.

Hamby Erby L, Rushton C, Geller G. "My son is still walking"; Stages of receptivity to discussions of advance care planning among parents of sons with Duchenne muscular dystrophy. *Semin Pediatr Neurol* 2006;**13**:132–40.

Lim LE, Rando TA. Technology insight: therapy for Duchenne muscular dystrophy – an opportunity for personalized medicine. *Nat Clin Pract Neurol* 2008;**4**:149–58.

Manzur AY, Kuntzer, Pike M, T et al. Glucocorticoid corticosteroids for Duchenne muscular dystrophy. *Cochrane Database Syst Rev* 2008;(**1**): CD003725.

Soltanzadeh P, Friez MJ, Dunn D, et al. Clinical and genetic characterization of manifesting carriers of *DMD* mutations. *Neuromusc Dis* 2010;**20**:499–504.

Van Deutekom JC, Janson AA, Ginjaar IB, et al. Local dystrophin restoration with antisense oligonucleotide PRO051 *N Engl J Med* 2007;**357**: 2677–86.

Limb–Girdle Dystrophies

Michela Guglieri and Kate Bushby

Institute of Genetic Medicine, International Centre for Life, Newcastle upon Tyne, UK

Proximal, limb–girdle muscle weakness is seen in a large number of patients with variable underlying diseases, among which muscular dystrophies (MDs) represent a rather rare occurrence. Therefore, approaching a patient with limb–girdle muscular dystrophy (LGMD) phenotype, more likely diagnoses, including acquired myopathies (e.g. drug effects, endocrine myopathies, inflammatory myopathies, myasthenia gravis) should always be considered first, due to their higher incidence and availability of treatment for some of these conditions. Within the inherited diseases presenting with limb–girdle weakness, each LGMD is relatively rare with an overall frequency of 1 in 100 000. More frequent inherited conditions, including dystrophinopathies, facioscapulohumeral muscular dystrophy (FSHD), myotonic dystrophies, and spinal muscular atrophy (SMA) types 2 and 3 should always be part of the differential diagnosis. Pompe's disease can be quickly excluded by relatively routine tests that might be worth performing before proceeding with further or invasive investigations, especially considering the availability of treatment. Bethlem myopathy, metabolic muscle disorders, mitochondrial diseases, myasthenic syndromes, central core disease, or other congenital myopathies may also present with an LGMD phenotype and may therefore be possible alternative diagnoses.

So far, 22 different LGMD forms have been described and genetically recognized (8 autosomal dominant and 14 autosomal recessive forms) but the list is continuously extended with the identification of new genes and proteins (Table 8.1). As well as this extensive genetic heterogeneity, LGMDs present considerable clinical variability, and the phenotypic spectrum of the different forms has been significantly broadened, including atypical or distal presentations, further complicating the diagnostic approach.

Diagnostic approach

Although, per definition, LGMDs are characterized by a common clinical phenotype of predominantly proximal muscle weakness, there is enormous variability in clinical presentation, course and progression of symptoms, inheritance patterns, genes responsible, and proteins involved among the different LGMDs, and often also within the same form. Achieving a precise diagnosis of a particular type of LGMD can therefore be challenging and requires a comprehensive, multidisciplinary approach (Figures 8.1 and 8.2).

Clinical approach

Age of onset, pattern of muscle involvement, additional clinical features (e.g. presence or absence of cardiac and/or respiratory involvement), and the presence of family history are all information that can be easily collected in clinic and are essential in directing the diagnosis and suggesting further investigations.

Neuromuscular Disorders, First Edition. Edited by Rabi N. Tawil, Shannon Venance.
© 2011 John Wiley & Sons, Ltd. Published 2011 by John Wiley & Sons, Ltd.

Table 8.1. Classification of the limb–girdle muscular dystrophies (LMGDs) and relative prevalence in different populations

Disease	Gene	Population	Other phenotypes
AD inheritance			
LGMD1A	MYO	Common mutation in all population	Myofibrillar myopathy
LGMD1B	LMNA	Present worldwide	Emery–Dreifuss muscular dystrophy; AD dilated cardiomyopathy with conduction system disease; pure AD dilated cardiomyopathy; Dunnigan-type familial partial lipodystrophy; AR axonal polyneuropathy (CMT2A); mandibuloacral dysplasia; Hutchinson–Gilford progeria
LGMD1C	CAV3	Present worldwide at low frequency	Dilated cardiomyopathy; asymptomatic hyperCKemia
LGMD1D	7q (7q36?)	Only a few families described	
LGMD1E	6q23	Only one French–Canadian family described	
LGMD1F	7q32	Only one Spanish family described	
LGMD1G	4q21	Only one white Brazilian family described	
LGMD1H	3p23-p25	Only one southern Italian family described	

AR inheritance

	Gene	Frequency/population	Associated phenotype
LGMD2A	CAPN3	Most frequent form worldwide (25–30% of LGMDs)	
LGMD2B	DYSF	Second most prevalent form in many populations (Italian, Brazilian, American, Australian, Dutch); less frequent in the UK (6%)	Miyoshi myopathy, distal muscular dystrophy with anterior tibial involvement (DMAT)
LGMD2C	γ-SG	Present worldwide; 100% of sarcoglycanopathy in northern Africa	
LGMD2D	α-SG	Present worldwide; most frequent sarcoglycanopathy in Europe and North America	
LGMD2E	β-SG	Present worldwide; more common in northern and southern Indiana Amish and Switzerland	
LGMD2F	δ-SG	Rarest sarcoglycanopathy worldwide; more common in African–Brazilian populations	Dilated cardiomyopathy
LGMD2G	TCAP	Present in different populations (Brazilian, Chinese, Moldavian) at very low frequency	Dilated cardiomyopathy 1N (CMD1N)
LGMD2H	TRIM32	Rare outside Hutterite population of Canada	Sarcotubular myopathy, Bardet–Biedl syndrome
LGMD2I	FKRP	Present worldwide; second most common LGMD in northern Europe (20% of the LGMD cases in the northern UK); founder mutation (C826A) identified in the Hutterite population and present worldwide with carrier frequency of 1 in 306.	Congenital muscular dystrophy (MDC1C)
LGMD2J	TTN	Only one Finnish family and a French sporadic case described	Distal myopathy (heterozygotes); dilated cardiomyopathy 1G (CMD1G) (heterozygotes)
LGMD2K	POMT1	Present worldwide at very low frequency	Congenital myopathy (Walker–Warburg syndrome)
LGMD2L	ANO5	Probably present worldwide: early to determine relative frequency, but there appears to be a common mutation in northern Europe/UK	
LGMD2M	Fukutin	Prevalent mutation in Japan	Congenital myopathy (Fukuyama muscular dystrophy)
LGMD2N	POMT2	Only few cases described	Congenital myopathy (Walker–Warburg syndrome)

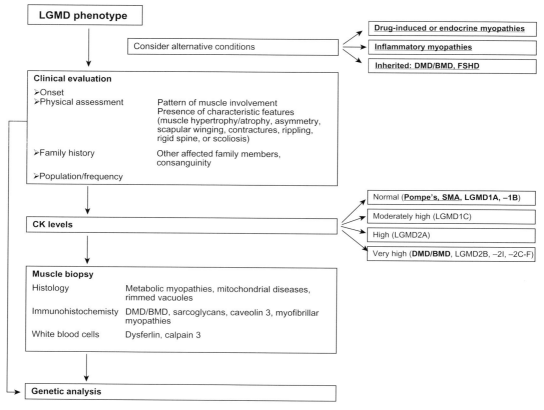

Figure 8.1. Diagnostic algorithm for achieving diagnosis in limb–girdle muscular dystrophies. CK, creatine Kinase; BMD, Becker muscular dystrophy; DMD, Duchenne muscular dystrophy; FSHD, facioscapulohumeral muscular dystrophy; LGMD limb–girdle muscular dystrophy; SMA, spinal muscular atrophy.

★ **TIPS AND TRICKS**

- LGMDs often show a high inter- and intrafamiliar variability in clinical presentation and course.
- Clinical phenotypes may range from almost asymptomatic cases to severely affected patients within the same genetic condition and sometime the same gene defect.
- Some of the genes involved in LGMDs are also responsible for different phenotypes which might be completely distinct or represent a continuous clinical spectrum.

Onset and medical history

The age of onset may vary between and within subtypes. Although a relatively well-defined age of onset has been reported in calpainopathies (onset in the early teens) and in dysferlinopathies (mean age of onset: 20 ± 5 years), a much wider age range has been described for most of the LGMDs. In general, dominant forms tend to present after the second decade of life and are usually slowly progressive, though even early childhood onset may be seen in laminopathy and LGMD1C. Early onset and relatively rapid progression are more common in sarcoglycanopathies, LGMD2I and the other LGMDs with abnormal α-dystroglycan glycosylation. A history of good sporting ability in childhood/early adulthood might suggest a diagnosis of LGMD2B or LGMD2L. Patients with dysferlinopathies are often misdiagnosed with an inflammatory myopathy due to a medical history of subacute onset of muscle pain and weakness not responding to steroids.

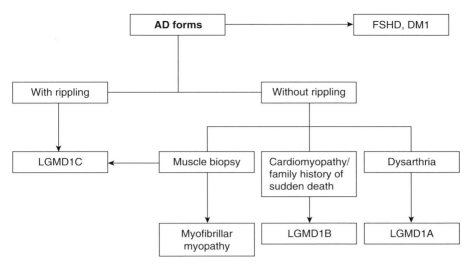

Figure 8.2. Diagnostic algorithm for autosomal dominant limb–girdle muscular dystrophies. AD, autosomal dominant; DM1, myotonic dystrophy type 1; FSHD, facioscapulohumeral muscular dystrophy; LGMD limb–girdle muscular dystrophy.

Muscle assessment and clinical phenotype

A comprehensive muscle strength assessment helps in identifying specific patterns of muscle involvement, sometimes putting forward a specific diagnosis. Relative preservation of hip abductors with prominent scapular winging might suggest a diagnosis of LGMD2A, whereas prominent involvement of the posterior leg muscles and biceps brachii is characteristic of dysferlinopathies. Associated features, which need to be specifically sought, include muscle hypertrophy and atrophy, asymmetry of muscle weakness and wasting, scapular winging, rigid spine, scoliosis, contractures, and muscle rippling (Table 8.2).

Calf hypertrophy is a common clinical feature in LGMD1C, sarcoglycanopathies, and LGMD2I. However, dystrophinopathies (including carrier status) should also be suspected in the presence of prominent calf hypertrophy.

Focal muscle wasting and calf hypotrophy are most common in LGMD2A and -2B respectively. Lower limb distal muscle weakness might be observed in association with the LGMD phenotype in patients with LGMD1A, -2B, -2G, and -2L. Presence of muscle rippling and percussion-induced repetitive contractures are almost pathognomonic for LGMD1C, although there are also acquired causes of rippling muscle disease.

> ★ **TIPS AND TRICKS**
>
> - LGMD1B is the only LGMD that may result in neonatal hypotonia.
> - Intellectual impairment is not characteristically seen in LGMDs and might suggest a differential diagnosis with dystrophinopathies.
> - Normal sporting ability, subacute onset with muscle pain suggest a diagnosis of LGMD2B.
> - Calf hypertrophy may frequently be observed in LGMD1C, -2C-F and -2I.
> - Joint contractures are common in LGMD1B and may be observed in LGMD2A.

Family history

A detailed family history is essential when an inherited condition is suspected. Identifying a pattern of inheritance or the presence of consanguinity can significantly narrow the differential diagnosis and simplify the diagnostic workup. Questions about personal and family history should always extend beyond the neuromuscular system because, with several forms of LGMD,

Table 8.2. Clinical features of limb–girdle muscular dystrophies (LMGDs)

Disease	Gene	Onset	Creatine kinase	Distinguishing clinical features	Atrophy/hypertrophy
LGMD1A	*MYO*	Adulthood	Normal to moderately high	Frequently associated distal weakness; possible facial weakness	Muscle atrophy
LGMD1B	*LMNA*	Any age	Normal to moderately high	Only late involvement of upper limbs; slowly progressive	–
LGMD1C	*CAV3*	Any age	Moderately high to very high	Rippling muscle disease; myalgia and muscle cramps; possible myoglobinuria; possible distal muscle weakness	Calf hypertrophy
LGMD1D	?	Adulthood	Normal to moderately high	Mostly lower limb involvement	–
LGMD1E	?	First to second decades	Normal to moderately high	Later onset in females; slowly progressive	Calf hypertrophy
LGMD1F	?	Any age	Normal to high	Faster progression in early onset cases; facial weakness (early onset cases); late distal muscle weakness	–
LGMD1G	?	Adulthood	Normal to very high	Only late involvement of upper limbs	Muscle atrophy (proximal lower limb muscles)
LGMD1H	?	Second to fifth decades	Normal to very high	Slowly progressive	Calf hypertrophy; upper and lower limb proximal muscle wasting
LGMD2A	*CAPN3*	8–15 years (earlier and later onset described)	High to very high	Prevalent involvement of posterior thighs and hips; relative preservation of hip abductors and quadriceps; toe walking	Posterior tight muscles atrophy; calf hypertrophy or atrophy
LGMD2B	*DYSF*	15–25 years (later onset described)	High to very high	Frequent subacute onset; myalgia (onset); possible distal weakness; only late involvement of upper limbs	Calf and biceps atrophy
LGMD2C - 2F	*SGs*	Usually childhood	High to very high	Dystrophinopathy-like phenotype; possible myoglobinuria; LGMD2D usually less severe	Calf hypertrophy
LGMD2G	*TCAP*	2–15 years (later onset described)	Moderately high to high	Associated distal weakness in the lower limbs	Calf hypertrophy

Scapular winging	Contractures	Cardiac involvement	Respiratory involvement	Scoliosis	Additional features
−	+(TA)	Arrhythmia	+	−	Dysarthria
−	+	Arrhythmia, sds; rarely DCM	+	−(rigid spine)	−
−	−	−	−	−	−
−	−	−	−	−	Dysphagia?
−	+(late onset)	DCM or arrhythmia; sds	−	−	−
+(early onset cases)	−	−	+(early onset cases)	+(early onset cases)	−
−	−	Not described	Not described	−	Progressive limitation of finger flexion
−	−	Not described	Not described	±	−
+	+	−	−	±(lumbar hyperlordosis)	−
−	−	−	−	−	−
+	+(secondary)	DCM	+(also in ambulant patients)	+	−
+	−	DCM	Not described	±(lumbar hyperlordosis)	−

(*Continued*)

Table 8.2. (*Continued*)

Disease	Gene	Onset	Creatine kinase	Distinguishing clinical features	Atrophy/ hypertrophy
LGMD2H	*TRIM32*	8–27 years (later onset described)	Normal to very high	Myalgia and fatigue (onset); only late involvement of upper limbs; possible distal weakness; possible late facial weakness	Calf hypertrophy
LGMD2I	*FKRP*	Any age	High to very high	High clinical variability; homozygotes for the common mutation have milder phenotype; axial and neck flexor muscles weakness; possible myoglobinuria	Muscle hypertrophy (calf, tongue); muscle atrophy (deltoids, pectoralis major)
LGMD2J	*Titin*	5–25 years	High to very high	Severe progression; possible distal weakness	Anterior tibial muscle atrophy
LGMD2K	*POMT1*	First decade	Very high	Slowly progressive; normal motor milestones	Muscle hypertrophy
LGMD2L	*ANO5*	Adulthood	Very high	Asymmetry; mainly lower limb involvement; possible distal lower limb weakness	Calf atrophy or hypertrophy; quadriceps atrophy
LGMD2M	*Fukutin*	Infancy (<1 year)	Very high	Acute deterioration after viral illnesses with good response to steroids; possible facial weakness; axial muscle involvement	Lower limb posterior muscle hypertrophy; generalized muscle atrophy
LGMD2N	*POMT2*	5 years	Very high	Possible response to steroids	Calf hypertrophy

Scapular winging	Contractures	Cardiac involvement	Respiratory involvement	Scoliosis	Additional features
+	–	±(subclinical EKG abnormalities)	+	–	Mild demyelinating polyneuropathic syndrome in some patients
–	–	DCM	+(also in ambulant patients)	±(lumbar hyperlordosis)	–
+	–	Not described	+(late onset)	–	–
–	+	Not described	Not described	+	Cognitive impairment; microcephaly; no structural brain abnormalities or white matter changes
±	±	Not described	Not described	–	–
–	+	DCM	Not described	+(rigid spine)	Normal intellectual development; no structural brain abnormalities or white matter changes
+	+	Not described	Not described	+(lumbar hyperlordosis)	Cognitive impairment (learning disability) in most cases; no structural brain abnormalities or white matter changes

The table summarizes the most common clinical features of each form of LGMD. However, it is important to emphasize that exceptions to these general rules may be seen. This is due to a well-recognized inter- and intrafamilial variability among the different forms and to limited described cases of some forms. Therefore the reported clinical characteristics should be used as guidelines only, and caution should be exercised when approaching a patient with LGMD in both differential diagnosis and management.

TA: Achilles tendons; DCM: dilated cardiomyopathy; sds: sudden death syndrome.
CK: normal <200 IU/L; mildly elevated 200-500 IU/L; moderately high = 500–1000 IU/L; high = 1000–2000 IU/L; very high = >1000 IU/L.

there may be multisystem disease. However, due to large intrafamilial variability and high occurrence of new mutations, especially in the autosomal dominant (AD) forms, a negative family history does not exclude the diagnosis of LGMD.

Epidemiology

It is now well recognized that LGMDs show variable patterns of disease frequency in different populations and therefore understanding the epidemiology of the condition in the population in question is helpful in outlining the differential diagnosis. The AD forms are rare, accounting for about 10% of cases. Calpainopathies seem to be the most common LGMD worldwide and LGMD2I appears to have a high prevalence in northern Europe. LGMD2L was only recently described and it seems to be relatively common in northern England and Germany. The availability of diagnostic genetic testing for anoctamin-5 may also confirm a high incidence of this form in other populations. The relative proportion of the other autosomal recessive (AR) forms varies from country to country (see Table 8.1).

Investigations

Serum creatine kinase

Serum creatine kinase (CK) represents a valuable, cheap, and noninvasive test, which helps in the differential diagnosis (see Table 8.2). As a rule of thumb, higher CK levels are observed in the AR compared with the AD forms, with the exception of LGMD1C. Within the AR LGMD, calpainopathies, dysferlinopathies, sarcoglycanopathies, and LGMD2I are usually associated with very to extremely high CK levels. Normal CK at onset of disease essentially excludes AR LGMD and is very unlikely even in the AD forms. It is important to note that, as with all forms of muscular dystrophy, CK levels fall with age and disease progression so in older patients CK levels may be normal or only minimally elevated.

Electrophysiology

Electromyography and nerve conduction studies are not likely to be of value in distinguishing the different forms of LGMD, but may be helpful in the differential diagnosis with other conditions such as SMA, myotonic dystrophies, and myasthenic syndromes.

Muscle magnetic resonance

Over the last few years, muscle magnetic resonance imaging (MRI) has been used to detect distinct patterns of muscle involvement in different neuromuscular conditions and may represent a promising noninvasive investigation in the diagnosis of the different forms of LGMD. However, reliable sequencing and protocols are so far available only in specialized centers and require highly qualified personnel with experience in muscle imaging and analysis. This expertise will hopefully become more widely available in the future.

Muscle biopsy

Despite continuous progress toward understanding the molecular basis of LGMDs, a diagnostic approach exclusively based on genetic testing is often inefficient and too expensive to be applicable in clinical practice. Although the prospect of new generation sequencing and "LGMD chips" offers promise, for now such technologies are not widely applicable in the diagnostic setting. The muscle biopsy is therefore unavoidable in most cases and continues to be a highly informative and relatively economic diagnostic step for many forms of MD. No studies have compared open versus needle or conchotome biopsies; however, immunohistochemical and immunoblotting procedures often require a substantial sample to allow meaningful interpretation. Muscle MRI may be useful before biopsy to identify muscle with sufficient preservation to yield useful results, especially in advanced disease.

Basic histology is of little value in discriminating between the different LGMD forms but might be useful in the differential diagnosis. AD forms might show a nonspecific myopathic pattern without clear dystrophic abnormalities. Inflammatory infiltrates are common in dysferlinopathies, whereas rimmed vacuoles might be seen in LGMD1A, -2G, and -2J although these changes are nonspecific. Muscle immunohistochemistry and immunoblotting are crucial in the diagnosis of the different forms of LGMD and in directing further genetic testing in most cases. If DMD/BMD has not been genetically excluded, demonstration of normal dystrophin expression is imperative, due to the higher incidence of dystrophinopathies compared with LGMDs. Immunoanalysis might show primary protein changes, clearly suggesting a specific genetic defect, such as caveolin 3 deficiency in LGMD1C. However, secondary protein deficiencies are commonly observed in some LGMDs, such as calpain 3 reduction in dysferlin deficiency and LGMD2J patients, and dystrophin reduction in all sarcoglycanopathies. Secondary reduction in caveolin 3 expression has also been described in patients with autoimmune rippling muscle disease. Moreover, normal protein expression on immunoanalysis can be observed in many LGMDs, including LGMD1A, -1B, and -2A (Table 8.3).

✋ CAUTION!

Caution also needs to be taken in the presence of very specific clinical features as, even where protein testing is usually highly predictive, there may be cases with mutations and normal protein on antibody analysis.

A blood-based assay to screen dysferlin expression in monocytes was suggested as a simple and less invasive procedure to identify patients with dysferlin deficiency. Although promising, this technique is not routinely available at present. Recently, a novel, tissue lysate, reverse-protein array approach was developed for the measurement and quantification of muscle proteins for the diagnosis of different MDs, including sarcoglycanopathies. This technology has the advantage of assessing expression of multiple muscle proteins in small amounts of muscle tissue; however, further studies are required to validate its applicability in other forms of LGMDs.

Considering the complexity of muscle biopsy analysis in the diagnosis of the different forms of LGMD, it should be undertaken in a laboratory with expertise in performing and interpreting these techniques.

Genetics

The identification of the causative mutation by molecular analysis remains the gold standard in the diagnosis of the different forms of LGMD.

✋ CAUTION!

Genetic analysis might be straightforward in some forms such as LGMD2I, where direct sequencing can be rapidly performed in a diagnostic laboratory and the common mutation (C826A) is readily tested in high prevalence populations (see Table 8.1). In other cases (e.g. LGMD2A and -2B) the large size of the involved gene makes the sequencing process more challenging and therefore available only in specialized centers. According to several studies, the location of the second expected mutation in *CAPN3* is difficult to identify in about 20–25% of the LGMD2A cases even in dedicated laboratories, partly due to the occurrence of deep intronic mutations or deletions. Finally, some of the genes responsible for the rarer forms of LGMD can be currently tested only on a research basis (*TCAP*, *TRIM32*, and *TTN*). Furthermore, even though the underlying genetic defect has been identified for many of the LGMDs and new genes are continuously discovered, a precise diagnosis cannot be reached in 25–50% of patients even in specialized centers.

⚜ SCIENCE REVISITED

As already noted, considering the genetic heterogeneity of LGMDs and the clinical overlap between the different forms, recently a new sensitive high-throughput DNA microarray ("gene chip") was developed and validated on a research basis for the diagnosis of different inherited neuromuscular disorders, including LGMDs (www.nmd-chip. eu). This technique represents a potentially important improvement in the diagnostic process of LGMDs because it allows simultaneous sequencing of multiple genes, reducing costs and lag times. Its worldwide clinical application in the future might change the diagnostic algorithm in LGMDs and other neuromuscular conditions, avoiding or reducing the need for other invasive procedures.

Table 8.3. Limb–girdle muscular dystrophies (LMGDs): muscle biopsy and diagnostic protein analysis

Disease	Protein involved	Histology	Primary protein abnormality (muscle biopsy)	Secondary protein abnormality (muscle biopsy)	Predictive value of protein abnormality on diagnosis[a]
LGMD1A	Myotilin	Myopathic, dystrophic, rimmed vacuoles, desmin accumulation	Possible myotilin accumulation	↓ laminin γ_1; possible desmin accumulation (histology)	Protein accumulation may indicate involvement of family of MF genes: precise gene involved not generally reliable
LGMD1B	Lamin A/C	Dystrophic	Normal lamin A/C	↓ laminin β1	None
LGMD1C	Caveolin 3	Dystrophic, myopathic	↓ caveolin 3	↓ dysferlin	Very high (immunohistochemistry and immunoblotting)
LGMD2A	Calpain 3	Dystrophic	Normal or ↓ calpain3 (immunoblotting)	Calpain 3 degradation	Variable. Absence of protein on immunoblotting should direct mutation testing unless obvious protein degradation; however, protein may be normal in presence of confirmed mutations.
LGMD2B	Dysferlin	Dystrophic, inflammatory	↓ dysferlin	Possible ↓ calpain 3 and/or caveolin 3	Very high when absence of protein on immunoblotting
LGMD2C	γ-Sarcoglycan	Dystrophic	↓ γ-sarcoglycan	↓ other sarcoglycans and dystrophin	Highly predictive of involvement of one of the sarcoglycan genes but not predictive of which sarcoglycan is involved
LGMD2D	α-Sarcoglycan	Dystrophic	↓ α-sarcoglycan	↓ other sarcoglycans and dystrophin	Highly predictive of involvement of one of the sarcoglycan genes but not predictive of which sarcoglycan is involved
LGMD2E	β-Sarcoglycan	Dystrophic	↓ β-sarcoglycan	↓ other sarcoglycans and dystrophin	Highly predictive of involvement of one of the sarcoglycan genes but not predictive of which sarcoglycan is involved

LGMD2F	δ-Sarcoglycan	Dystrophic	↓ δ-sarcoglycan	↓ other sarcoglycans and dystrophin	Highly predictive of involvement of one of the sarcoglycan genes but not predictive of which sarcoglycan is involved
LGMD2G	Telethonin	Dystrophic, rimmed vacuoles	↓ telethonin		High
LGMD2H	TRIM32	Myopathic, dystrophic, rimmed vacuoles	TRIM32 antibodies not in use		None
LGMD2I	FKRP	Dystrophic	FKRP antibodies not in use	↓ α-dystroglycan and laminin α2	Secondary changes may be suggestive but are not specific as involvement of many genes may alter α-dystroglycan
LGMD2J	Titin	Myopathic, dystrophic, rimmed vacuoles	↓ titin	↓ calpain 3	Unknown – secondary calpain 3 deficiency has been reported
LGMD2K	POMT1	Dystrophic	POMP1 antibodies not in use	↓ α-dystroglycan and laminin α2	Secondary changes may be suggestive but are not specific as involvement of many genes may alter α-dystroglycan
LGMD2L	Anoctamin 5	Myopathic, dystrophic	ANO5 antibodies not in use		None
LGMD2M	Fukutin	Dystrophic	Fukutin antibodies not in use	↓ α-dystroglycan and laminin α2	Secondary changes may be suggestive but are not specific as involvement of many genes may alter α-dystroglycan
LGMD2N	POMT2	Dystrophic, inflammatory	POMPT2 antibodies not in use	↓ α-dystroglycan and laminin α2	Secondary changes may be suggestive but are not specific as involvement of many genes may alter α-dystroglycan

aNote that the absence of abnormality of protein expression can in itself be a pointer to the diagnosis of LGMD1B, -2A, -2L, and (the much rarer conditions) -2H and -2J.

As already noted, considering the genetic heterogeneity of LGMDs and the clinical overlap between the different forms, recently a new sensitive high-throughput DNA microarray ("gene chip") was developed and validated on a research basis for the diagnosis of different inherited neuromuscular disorders, including LGMDs (www.nmd-chip.eu). This technique represents a potentially important improvement in the diagnostic process of LGMDs because it allows simultaneous sequencing of multiple genes, reducing costs and lag times. Its worldwide clinical application in the future might change the diagnostic algorithm in LGMDs and other neuromuscular conditions, avoiding or reducing the need for other invasive procedures.

Management

MDs are often multisystemic disorders. The presence or absence of complications, including contractures, heart and respiratory involvement, helps narrow the differential diagnosis, but more importantly understanding risks in a particular patient allows adequate follow-up to be put in place. An efficient workup and early diagnosis are key in the management of patients with LGMDs. This allows precise genetic counseling and the recognition and management of any specific complications that the patient is at risk for. Prevention and accurately timed symptomatic treatment of complications, in particular cardiac and respiratory dysfunction, are crucial to improve quality of life and prolong survival. As a general rule, patients in whom the underlying genetic diagnosis is unknown should be monitored and managed for cardiovascular and other associated consequences. In this scenario, even in the absence of a positive family history, AR inheritance cannot be assumed and so the risk of recurrence cannot be accurately assessed.

Muscle, joint, and spine assessment

Although universally agreed guidelines are not available, physiotherapy input is recommended in LGMDs. Effective exercises including active stretching, active-assisted stretching, and passive stretching on ankles, knees, hips, and elbows should be done on a regular basis (4–6 days a week) to prevent or minimize joint contractures. This is particularly important in those LGMDs that are known to be associated with contractural phenotypes at early stages (LGMD1B, -2A, -2I, and sarcoglycanopathies) but are otherwise recommended in all patients with reduced mobility. Ankle–foot orthoses used at night can further help prevent contractures, while surgical interventions, such as Achilles tendon lengthening, should be considered on an individual basis. Regular submaximal exercise and low-resistance strength training are recommended to avoid disuse atrophy and other complications, but high-resistance strength training and eccentric exercise are inappropriate. Significant muscle pain and myoglobinuria should be considered as signs of overexertion, to be avoided in patients with MDs. Rehabilitation and early mobilization are essential in the event of bone fractures to allow functional recovery. Surgical fixation should be considered in patients with neuromuscular diseases because it might allow shorter convalescence and earlier mobilization. Spine deformities and scoliosis might be observed in some patients and should be clinically monitored. Spinal surgery might be considered in case of severe spinal deformities. These complications are more typically seen in cases where there is childhood onset and severe muscle weakness. Spinal rigidity can be an important complication in LGMD1B. Appropriate and timely aids and adaptations should aim to guarantee independence and improve quality of life. Manual or powered wheelchairs should be considered in advance and provided when functional ambulation declines.

Respiratory function

Respiratory muscle weakness should be monitored in all LGMDs, especially in severely affected patients, due to the risk of infection, hypoventilation, and respiratory failure. However, some forms of LGMDs are more likely to be associated with respiratory impairment than others and more careful follow-up is required (see Table 8.2). Particular attention should be paid in LGMD2I because patients may develop respiratory insufficiency even while ambulant, due to substantial diaphragmatic involvement. In other forms of LGMDs, respiratory insufficiency is much rarer and is typically seen only very late in the disease course, associated with significant generalized muscle weakness. Symptoms of respiratory insufficiency and nocturnal hypoventilation (frequent chest infections, morning headaches, poor appetite, extreme tiredness, and sleepiness) should be monitored. Forced vital capacity (FVC), checked in a sitting and a supine position, should be measured annually or more often in patients with LGMD forms associated with respiratory involvement. In the presence of symptoms or signs (FVC <60% of the predicted value per sex, age, and height) of respiratory muscle weakness, an overnight pulse oximetry should be organized and referral to a respiratory specialist for assessment and introduction of nocturnal noninvasive ventilation if indicated. Annual flu immunization should be provided in this population and chest infections should be treated promptly with antibiotics. Cough assist devices might be helpful for patients with severe respiratory impairment and frequent infections.

Cardiac function

Regular cardiac evaluation will identify early signs of contractile and rhythm involvement, and allow prompt treatment when indicated. Generally, annual EKG and echocardiogram are recommended in all patients at risk of cardiomyopathy (see Table 8.2) and more frequent assessments, and a referral to a specialist with experience in MDs are required if any abnormality is observed. Cardiac surveillance is not indicated routinely in LGMD2A, -2B, -2G, -2H, -2J, and -1C, but baseline cardiac investigations might be useful at diagnosis and when patients lose independent ambulation.

Dilated cardiomyopathy with reduced ejection fraction is typically associated with LGMD2I and sarcoglycanopathies, with the exception of LGMD2D. Management of impaired left ventricular function is usually with angiotensin-converting enzyme inhibitors and/or β blockers. Careful cardiac surveillance is mandatory in LGMD1B and other AD forms, due to the high risk of ventricular arrhythmias and sudden death, which may present at onset or develop at any time. Management of cardiomyopathy and rhythm abnormalities may be life saving for these patients. The consensus recommendation at present is that implantable defibrillators may be more appropriate because sudden ventricular tachyarrhythmias would not be adequately treated by pacemaker alone. As management of these cases is complex, monitoring in specialized centers is highly recommended.

Genetic counseling

Once the molecular diagnosis has been established genetic counseling is always appropriate. Among the AD cases, the known reproductive risk of 50% might be complicated by nonpenetrant cases, germline mosaicism, and late onset of the disease in some family members. Moreover, private mutations and new changes are relatively common, and determination of the pathogenicity might be difficult. The AR LGMDs are rare conditions, so the probability of a carrier having a child with another carrier in the general population is very low. However, the occurrence risks increase within populations with founder mutations and where there is consanguinity. Experienced counseling becomes particularly important in these situations. Currently, a specific genetic diagnosis is not achievable in about 25–50% of cases. Prenatal diagnosis is possible in case of known mutations but is generally offered only in cases of high recurrent risk. A preclinical diagnosis is recommended only when prevention and early treatment of complications are possible, such as cardiac arrhythmia in LGMD1A and -1B, or if this information can play a role in reproductive decisions.

Therapy

Currently there is no curative treatment for any of the LGMD forms. Corticosteroids have been empirically used in sarcoglycanopathies and α-dystroglycanopathies with reported improvement. However no randomized, placebo-controlled trials have been conducted so far and further studies are required before their routine clinical application. A phase 2/3 clinical trial with deflazacort in dysferlinopathies has been completed and early results suggest that there is no benefit. A phase 1/2 clinical trial with MYO-029 failed to achieve clinical efficacy, but other pharmacological agents to increase muscle mass are currently under investigation as possible therapeutic approaches in different MDs, including LGMDs. Different novel strategies, including gene replacement, stem cell transplantation, and pharmacological agents to impact the genetic defect or its downstream effects, are currently under development, many working in parallel with efforts in other muscular dystrophies. A gene transfer therapy has been developed as one possible approach in sarcoglycanopathies and is currently in a phase 1 clinical trial in LGMD2D. Exon skipping using antisense technology has been suggested as a possible therapeutic strategy in dysferlinopathy. A phase 2/3 clinical trial with coenzyme Q10 and lisinopril in different types of MD, including some LGMDs, has recently started recruitment in the USA (www.clinicaltrials.gov).

✭ TIPS AND TRICKS

Natural history studies provide invaluable information regarding disease progression and complications of each form of LGMD. However, in clinical practice involving individual patients, they should be used only as guidelines.

✋ CAUTION!

Patients with LGMDs may have an increased anesthetic risk because of possible respiratory and/or heart involvement in some (LGMD2I). Moreover, malignant hyperthermia after general anesthesia has been reported in LGMD2I patients. The anesthetist has therefore to be informed about the muscle condition of the patient before planning procedures under general anesthesia.

Patients with LGMDs do not have an increased risk with local anesthesia.

GENERAL POINTS TO REMEMBER

- Complete cardiac and respiratory preoperative assessments are essential to predict anesthetic risk and prevent complications.
- Inhalational anesthetics, hypnotic agents with slow metabolism (thiopental), and opiates should be avoided.
- Propofol and fentanyl are preferred for induction.
- Short-acting, non-depolarizing muscle relaxants in small doses can be used if necessary, but be aware that recovery may be prolonged.
- Paralytic muscle relaxants (e.g. succinylcholine) should be avoided.
- EKG monitoring should be kept in the peri- and postoperative period because of increased tendency to dysrhythmia.
- Respiratory monitoring and early postoperative chest physiotherapy are essential in patients with respiratory involvement.

Conclusions

Over the last 15 years, our knowledge of LGMDs has been impressively enlarged. New genes are continually being discovered and several studies have reported that a precise diagnosis can be reached in 50–75% of cases in different parts of the world. However, achieving a diagnosis of a specific form of LGMD is a complex process, which requires a multidisciplinary approach and combined clinical and laboratory evaluations.

It has been long argued that there is little practical relevance to reaching a molecular diagnosis because no therapeutic approaches are currently available. However, it is becoming clear that a precise diagnosis is necessary for patients to allow form-specific management of complications and appropriate genetic counseling, and in the future as new gene- and protein-specific therapies are becoming a reality.

An integrated clinical and research approach with international collaborations is essential to increase diagnosis, facilitate the investigative approach, and enable translational research in these rare disorders.

National or global patient registries are developing around the world with the aim of enlarging our current knowledge about the natural course and management of the different LGMDs and to promote translational research. These efforts will be essential to improve quality of life and survival, and to expedite treatment development for this patient group.

Bibliography

Bushby K. Diagnosis and management of the limb girdle muscular dystrophies. *Pract Neurol* 2009;**9**:314–23.

Guglieri M, Magri F, D'Angelo MG, et al. Clinical, molecular, and protein correlations in a large sample of genetically diagnosed Italian limb girdle muscular dystrophy patients. *Hum Mutat* 2008;**29**:258–66.

Hicks D, Sarkozy A, Muelas N, et al. A founder mutation in Anoctamin 5 is a major cause of limb girdle muscular dystrophy. *Brain* 2010; **133**:2528.

Lo HP, Cooper ST, Evesson FJ, et al. Limb-girdle muscular dystrophy: diagnostic evaluation, frequency and clues to pathogenesis. *Neuromusc Disord* 2008;**18**:34–44.

Manzur AY, Muntoni F. Diagnosis and new treatments in muscular dystrophies. *Postgrad Med J* 2009;**85**:622–30.

Mercuri E, Pichiecchio A, Allsop J, et al. Muscle MRI in inherited neuromuscular disorders: past, present, and future. *J Magn Reson Imaging* 2007;**25**:433–40.

Moore SA, Shilling CJ, Westra S, et al. Limb-girdle muscular dystrophy in the United States. *J Neuropathol Exp Neurol* 2006;**65**:995–1003.

Norwood F, de Visser M, Eymard B, et al. EFNS guideline on diagnosis and management of limb girdle muscular dystrophies. *Eur J Neurol* 2007;**14**:1305–12.

Norwood FL, Harling C, Chinnery PF, et al. Prevalence of genetic muscle disease in Northern England: in-depth analysis of a muscle clinic population. *Brain* 2009;**132**(Pt 11):3175–86.

Paradas C, Llauger J, Diaz-Manera J, et al. Redefining dysferlinopathy phenotypes based on clinical findings and muscle imaging studies. *Neurology* 2010;**75**:316–23.

Rocha CT, Hoffman EP. Limb-girdle and congenital muscular dystrophies: current diagnostics, management, and emerging technologies. *Curr Neurol Neurosci Rep* 2010;**10**:267–76.

Sáenz A, Leturcq F, Cobo AM, et al. LGMD2A: genotype-phenotype correlations based on a large mutational survey on the calpain 3 gene. *Brain* 2005;**128**(Pt 4):732–42.

Straub V, Bushby K. Therapeutic possibilities in the autosomal recessive limb-girdle muscular dystrophies. *Neurotherapeutics* 2008;**5**:619–26.

Vainzof M, Bushby K. Muscular dystrophies presenting with proximal muscle weakness. In: *Disorders of Voluntary Muscles*, 8th edn. Cambridge: Cambridge University Press, 2010.

van der Kooi AJ, Frankhuizen WS, Barth PG, et al. Limb-girdle muscular dystrophy in the Netherlands: gene defect identified in half the families. *Neurology* 2007;**68**:2125–8.

Facioscapulohumeral Dystrophy

Constantine Farmakidis[1] and Rabi Tawil[2]

[1]Columbia University Medical Center, Neurological Institute, New York, NY, USA
[2]Neuromuscular Disease Unit, Fields Center for FSHD and Neuromuscular Research, University of Rochester Medical Center, Rochester, NY, USA

Facioscapulohumeral dystrophy (FSHD) is an autosomal dominant neuromuscular disorder that affects about 1 in 20 000. It is the third most common form of muscular dystrophy after Duchenne muscular dystrophy, which causes relentlessly progressive weakness in boys, and myotonic dystrophy, which causes gradually progressive weakness and stiffness in men and women. As the name suggests, FSHD has a fairly specific distribution of weakness at onset that allows the practitioner to make an accurate bedside diagnosis.

A prompt diagnosis, confirmed by genetic testing, can avoid unnecessary tests, allow for timely genetic counseling and provide the patient with appropriate prognostic information. This last point is of particular importance because FSHD, on average, carries a substantially better prognosis than the diseases in its differential diagnosis.

Clinical presentation

FSHD has a very broad clinical spectrum of age at onset and severity. Symptom onset occurs most commonly in the second decade but ranges from infancy, for the most severe forms of FSHD, to late adulthood. FSHD runs in families with an autosomal dominant pattern of inheritance,

although new mutations, presenting as sporadic cases, are common.

Despite the variability in severity and age at symptom onset, the characteristic distribution of weakness is broadly retained and remains the most important identifying feature in making a clinical diagnosis. The disease's name, facioscapulohumeral dystrophy, is a useful device for recalling the distinctive pattern of weakness seen most reproducibly in the earlier stages of FSHD. Initially weakness is restricted to the face and can be quite subtle and typically asymptomatic. Facial weakness is commonly followed by weakness of muscles around the scapula, manifesting with difficulty raising the arms above shoulder level and is associated with scapular winging. As facial weakness is most often asymptomatic, most patients present when shoulder weakness sets in. The humeral component of FSHD refers to weakness of biceps and triceps with notable sparing of the deltoid muscle.

Facial weakness, as subtle and asymmetric as it may be, remains, along with the characteristic appearance of the shoulders, the most distinctive feature of FSHD. On inspection FSHD patients can have widened palpebral fissures, decreased facial expression, and pouty lips. Examination confirms bifacial, typically asymmetric weakness

Neuromuscular Disorders, First Edition. Edited by Rabi N. Tawil, Shannon Venance.
© 2011 John Wiley & Sons, Ltd. Published 2011 by John Wiley & Sons, Ltd.

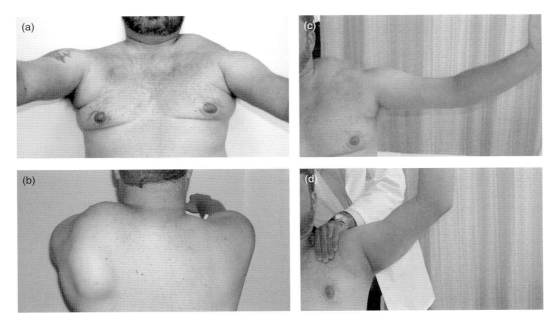

Figure 9.1. The left panel shows typical shoulder profile with straight clavicles, axillary creases due to pectoral muscle atrophy (a), and asymmetric winging (b). The right panel shows limited arm shoulder abduction to about 90° (c) with improvement to about 130° with manual fixation of the scapula (d). (Reproduced from Tawil R, van der Maarel SM. Facioscapulohumeral muscular dystrophy. *Muscle Nerve* 2006;**34**:1–15, with permission from Wiley-Blackwell.)

with a horizontal smile, and an inability to purse the lips and bury the eyelashes. Shoulders typically show asymmetric winging on attempted shoulder abduction or forward flexion, straight clavicles, forward sloping of the shoulders at rest, and axillary creases reflecting pectoral muscle wasting (Figure 9.1).

Although weakness is initially proximal in the upper limbs, weakness in the lower limbs most often begins in more distal muscles such as tibialis anterior, producing a foot drop. Core muscle weakness in the abdomen and back is an early, common, and often under-appreciated feature of FSHD. Weak abdominal muscles may result in a distended abdomen, out of proportion to body habitus, and in difficulty doing a sit-up. Paraspinal muscle weakness may also cause an exaggerated lumbar lordosis. On physical examination, selective involvement of the lower abdominal muscles may produce a striking upward displacement of the umbilicus with neck flexion in a supine position. This is known as Beevor's sign and, in the setting of a suggestive history, is supportive of an FSHD diagnosis.

Weakness in FSHD tends to be asymmetric and the presence of striking asymmetry supports the FSHD diagnosis. Extraocular and bulbar muscles are typically spared. Respiratory failure due to neuromuscular weakness occurs in less than 5% of patients with FSHD, typically in wheelchair-bound patients with progressive kyphoscoliosis.

The most likely initial symptom is difficulty reaching above shoulder level, more pronounced on one side than the other. Foot drop is a less common presentation although invariably such patients have unnoticed shoulder weakness and scapular winging. Overall, deficits in FSHD tend to be chronic and slowly progressive, and consequently patients learn to adapt to significant weakness.

Extramuscular manifestations

The two most common extramuscular manifestations in FSHD are: high-frequency hearing loss, occurring in 75% of affected individuals, and retinal vascular abnormalities, occurring in 60% of patients. In most patients neither the retinal nor the auditory involvement results in clinically significant impairment; however, recognition of their occurrence is important for physicians participating in the long-term care of these patients. Hearing loss, which is most frequently asymptomatic, may be severe in children with infantile-onset disease and thus require prompt intervention with hearing aids to avoid developmental delays in language. Also, in some of the most severely affected FSHD patients, the retinal vascular abnormalities may progress into an exudative retinopathy and resulting visual loss, a clinical sequence known as Coat's syndrome. Screening of such patients with indirect ophthalmoscopy and treatment of significant vascular aneurysmal dilations can help arrest or prevent visual loss.

Prognosis

Prognosis tends to be inversely related to age of symptom onset. A child with significant periscapular weakness carries a worse prognosis than a 20 year old with only subtle facial weakness. In FSHD, the rate of progression is slow and typically remains steady. A subset of patients, however, reports a stepwise course where quiet intervals are followed by sentinel pain and then rapid deterioration in the involved muscles.

Individuals develop variable degrees of disability, with 20% of patients eventually becoming wheelchair bound. Patients with infantile-onset disease are frequently severely disabled, with the potential additional burden of hearing loss and visual loss compounding their limb weakness.

Life expectancy in FSHD is said to be normal because severe bulbar, respiratory, and cardiac involvement is rare. Nevertheless, unrecognized and untreated respiratory failure can lead to unexpected early mortality.

Genetics

Understanding the genetic mechanism of FSHD has been a challenge since 1992, when FSHD was first associated with a deletion of what appeared to be transcriptionally silent repetitive DNA elements in the subtelomeric region of chromosome 4q35. In over 95% of individuals with FSHD, there is a deletion of an integral number of macrosatellite repeats on 4q35. Normal individuals have 11–100 repeats, whereas patients with FSHD have 1–10 D4Z4 repeats. The absence of signs of FSHD in individuals with large deletions of 4q35 involving all D4Z4 repeats and the need to have at least one residual repeat in FSHD suggest a deleterious gain of function rather than a loss of function. Moreover, although D4Z4 contractions are necessary to cause FSHD, the contraction has to occur on a specific chromosomal background, known as A161, with specific DNA-sequence variations proximal and distal to the repeats. Moreover, contraction on this permissive background is also associated with a change in the chromatin state in the D4Z4 region from a nonpermissive to a permissive chromatin conformation. Recently, evidence for a unifying genetic model of FSHD was published.

> ### ⚙ SCIENCE REVISITED
>
> Two prevailing models for FSHD were pursued. One postulated that the D4Z4 contraction resulted in a change is expression of a gene from within the repeats. Indeed an open reading frame for a gene, DUX4, was present in each repeat, but it was difficult to demonstrate whether it was an expressed gene or a pseudogene. In the second model, contraction of the repeats influenced the expression of genes proximal to the deletion. Recent evidence supports the former model. The current model of FSHD pathogenesis is

as follows: contraction of a critical number of D4Z4 repeats changes the chromatin structure to a euchromatic conformation which is more permissive of gene expression; the 4qA161 background contains a polyadenylation (poly(A)) sequence just distal to the last copy of the DUX4 gene. This poly(A) tail is essential in stabilizing mRNA for translation into protein. Thus, contraction of D4Z4 on a 4qA161 background triggers expression of a stable DUX4 mRNA and protein. The function of DUX4 remains uncertain, although early experiments indicate that it can interfere with muscle regeneration and make cells more susceptible to oxidative stress, leading to apoptosis.

Clinical diagnosis

For practitioners who are not neuromuscular specialists, the challenge of a bedside FSHD diagnosis tends to be in the rarity of the disease rather than an absence of distinctive clinical features. The presence of the cardinal features of FHSD – slowly progressive muscular weakness with prominent facial weakness and scapular winging, in the setting of a positive family history – should raise FSHD in the differential diagnosis. Whereas the clinical symptoms of weakness in FSHD may appear to be acute or subacute, raising the possibility of an acquired myopathy, a careful history will uncover longstanding signs of muscle weakness. Evidence for pre-existing facial weakness is suggested by the patient's inability to whistle or drink through a straw or by reports from parents that the patient sleeps with eyes slightly open. Longstanding difficulty doing pushups, climbing ropes, or using a jungle gym may indicate the presence of shoulder–girdle weakness.

On physical examination, perhaps the most distinctive feature of FSHD is the combination of facial and shoulder weakness. The shoulders have a characteristic appearance with forward sloping of the shoulder, straight clavicles, and asymmetric scapular winging. In more advanced cases, hip–girdle, quadriceps, hamstring, and foot dorsiflexor weakness can also be seen. Extraocular and pharyngeal weakness, promi-nent contractures, or early respiratory compromise is not seen in FSHD and their presence suggests an alternative diagnosis.

Laboratory diagnostic testing

Routine laboratory testing is helpful in ruling out other diseases from the differential diagnosis. Creatine kinase (CK) levels are normal to slightly elevated (three to five times normal); CK levels that are elevated more than ten times normal suggest an alternative diagnosis. When difficulty arises in differentiating a myopathic from a neuropathic process, such as when patients present with unilateral scapular winging, mimicking a long thoracic nerve injury, needle electromyography is helpful and shows nonspecific changes of active and chronic myopathy, more prominent in weak muscles. Muscle biopsy in FSHD shows nonspecific myopathic changes and up to a third can show variable inflammatory features. A muscle biopsy is not needed where genetic testing is available. If genetic testing is negative, a muscle biopsy is helpful in pursuing and establishing an alternative diagnosis. A number of conditions can at times mimic the clinical presentation of FSHD.

★ **TIPS AND TRICKS**

CONDITIONS THAT CAN MIMIC FSHD

- Myofibrillar myopathy
- Polymyositis
- Adult-onset acid maltase deficiency
- Inclusion body myositis
- Mitochondrial myopathy
- Congenital nemaline and centronuclear myopathy
- Neuralgic amyotrophy
- Limb–girdle muscular dystrophy
- Emery–Dreifuss muscular dystrophy

Molecular genetic diagnosis

Clinical genetic testing identifies the presence of contraction in the chromosome 4 repetitive sequences (D4Z4) associated with FSHD. DNA from a blood sample undergoes Southern blot analysis using a macrosatellite probe after double digestion with *Eco*RI/*Bln*I restriction enzymes, which cut the DNA on either end of the D4Z4 repeats. Unaffected individuals typically have two allele sizes of more than 50 kilobases, whereas affected individuals have one allele in the normal range and one deletion-containing allele of reduced size between 10 and 38 kilobases. This test is both highly sensitive and specific (>95% and >95%); however, approximately 5% of patients with a clinical diagnosis of FSHD will have negative DNA analysis and referral to a neuromuscular center could be considered. In all patients, a genetics referral for counseling is appropriate.

Management

The identification of a specific overexpressed gene as the causal mechanism for FSHD has given scientists, for the first time, a target for the development of a disease-specific treatment for FHSD. However, at present, there are no medical treatments known to reverse, stop, or delay progression of muscle weakness and atrophy in FSHD. Nevertheless, there are a number of interventions that can provide symptomatic and functional improvement in many patients.

In general FSHD produces small functional deficits at onset. As the disease is slowly progressive, individuals most often are able to develop adaptive strategies to compensate, and frequently remain highly functional despite having significant muscular weakness. Other than the specific management issues discussed below, patients with FSHD often have pain-related changes in posture in the shoulders and back, and overuse pain around joints supported by weak muscles. The management of such pain must be individualized but should involve a combination of range of motion exercises, physical therapy, and pharmacological agents such as nonsteroidal anti-inflammatory drugs for acute pain, in a addition to medications used in the management of chronic pain.

Assistive devices

Foot drop is a frequent early manifestation of FSHD in the lower extremity and patients can benefit from the use of a molded ankle–foot orthosis (AFO). If quadriceps weakness is also present, fixed AFOs hinder walking by preventing hyperextension and locking of the knee. A more preferable brace in such situations is a floor reaction ankle–foot orthosis, because it can provide extension support to the knee upon floor contact, preventing buckling of the knee.

Role of exercise

Unlike other dystrophies with friable muscle membranes, such as Duchenne muscular dystrophy, where there is concern that exercise may actually hasten progression, studies in FSHD have shown that aerobic exercise is safe and beneficial.

Scapular fixation surgery

Inability to raise the arm to or above shoulder level is both a cardinal manifestation and one of the major sources of functional disability in FSHD. Surgical scapular fixation can improve shoulder range of motion but it has not been studied in a prospective manner. Nevertheless, recent case series suggest that scapular arthrodesis is effective and safe. Currently surgical intervention can be considered in patients with slowly progressive disease, fairly preserved strength in the shoulder, and in whom manual scapular fixation on physical examination shows an increase in shoulder range of motion.

Extramuscular manifestations

Hearing loss in FSHD, although common, is predominantly asymptomatic and requires no intervention. In infantile-onset FSHD, hearing loss can frequently be more severe and, if not addressed with hearing aids, can interfere with cognitive development. For this reason, audiograms should be performed on all children diagnosed with infantile FSHD.

Retinovascular abnormalities

Mild retinovascular abnormalities are also very common in FSHD, and in the vast majority of cases remain clinically silent. Rarely, however, severely affected infantile-onset FSHD can develop an exudative retinopathy, resulting in visual loss. Screening all infantile-onset FSHD patients at diagnosis with indirect ophthalmoscopy is essential because early laser photocoagulation can prevent Coat's syndrome and visual loss.

Bibliography

Eger K, Jordan B, Habermann S, Zierz S. Beevor's sign in facioscapulohumeral muscular dystrophy: an old sign with new implications. *J Neurol* 2010;**257**:436–8.

Fitzsimons RB, Gurwin EB, Bird AC. Retinal vascular abnormalities in facioscapulohumeral muscular dystrophy. A general association with genetic and therapeutic implications. *Brain* 1987;**110**(Pt 3):631–48.

Lemmers RJ, van der Vliet PJ, Klooster R, et al. A unifying genetic model for facioscapulohumeral muscular dystrophy. *Science* 2010;**329**:1650–3.

Orrell RW, Copeland S, Rose MR. Scapular fixation in muscular dystrophy. *Cochrane Database Syst Rev* 2010;(**1**):CD003278.

Padberg GW. *Facioscapulohumeral Disease.* Leiden: University of Leiden, 1982.

Snider L, Geng LN, Lemmers RJLF, et al. *Facioscapulohumeral dystrophy: incomplete suppression of a retrotransposed gene.* 2010; **6**:e1001181.

Tawil R. Facioscapulohumeral muscular dystrophy. *Neurotherapeutics* 2008;**5**:601–6.

Tawil R, van der Maarel SM. Facioscapulohumeral muscular dystrophy. *Muscle Nerve* 2006;**34**: 1–15.

Tawil R, van der Maarel S, Padberg GW, van Engelen BG. 171st ENMC international workshop: Standards of care and management of facioscapulohumeral muscular dystrophy. *Neuromusc Disord* 2010;**20**:471–5.

Trevisan CP, Pastorello E, Ermani M, et al. Facioscapulohumeral muscular dystrophy: a multicenter study on hearing function. *Audiol Neurootol* 2008;**13**:1–6.

van der Kooi EL, Vogels OJ, van Asseldonk RJ, et al. Strength training and albuterol in facioscapulohumeral muscular dystrophy. *Neurology* 2004;**63**:702–8.

Wijmenga C, Hewitt JE, Sandkuijl LA, et al. Chromosome 4q DNA rearrangements associated with facioscapulohumeral muscular dystrophy. *Nat Genet* 1992;**2**:26–30.

Myotonic Dystrophies

Nicholas Johnson and Chad R. Heatwole

Department of Neurology, University of Rochester Medical Center, NY, USA

Epidemiology

Myotonic dystrophy type 1 (DM1) is the most common adult muscular dystrophy in the world with an estimated prevalence of 5–20 per 100 000. The exact prevalence of myotonic dystrophy type 2 (DM2) is not known; however, it is likely that this disorder is both under-recognized and frequently misdiagnosed. The gene mutation for DM2 appears to have come from a northern European founder and may be more common in those with northern European ancestry.

Genetics

DM1 is the result of a gene defect on chromosome 19q13.3 consisting of an unstable CTG trinucleotide repeat expansion in the untranslated region of the *DMPK* gene. DM2 results from a tetranucleotide expansion CCTG in intron 1 of the zinc finger protein 9 gene on chromosome 3q21.

Clinical features

Myotonic dystrophy type 1

The cardinal features of DM1 are cataracts before age 50, weakness, and myotonia (impaired muscle relaxation after voluntary contraction). Diagnosis is often aided by a characteristic appearance consisting of male pattern baldness, temporal wasting, prominent facial musculature weakness, and atrophy of the forearm flexor muscles (Table 10.1). The range of symptom onset and severity is large. Some patients present later in life with baldness, mild myotonia, and cataracts, whereas other patients may present in their 20s or 30s with dysarthria, dysphagia, cognitive symptoms, sleep disturbances, fatigue, cardiac conduction disturbances, hypogonadism, hypotension, insulin resistance, and weakness. Still other patients present at birth (congenital myotonic dystrophy) with more severe and potentially life-threatening clinical symptoms.

Weakness

Typically, muscle weakness in DM1 includes the facial muscles, long flexors of the fingers (flexor profundus muscles), intrinsic hand muscles, and dorsiflexors of the feet (tibialis anterior, extensor hallucis longus, and extensor digitorum longus). Less frequently, DM1 patients have proximal upper extremity weakness including the shoulder stabilizing and abduction muscles. In advanced cases, respiratory muscles may be impaired, placing patients at risk for respiratory failure and aspiration.

Neuromuscular Disorders, First Edition. Edited by Rabi N. Tawil, Shannon Venance.
© 2011 John Wiley & Sons, Ltd. Published 2011 by John Wiley & Sons, Ltd.

Table 10.1. Comparative features of myotonic dystrophies

Clinical features	Myotonic dystrophy type 1	Myotonic dystrophy type 2
Gene defect	Chromosome 19 *DMPK*, CTG expansion	Chromosome 3 Zinc finger protein 9, CCTG
Inheritance	Autosomal dominant	Autosomal dominant
Age of onset	Infancy – adulthood, varies with severity and number of repeats	Childhood –adulthood, varies with severity and number of repeats
Typical pattern of myopathy	Face, forearms, finger flexors, distal legs	Neck flexors, thighs and hips; more mild weakness
Clinical myotonia	Prominent, primarily hand, forearm muscles and tongue; can affect both smooth and skeletal muscle	Mild, primarily hands and thighs; can affect both smooth and skeletal muscle. Patients may have atypical muscle pain

Myotonia

Myotonia is commonly demonstrated in the hands, forearms, and grip of patients with DM1. Often patients develop this symptom before they develop weakness and present with "locking or stiffness" of the hands. Although percussion myotonia can also be demonstrated at a patient's tongue, this test is uncomfortable to patients and does not have obvious advantages over testing the extremities.

Cardiac involvement

Life-threatening progressive cardiac arrhythmias and sudden death may occur in DM1. Cardiac conduction abnormalities are more likely with increased age and with more severe neuromuscular symptoms. Screening echocardiograms may reveal global diastolic dysfunction and reduced systolic function. Progressive heart block, prolongation of the QRS and P–R intervals, sinus node dysfunction, atrial or ventricular tachycardia or fibrillation, and atrial flutter occur. Higher rates of sudden death are associated with the presence of atrial tachyarrhythmias and other severe EKG abnormalities.

Gastrointestinal symptoms

Some DM1 patients experience gastrointestinal symptoms including dysarthria, dysphagia, gastric regurgitation, constipation, diarrhea, and insulin resistance. These symptoms can be severe and cause a substantial disruption to a patient's life.

Cognitive symptoms

Cognition may be impaired in DM1. Impaired executive function, difficulty with visual spatial processing, depression, apathy, and avoidant personality disorders are reported. Radiologically, these symptoms may correspond with increased cerebral atrophy at the bifrontal and parietal lobes, bilateral middle temporal gyrus, and left superior and occipital gyri.

Sleep disturbance

Excessive daytime sleepiness is seen in approximately a third of DM1 patients and tends to be proportional to the degree of weakness. In addition, patients often report excessive sleep requirements (more than 10 hours), irregular sleep patterns, extensive daytime naps, insomnia, and somnolence after meals.

Vision and hearing

Over time cataracts develop and impede vision. Cataracts may be the initial or only findings of DM1. Patients may also develop corneal abrasions secondary to the inability to fully close their eyelids at night. Sensorineural hearing loss occurs in DM1 and may impair a patient's ability to communicate effectively.

Laboratory abnormalities in DM1

Multiple laboratory abnormalities are common in DM1 and reflect the multisystemic involvement. Among these, creatine kinase levels, liver function tests, and cholesterol panels often demonstrate elevated values whereas albumin, and red and white blood cell counts are frequently low.

Congenital myotonic dystrophy

DM1 may present as a congenital form. As CTG repeat lengths increase from one generation to the next, a parent with minimal symptoms may have a child with congenital DM1 with severe clinical features. Congenital DM1 should be considered in infants with any of the following: hypotonia, generalized weakness, respiratory failure, failure to thrive, feeding difficulties, clubfoot deformity, or a history of reduced fetal movement with polyhydramnios. Newborns with congenital myotonia do not have clinical myotonia on examination. Patients requiring prolonged ventilation have a 25% mortality rate in the first year. Congenital DM1 patients who survive may have cognitive symptoms ranging from mild learning difficulties to behavioral issues to severe learning difficulties. Although some patients experience both physical and cognitive improvement during childhood, the progressive weakness and symptoms consistent with adult-onset DM1 may occur and progress in the second and third decades.

Myotonic dystrophy type 2

MD2 (also referred to as proximal myotonic myopathy) typically presents in adulthood, usually between 20 and 75 years of age. As with DM1, the cardinal symptoms of DM2 are early cataracts (age <50 years), weakness, and myotonia; however, in comparison with DM1, DM2 may have a more benign phenotype with less widespread weakness, muscle atrophy, and lower rates of systemic complications (see Table 10.1). Patients with an early age of onset are more likely to have more severe weakness and a broader spectrum of symptoms. In contrast to DM1, DM2 patients tend to experience more proximal extremity pain and stiffness with variable degrees of clinical myotonia.

Weakness

The distribution of weakness in DM2 is more proximal than in DM1 and often involves the neck flexors, hip flexors, hip extensors, and long flexors of the fingers. In general, facial weakness and muscle wasting are not as severe as in DM1, although some patients may experience mild hypertrophy at their gastrocnemius muscles.

Myotonia

The presence of myotonia may be tested for and detected in DM2. In late-onset DM2 cases, myotonia may be present only electrodiagnostically, or may be absent entirely.

Pain

Pain is a prominent and disabling feature in DM2. Patients often describe this symptom as cramping, stiffness, or an aching sensation that fluctuates in intensity and distribution over the limbs. Occasionally this symptom is inappropriately attributed to sciatica, fibromyalgia, or a statin-induced myopathy while exacerbating factors may include exercise, palpation, and temperature.

> ### ★ TIPS AND TRICKS
>
> - One of the most useful bedside tests for myotonia is percussion, particularly of the thenar and forearm extensor muscles. After gentle percussion with a reflex hammer, these muscles may demonstrate continuous contractions lasting several seconds. Grip myotonia can also be demonstrated by having a patient make a fist followed by a request to quickly open the hand. In affected patients this process can sometimes take several seconds to accomplish. In DM1, an effect known as a "warm-up phenomenon" is demonstrated where the presence of grip myotonia diminishes after several repetitions.
> - Myotonia in DM2 is best tested with percussion of the thenar or forearm extensor muscles. When present, grip myotonia in DM2 may have a jerky quality that distinguishes it from DM1 or the nondystrophic myotonias.

Cognitive symptoms

DM2 patients have similar deficits to DM1 patients on neuropsychological testing, with decreased frontal lobe function, decreased visual spatial processing, and increased prevalence of avoidant personality disorders.

Sleep disturbance

DM2 patients have impaired sleep quality and fatigue. Compared with DM1, pain appears to have a major role in the sleep disturbance of DM2 patients whereas daytime sleepiness is less frequently reported and comparable to normal controls.

> ✋ **CAUTION!**
>
> Both pregnancy and hypothyroidism can unmask myotonia and weakness. Muscle stiffness, pain, weakness, and delayed muscle relaxation may be erroneously ascribed to either hypothyroidism or the hormonal changes associated with pregnancy.

Cardiac symptoms

Cardiac conduction disturbances occur in DM2 but are less common than in DM1. Despite this, sudden cardiac death is a possibility in this population and dilated cardiomyopathies and cardiac arrhythmias may occur.

> ✋ **CAUTION!**
>
> Patients with myotonic dystrophy may not tolerate anesthesia and can experience apnea after anesthesia. Undiagnosed patients may present with a "failure to wean" from a ventilator after an illness or surgical procedure.

Diagnostic evaluation

The gold standard test to confirm the diagnosis of DM1 and DM2 is leukocyte DNA testing. In DM1, expanded CTG repeats on 19q13.3 can be detected. In DM2 expanded CCTG repeats occur on the zinc finger protein 9 gene on chromosome 3q21. Genetic testing is not required for patients with a clear clinical phenotype and a first-degree relative with a positive genetic test.

Electrodiagnostic testing is a useful tool during the initial evaluation of a patient with suspected myotonic dystrophy. Electrical myotonia is commonly elicited from muscles tested in DM1 and has a characteristic waxing–waning pattern. In infants with DM1 this finding may be absent. In DM2, electrical myotonia occurs; however, this finding may be absent in select muscles or only elicit waning features. In muscles where electrical myotonia is not overriding, nonspecific myopathic electromyographic features may be observed.

Muscle biopsy is not necessary to make the diagnosis of DM1 or DM2.

Management

Treatment for the myotonic dystrophies is symptomatic or preventive, and best conducted using a multidisciplinary approach.

Ambulation

DM patients fall more frequently then healthy individuals. Involvement of physical therapy, occupational therapy, and orthopedics is helpful to ascertain disability and obtain assistive devices to compensate for leg weakness and balance impairment. Patients may benefit from ankle–foot orthoses, high top shoes, or wheelchairs depending on the location and severity of their weakness. Prescribed low-impact aerobic exercise may also assist patients in developing better overall fitness and improved oxygen uptake.

Myotonia

Muscle stiffness, impaired leg, arm, and hand function, altered speech, pain, gastrointestinal symptoms, and impaired swallowing can be attributed to skeletal or smooth muscle myotonia. A recent, randomized, double-blind, placebo-controlled, crossover trial demonstrated the utility of mexiletine as a potential treatment for myotonia in DM1. DM1 patients were found to have significant reductions in grip relaxation time with both 150 mg (three times a day) and 200 mg (three times a day) dosages without serious adverse effects or prolongation of the Q–Tc, P–R interval, or of QRS duration. Other antimyotonic agents used empirically include phenytoin, acetazolamide, clomipramine, imipramine, and taurine.

Cardiac and respiratory monitoring

Given the potential for life-threatening cardiac arrhythmias and progressive cardiac conduction block, patients should receive annual electrocardiogram (EKG) monitoring for progressive P–R interval lengthening and cardiac block, or other potentially life-threatening arrhythmias. When warranted, placement of a pacemaker can be life saving. Although the data for widespread prophylactic placement of pacemakers or defibrillators in all patients cannot be supported at this time, most patients benefit from being followed by a cardiologist. Patients should also receive serial monitoring of their respiratory function. Supine and sitting forced vital capacity measurements are essential to detect and monitor early respiratory and diaphragmatic decline, with referral to a pulmonologist as appropriate. A low threshold for empiric antibiotics is warranted in the presence of chronic respiratory failure.

Cataract and hearing assessments

Patients should be monitored for cataracts and referred for surgery once these become symptomatic. Slit-lamp examination is useful to detect the multicolored, iridescent, punctuate opacities in the anterior and posterior subcapsular regions. Corneal abrasions are treated with nocturnal eyelid taping or protective ophthalmological ointments. Given the possibility of impaired hearing, symptomatic patients should also receive audiometric evaluations and hearing aids as appropriate.

Sleep disturbances

Myotonic dystrophy patients should be questioned about their sleep requirements, daytime somnolence, and insomnia. Patients with daytime somnolence may respond well to modafinil or methylphenidate. In some cases, patients may have superimposed sleep apnea warranting a referral for a polysomnogram. If sleep apnea is detected, a patient's fatigue may benefit from positive airway pressure, behavior modification, or other therapeutic interventions.

Endocrine assessment

Given the prevalence of endocrine dysfunction, DM patients should be periodically assessed for testosterone deficiency, insulin resistance, elevated cholesterol levels, and thyroid abnormalities.

Reproductive counseling

All patients considering having children should be referred to a genetic counselor. Early screening processes are currently available and an accurate prenatal assessment of DM1 can be obtained.

Gastrointestinal symptoms

Patients who experience diarrhea may benefit from dietary readjustment with small low-fat meals. Patients with gastroesophageal reflux can be treated with an avoidance of late meals, keeping the head of the bed elevated, and appropriate medications. For patients with abdominal pain, a trial of an antimyotonic therapy may prove beneficial.

Anesthesia

In DM1, there can be a paradoxical reaction to muscle depolarizing agents and these patients may be sensitive to sedating medications such as opiates and barbiturates. Patients with DM1 are also at increased risk for sudden arrhythmias or hypotension during anesthesia and may experience postoperative apnea or atelectasis, or require a prolonged ventilator wean if there is preexisting respiratory insufficiency. Close monitoring for these complications with 24 hours of monitored pulse oximetry is advised, as is noninvasive ventilation use and aggressive pulmonary physical therapy.

Pregnancy

During pregnancy a number of complications are reported including spontaneous abortion, hydramnios, prolonged first stage of labor, retained placenta, and postpartum hemorrhage. With these risks and the risks of anesthesia, DM patients require close monitoring throughout pregnancy.

Additional management points regarding congenital DM1

Depending on the severity of the disease, patients with congenital DM1 may require ventilation, feeding tubes, and potentially bracing and orthopedic surgery if foot deformities are present.

Congenital DM1 patients should be serially screened for hearing and cardiac conduction abnormalities. During childhood, patients with behavioral problems may respond to both medication and counseling.

Additional management points regarding DM2

There is significant overlap between the management strategies of DM1 and DM2. In general, with the possible exception of pain and proximal weakness, the symptoms of DM2 are less severe than in DM1. Cardiac monitoring in the form of serial EKGs is required, although disturbances in cardiac rhythms appear to be less frequent in DM2. Endocrine abnormalities, including hypogonadism and insulin resistance, may occur and require appropriate treatment. Clinical myotonia is often less severe and more proximal than in DM1 but may be responsive to antimyotonic therapy. Similarly, pain may be responsive to this class of medications or to nonsteroidal anti-inflammatory therapies.

Woman with DM2 patients can experience their initial presentation during pregnancy, or may develop progressive myotonia and weakness in the later stage of their pregnancies. Reports suggest that the symptoms that develop during pregnancy may reverse after delivery.

Although one study suggested that patients with DM2 do not appear to have disease-specific anesthesia complications, more research is needed in this area and caution should be implemented during anesthetic procedures.

⚙ SCIENCE REVISITED

EXPERIMENTAL THERAPEUTICS IN NYOTONIC DYSTROPHY

One encouraging recent development is the development of antisense oligonucleotides (AONs) as potential therapeutics for DM1. Using an AON, CAG 25, researchers have been able to demonstrate that specific derangements of myotonic dystrophy can be limited in a mouse model by inhibiting the interaction between critical body proteins and the pathogenic RNA associated with DM1. It has also been shown that a $2'-O$-methyl-phosphorothioate-modified $(CAG)7$ AON can reduce levels of toxic (CUG) RNA in DM1 mouse models. Although additional translational research is needed, these approaches show promise as future therapeutic mechanisms for DM1 patients.

The myotonic dystrophies are disorders that are genetically characterized by tri- or tetranucleotide repeat expansions inherited in an autosomal dominant fashion. Although characterized by cataracts, weakness, and myotonia, many additional organ systems in the body may be affected and be amendable to a multidisciplinary therapeutic approach.

Bibliography

Brook JD, McCurrach ME, Harley HG, et al. Molecular basis of myotonic dystrophy: expansion of a trinucleotide (CTG) repeat at the 3′ end of a transcript encoding a protein kinase family member. *Cell* 1992;**68**:799–808.

Day JW, Ricker K, Jacobsen JF, et al. Myotonic dystrophy type 2: molecular, diagnostic and clinical spectrum. *Neurology* 2003;**60**:657–64.

Groh WJ, Groh MR, Saha C, E et al. Electrocardiographic abnormalities and sudden death in myotonic dystrophy type 1. *N Engl J Med* 2008;**358**:2688–97.

Harper PS. *Myotonic Dystrophy*, 3rd edn. London: WB Saunders, 2001.

Heatwole CR, Miller J, Martens B, Moxley RT 3rd. Laboratory abnormalities in ambulatory patients with myotonic dystrophy type 1. *Arch Neurol* 2006;**63**:1149–53.

Liquori CL, Ricker K, Moseley ML, et al. Myotonic dystrophy type 2 caused by a CCTG expansion in intron 1 of ZNF9. *Science* 2001;**293**:864–7.

Logigian EL, Martens WB, Moxley RT 4th, et al. Mexiletine is an effective antimyotonia treatment in myotonic dystrophy type 1. *Neurology* 2010;**74**:1441–8.

Meola G, Sansone V, Perani D, et al. Executive dysfunction and avoidant personality trait in myotonic dystrophy type 1 (DM-1) and in proximal myotonic myopathy (PROMM/DM-2). *Neuromusc Disord* 2003;**13**:813–21.

Ricker K, Koch MC, Lehmann-Horn F, et al. Proximal myotonic myopathy. Clinical features of a multisystem disorder similar to myotonic dystrophy. *Arch.Neurol* 1995;**52**:25–31.

Rudnik-Schoneborn S, Schneider-Gold C, Raabe U, Kress W, Zerres K, Schoser BG. Outcome and effect of pregnancy in myotonic dystrophy type 2. *Neurology* 2006;**66**:579–80.

Weingarten TN, Hofer RE, Milone M, Sprung J. Anesthesia and myotonic dystrophy type 2: a case series. *Can J Anaesth* 2010;**57**:248–55.

Wheeler TM. Myotonic dystrophy: therapeutic strategies for the future. *Neurotherapeutics* 2008;**5**:592–600.

Young NP, Daube JR, Sorenson EJ, Milone M. Absent, unrecognized, and minimal myotonic discharges in myotonic dystrophy type 2. *Muscle Nerve* 2010;**41**:758–62.

Oculopharyngeal Muscular Dystrophy

Annie Dionne and Jean-Pierre Bouchard

Department of Neurological Sciences, Université Laval, CHA Hôpital
Enfant-Jésus, Québec, Canada

Clinical features

Oculopharyngeal muscular dystrophy (OPMD) is a late-onset, dominantly inherited myopathy that has two cardinal symptoms: eyelid ptosis and dysphagia.

The eyelid ptosis usually presents first in the fifth decade (mean age of onset 48.1 years). It is often symmetric and defined as at least one palpebral fissure measuring <8 mm at rest. Wrinkling of the frontalis muscle, raising of the eyebrows, and backward tilting of the head are often noted as a way of compensating for the eyelid ptosis, causing limitation of the visual field (Figure 11.1).

Dysphagia usually follows ptosis by a few years, although it may precede ptosis in some patients. It tends to be more severe for solids than for liquids and can be assessed with a simple bedside test. A time for swallowing 80 mL ice-cold water >7 s is considered positive for dysphagia. Nasal regurgitation is often present as the disease progresses. Untreated, dysphagia may lead to choking, aspiration pneumonia, and cachexia. It is a significant cause of morbidity and mortality in OPMD patients.

EVIDENCE AT A GLANCE

OPMD is a late-onset, highly penetrant muscular dystrophy. Penetrance per decade of age for ptosis and dysphagia is 1% in those aged <40 years, 6% for those aged between 40 and 49, 31% for those aged between 50 and 59, 63% fro those aged between 60 and 69, and 99% for those aged >69 years.

As the disease progresses, other muscle groups may become involved. Extraocular movements may become limited, especially for upward gaze. When present, horizontal gaze limitation is often discrete. Diplopia is usually not a complaint because of the slowly progressive course of the disease.

Limb–girdle weakness is eventually noted in over two-thirds of patients, and more frequently involves the lower than the upper extremities. In a study of 72 patients, proximal lower limb weakness was found in 71% of patients and upper extremity weakness in 38% of patients. Lower limb weakness is often limited to hip flexion, although hip abduction, adduction, and extension may be involved as the disease progresses. Upper limb weakness tends to involve the deltoid and biceps muscles more prominently. A large percentage of patients will use either a cane or a walker late in the course of the disease. The occasional, more severely affected patient will require a wheelchair, mainly to cover long distances.

Among other clinical features, weakness of facial muscles (43%), weakness and/or atrophy of the tongue (82%), and voice changes such as

Neuromuscular Disorders, First Edition. Edited by Rabi N. Tawil, Shannon Venance.

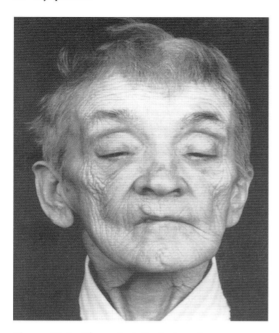

Figure 11.1. Characteristic facies of oculopharyngeal muscular dystrophy: bilateral ptosis, raised eyebrows, and wrinkling of the forehead.

hoarseness and hypernasality due to palatal weakness (67%) may be observed.

The disease has a slowly progressive course and life expectancy is not diminished when swallowing is managed appropriately. With progress in the treatment of dysphagia, prognosis and quality of life are much improved.

Homozygotes for OPMD (children of two carrier parents) have been reported and compared with their heterozygote siblings. The onset of symptoms is on average 18 years earlier, the disease progresses faster, and death usually occurs in the sixth decade. In addition, cognitive decline, psychotic episodes, and depression are observed in homozygote patients.

Epidemiology

Although OPMD has now been reported in over 35 countries, a founder effect is responsible for a high prevalence of OPMD in the province of Québec (Canada) where the prevalence is estimated at 1 in 1000. A higher concentration of cases is also seen in the south-western states of the USA as well as in Bukhara Jews living in Israel.

Diagnosis

The diagnosis of OPMD can be easily confirmed by genetic testing. It is caused by variable size expansion of GCG triplets coding for alanine in a gene called polyadenylation-binding protein nuclear 1 (*PABPN1*) (Brais 2003). The test has 99% sensitivity and specificity, and is available in many commercial laboratories worldwide. A point mutation in the first exon of the gene may account for cases without GCG triplet expansion, so sequencing of the first exon may be ordered when the diagnosis is strongly suspected on clinical grounds, but the genetic test for *PABPN1* expansions is negative.

A rarer recessive form allelic to the dominantly inherited OPMD has also been reported with either a milder or a more severe phenotype.

Although OPMD is caused by triplet expansions, there is no correlation between expansion size and age of onset or severity of clinical manifestations. Unlike myotonic dystrophy, another triplet repeat disease, there is no anticipation through generations as the expansion size is mitotically stable.

With genetic testing readily available, muscle biopsy is not indicated. If performed, rimmed vacuoles and intranuclear inclusions are the two main abnormalities observed. Rimmed vacuoles are readily detected by light microscopy but are not specific, being observed in other myopathies, mainly inclusion body myositis. Electron microscopy shows the intranuclear inclusions comprising tubular filaments. Other nonspecific findings that are common to many muscular dystrophies are atrophied, small, angulated, muscle fibers, type 1 fiber predominance, variation in fiber size, degenerating and regenerating fibers, and an increased percentage of internal nuclei.

✋ CAUTION!

Rimmed vacuoles are also seen in inclusion body myositis, a late-onset acquired inflammatory myopathy.

The creatine kinase (CK) levels may be normal or elevated to two to five times the upper limit of normal. Electromyography (EMG) may show a mixture of both myopathic motor unit action potentials (MUAPs: low-amplitude, short-duration, polyphasic potentials) and neurogenic MUAPs (increased-amplitude polyphasic potentials). No spontaneous activity is found.

Dysphagia can be assessed by a barium swallow. The pharynx usually shows weak or nonexistent contractions against the upper esophageal sphincter which relaxes incompletely or late. Consequently, laryngeal pooling may induce aspiration and repeated swallowing is necessary to empty the pharynx of its contents.

⬡ SCIENCE REVISITED

The expansion of GCG repeats probably results in abnormal folding of the polyalanine domains of *PABPN1*. The misfolded proteins are resistant to degradation and accumulate as the intranuclear inclusions seen on electron microscopy. Those aggregates may lead to disruption of cell function, in turn leading to cell death.

Differential diagnosis

Myasthenia gravis is associated with ptosis, restriction of extraocular movements, and dysphagia, but is differentiated from OPMD by a subacute rather than a chronic onset, the presence of diplopia, and the fluctuating nature of the symptoms, being more marked at the end of the day. The family history should be negative except in the rare instances of congenital myasthenia gravis.

Mitochondrial myopathies, mainly chronic progressive external ophthalmoplegia (CPEO) and Kearns–Sayre syndrome, have to be considered in the differential diagnosis of patients presenting with ptosis and restriction of extraocular movements. Ophthalmoplegia is more marked in mitochondrial myopathies than in OMPD, and dysphagia is not as prominent as in OPMD. In addition, CPEO usually affects sporadic cases but can be maternally transmitted, or recessively or dominantly inherited. Kearns–Sayre syndrome is usually sporadic and symptom onset is before the age of 20. Additional features such as a sensory ataxia, seizure, deafness, pigmentary retinopathy, or parkinsonism may be observed in mitochondrial cytopathies.

Finally, ptosis, restriction of extraocular movements, and dysphagia are also encountered in myotonic dystrophy. Associated signs such as myotonia, presence of distal weakness, and multisystemic involvement will help to clinically differentiate the two disorders.

★ TIPS AND TRICKS

Having the patient look upward for a minute may elicit or worsen ptosis or ocular malalignment in myasthenia gravis whereas the ptosis and extraocular movement abnormalities are not fatigable in OPMD or mitochondrial myopathies.

Cogan's sign may also help to distinguish myasthenia gravis from a myopathy. The patient is instructed to look downward for a few seconds and then back to the primary position of gaze. A positive Cogan sign refers to a brief overshoot of the upper lid followed by a rapid return of ptosis. It is fairly specific for myasthenia gravis.

Treatment

Treatment of OPMD is symptomatic. When eyelid ptosis interferes with vision, surgical treatment can be offered to the patient. Either resection of the levator palpebral aponeurosis or frontal suspension of the eyelids may be performed. The latter is more durable than resection of the former, and is usually the favored treatment. Few complications are reported with either procedure. Mild superficial exposure keratitis occurs in virtually every case, with resolution over a 4- to 6-week period. Alternatively, eyelid crutches on glasses can be used if there is a contraindication to blepharoplasty such as marked ophthalmoplegia (unusual in OPMD), dry-eye syndrome, or poor orbicularis function.

With regard to dysphagia, dietary modifications need to be made when difficulties are noted by the patient. Cutting food into small pieces, thickening liquids, and eating slowly are the first steps to management of dysphagia. Encouraging patients to have a high-protein diet is particularly important because patients tend to avoid eating meat, which is especially difficult to swallow. When dysphagia becomes severe and weight loss or recurrent pneumonia occurs, surgery needs to be considered. In OPMD, the upper esophageal sphincter acts as a barrier to the pharyngoesophageal transit because the weakened pharynx is unable to push the bolus into the esophagus. Therefore, cricopharyngeal myotomy helps to relieve this functional obstruction. In the short term, it has been reported to improve the symptoms in 75% of patients with OPMD. However, reappearance of symptoms with time is seen with progression of the disease. Severe dysphonia and lower esophageal sphincter incompetence are contraindications to cricopharyngeal myotomy.

Alternatively, upper esophageal sphincter dilation using endoscopy may be considered because it is a less invasive procedure and does not require general anesthesia. In a series of 17 patients, the improvement rate was 64% at 3 months, but it dropped to 55% after 18 months. Repetitive dilations then become necessary. Botulinum toxin injections of the upper esophageal sphincter cricopharyngeal muscle has been performed but is not yet considered a standard treatment.

Future perspectives

Intranuclear aggregates are believed to be central to OPMD pathogenesis. Recently, doxycycline was shown to reduce intranuclear aggregates and delay toxicity of the OPMD mutation in transgenic mice. This may eventually represent a promising therapy for OPMD as well as other aggregate-associated disorders.

Bibliography

Blumen SC, Bouchard JP, Brais B, et al. Cognitive impairment and reduced life span of oculopharyngeal muscular dystrophy homozygotes. *Neurology* 2009;**73**:596–601.

Bouchard JP, Brais B, Brunet D, Gould PV, Rouleau GA. Recent studies on oculopharyngeal muscular dystrophy in Quebec. *Neuromusc Disord* 1997;**7**(suppl 1):S22–9.

Brais B. Oculopharyngeal muscular dystrophy: a late-onset polyalanine disease. *Cytogenet Genome Res* 2003;**100**:252–60.

Brais B, Bouchard JP, Gosselin F, et al. Using the full power of linkage analysis in 11 French Canadian families to fine map the oculopharyngeal muscular dystrophy gene. *Neuromusc Disord* 1997;**7**(suppl 1):S70–4.

Codere F, Brais B, Rouleau G, Lafontaine E. Oculopharyngeal muscular dystrophy: What's new? *Orbit* 2001;**20**:259–66.

Davies JE, Wang L, Garcia-Oroz L, et al. Doxycycline attenuates and delays toxicity of the oculopharyngeal muscular dystrophy mutation in transgenic mice. *Nat Med* 2005;**11**:672–7.

Duranceau A. Cricopharyngeal myotomy in the management of neurogenic and muscular dysphagia. *Neuromusc Disord* 1997;**7**(suppl 1):S85–9.

Duranceau AC, Beauchamp G, Jamieson GG, Barbeau A. Oropharyngeal dysphagia and oculopharyngeal muscular dystrophy. *Surg Clin North Am* 1983;**63**:825–32.

Karpati GH-J, Bushby K, Griggs RC. *Disorders of Voluntary Muscle*, 8th edn. New York: Cambridge University Press, 2010.

Mathieu J, Lapointe G, Brassard A, et al. A pilot study on upper esophageal sphincter dilatation for the treatment of dysphagia in patients with oculopharyngeal muscular dystrophy. *Neuromusc Disord* 1997;**7**(suppl 1):S100–4.

Rodrigue D, Molgat YM. Surgical correction of blepharoptosis in oculopharyngeal muscular dystrophy. *Neuromusc Disord* 1997;**7**(suppl 1):S82–4.

Tome FM, Chateau D, Helbling-Leclerc A, Fardeau M. Morphological changes in muscle fibers in oculopharyngeal muscular dystrophy. *Neuromusc Disord* 1997;**7**(suppl 1):S63–9.

Distal Myopathies

Bjarne Udd

Neuromuscular Research Center, University of Tampere and Tampere University Hospital, Tampere; Folkhalsan Institute of Genetics, University of Helsinki, Helsinki; and Department of Neurology, Vasa Central Hospital, Vasa, Finland

Distal myopathies are a diverse group of inherited disorders of muscle (Table 12.1) characterized by early, predominant involvement of distal limb muscles. In many autosomal dominant distal myopathies, symptom onset is in the fifth or sixth decade of life. Symptoms typically relate to functional difficulties in the hand or leg muscles depending on the particular form of distal myopathy. Many of the clinically and genetically defined distal myopathies have characteristic patterns of muscle involvement early in the disease process, which can help narrow the differential diagnosis. For example, early involvement of hand and finger extensors in a late-onset form favors Welander distal myopathy, whereas weakness of the posterior leg compartment and very high creatine kinase (CK) levels might favor Miyoshi myopathy or the new distal anoctaminopathy.

Diagnostic workup

When should a distal myopathy be considered in a patient? Distal myopathy is one diagnostic alternative whenever insidious distal muscle weakness and atrophies are found without sensory symptoms and signs. As neurogenic causes are more frequent than myopathic ones, the next step is to check CK levels and to have a comprehensive nerve conduction and electro-myographic investigation. Neurogenic distal atrophies rarely raise CK levels above twice the upper normal limit. If no definite electrophysiological evidence of neurogenic abnormality can be obtained, the probability of a myopathic condition is very high.

> ### ★ TIPS AND TRICKS
>
> - Distal myopathies are frequently confused with inherited sensorimotor neuropathies.
> - Consider a distal myopathy when:
>
> there is insidious onset of distal weakness without sensory symptoms
> the extensor digitorum brevis muscles are intact in bulk while anterior leg compartment muscles are atrophic.

When a decision is taken that one is dealing with a distal myopathy, the pattern of weakness and mode of inheritance may further help narrow the diagnosis to a fraction of the list shown in Table 12.1. However, ultimately, a specific diagnosis will rely on histopathological findings on muscle biopsy and confirmation of the diagnosis by genetic testing. As different muscles can be very differently affected in distal myopathies,

Neuromuscular Disorders, First Edition. Edited by Rabi N. Tawil, Shannon Venance.

Table 12.1. Currently identified distal myopathy entities grouped by inheritance pattern and age at onset

Disease entities	Presenting weakness	Other features
Late adult-onset autosomal dominant forms		
Welander distal myopathy	Hands	
Tibial muscular dystrophy (TMD, Udd myopathy)	Anterior leg	
Distal myotilinopathy	Ankles	
Zaspopathy (Markesbery–Griggs type)	Ankles	Later hands
Matrin-3 distal myopathy (VCPDM, MPD2)	Anterior leg	Bulbar
VCP-mutated distal myopathy	Anterior leg	
αB-crystallin mutated Distal myopathy	Anterior leg	Cataracts
Oculopharyngeal distal myopathy (OPDM)	Ankles	Ptosis, bulbar
Adult-onset autosomal dominant forms		
Desminopathy	Anterior leg	Cardiomyopathy
Finnish-MPD3	Ankles	
Italian 19p13-linked distal myopathy	Anterior leg	Pes cavus
Australian Victoria-family	Hands, calves	
Early onset autosomal dominant forms		
Myosinopathy MYH7 (Laing)	Anterior leg Finger extension	Neck flexion
Early onset autosomal recessive forms		
Distal nebulin myopathy	Anterior leg	
Oculopharyngeal distal myopathy (OPDM)	Anterior leg	Ptosis, facial Progressive
Early adult-onset autosomal recessive forms		
Dysferlinopathy (Miyoshi myopathy)	Calf atrophy	High CK
Miyoshi myopathy-like anoctaminopathy	Calf atrophy	Asymmetric
Distal myopathy with rimmed vacuoles (DMRV, Nonaka myopathy, HIBM)	Anterior leg	Progressive
Adult-onset autosomal recessive form		
Miyoshi myopathy-like non-DYSF/ANO5	Calf atrophy	Moderate CK

ANO5, anoctamin-5; CK, creatine kinase; DMRV, distal myopathy with rimmed vacuoles; DYSF, dysferlin; HIBM; hereditary inclusion body myopathy; MPD, myopathia distalis; MYH7, myosin heavy chain 7; TMD, tibial muscular dystrophy, Nonaka myopathy, HIBM; VCP, valosin-containing protein; VCPDM, vocal cord and pharyngeal distal myopathy; ZASP, Z-disk alternatively spliced PDZ-domain containing protein.

with pathology ranging from normal to end-stage, the site of biopsy has to be carefully evaluated. Muscle magnetic resonance imaging (MRI) is the preferred method to target which muscle will likely give the optimal yield on pathology. Moreover, MRI provides excellent additional diagnostic clues due to the distinct patterns of muscle involvement in the different distal myopathies.

After MRI and muscle biopsy (Figure 12.1), molecular genetic testing is needed to establish a final diagnosis. Distal dysferlinopathy (Miyoshi myopathy) can be diagnosed by protein immunohistochemistry and western blotting of the muscle sample, and the group of myofibrillar myopathy causing distal myopathies can be assessed by staining with antibodies against the accumulating mutant proteins such as desmin, myotilin, and αB-crystallin. See Table 12.1 for the list of currently identified distal myopathies.

Clinical features

Welander distal myopathy usually causes reduced finger extension after the age of 50, followed by lower leg weakness and finger flexor weakness. Onset of symptoms in the lower legs occurs in a minority of patients. Walking is preserved and lifespan is intact.

Tibial muscular dystrophy (Udd myopathy or TMD) starts with ankle dorsiflexion weakness after the age of 30–50, with slow progression to moderate foot drop 10–15 years after onset. Walking is usually preserved until age 85 and there is no reduction of lifespan.

Distal myotilinopathy also starts even later, usually after the age of 50, showing reduced plantar flexion and in some patients dysphonia. The progression is, however, more rapid and may lead to loss of ambulation within 10 years.

Zaspopathy (Markesbery–Griggs type) is very similar to distal myotilinopathy, although first symptoms are both dorsal and plantar flexion weakness, the progression is slower, including atrophies of intrinsic hand muscles, and cardiomyopathy may develop at late stages.

Matrin-3 mutated VCPDM (vocal cord and pharyngeal distal myopathy) is very late onset with ankle dorsiflexion weakness, foot drop, and clinical symptoms of dysphonia and dysphagia as additional features. The progression is slow.

VCP (valosin-containing protein)-mutated myopathies usually cause proximal or scapuloperoneal phenotypes. Nevertheless, in some families scapular or proximal involvement is not present and, in such cases with distal muscle weakness only, the clinical phenotype may be indistinguishable from Udd or Welander myopathy.

Desminopathy has an earlier onset than the previous disorders, starting usually before the age of 30 years. The first symptoms and signs are either cardiac weakness or distal weakness in the ankles. Progression to proximal muscles and severe disability usually occur within 10 years. Cardiomyopathy may be present many years before the skeletal myopathy, and involvement of respiratory muscles is common.

Patients with the distal myopathy of the type described in the Australian family from Victoria

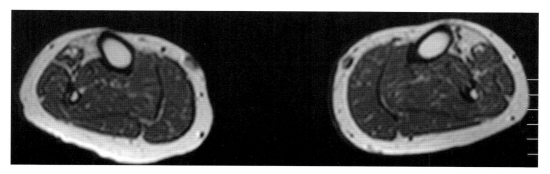

Figure 12.1. Muscle magnetic resonance imaging shows highly selective fatty degeneration of tibialis anterior and minor early changes in long toe extensors in distal titinopathy (Udd myopathy, TMD).

had first signs of weakness in the hand grip as young adults. There was slow progression to thenar atrophy and posterior calf atrophies, with subsequent plantar flexion weakness without total loss of ambulance even in the late 70s.

Laing distal myopathy is very early onset; sometimes reduced ankle dorsiflexion is present from the first years of walking. Slow progression to finger extension weakness and neck flexor weakness is the rule, whereas late generalized muscle weakness and severe disability are unusual. Cardiomyopathy may occur but is rare. So-called new mutations are frequent, which means that many patients present as sporadic cases without any family history.

Miyoshi myopathy (MM) was long thought to have a pathognomonic phenotype with early adult onset of calf muscle atrophy and weakness combined with very high CK levels, usually 50–100 times the upper normal limit. The disease progression is moderate with involvement of proximal muscles and disabilities 10–15 years after onset.

A subset of patients may present with a similar phenotype to MM, albeit with no loss of dysferlin protein in the muscle biopsy (dysferlin is mutated in MM). Recently another gene defect, anoctamin-5, was identified to cause a similar clinical phenotype, with the exception that MM is usually very symmetric whereas anoctaminopathy frequently causes asymmetric muscle involvement.

Nonaka distal myopathy also presents in early adulthood, with clear ankle dorsiflexion weakness as the first sign. The progression to involvement of proximal muscles is moderate to severe, causing loss of ambulation 12–15 years after the onset of symptoms.

There are, however, other myopathies that may present with distal weakness that can be mistaken for distal myopathies. Myotonic dystrophy type 1 (DM1) typically causes distal weakness in the hands and ankles, with no major proximal limb muscle weakness in the early stages of the disease. However, when distal weakness is present, the DM1 patient usually shows facial weakness and myotonia, leading to the correct diagnosis. Late-onset cases of sporadic inclusion body myositis (s-IBM) may mimic a distal myopathy because one hallmark of the disease is finger flexor weakness. In s-IBM, distinct quadriceps weakness and atrophy should be present. Quadriceps atrophy in s-IBM is in direct contrast to the quadriceps sparing in hereditary inclusion body myopathy/Nonaka distal myopathy (HIBM), which is an early adult-onset, autosomal recessive form of distal myopathy. Facioscapulohumeral muscular dystrophy (FSHD) usually presents with characteristic weakness and atrophy of facial and proximal upper limb muscles, with scapular winging, but it may rarely present with ankle dorsiflexion weakness with no obvious scapular or facial weakness.

★ TIPS AND TRICKS

- Muscle MRI is extremely valuable for assessment of the pattern of muscle involvement as well as for targeting the optimal muscle for biopsy.
- Of the distal myopathies, only desminopathy causes major involvement of heart and respiratory muscles.
- Many underlying gene defects occur as new mutations and therefore lack any family history.

Causes and pathomechanisms of distal myopathy

Practically all distal myopathies are dystrophies, which means that they are genetic disorders caused by gene defects. To date, some 15 different genes have been identified underlying these disorders, and strikingly many of these genes code for proteins that are parts of the sarcomeric contractile machinery, in the thin, thick, and third filaments, intermediate filaments, and proteins located in the Z-disc of the sarcomere. Most of the distal myopathies also share the morphological pathology of rimmed vacuolar degenerative changes in the muscle fibers, similar to the changes in sporadic IBM, although without generalized inflammatory changes. This is why the quadriceps-sparing myopathy, first described in the Middle East and later proved to be the same disease as Nonaka distal myopathy, is called hereditary inclusion body myopathy.

Management

Most late-onset distal myopathies are relatively benign disorders compared with other muscular dystrophies. They are not life threatening and usually cause mild-to-moderate disability. The weakness in the hands, fingers, and ankles can be severe and cause considerable functional limitations in activities of daily living. The use of orthoses, such as neutral wrist splints in patients with wrist and finger extension weakness and ankle foot orthoses for foot drop, may be helpful. In cases with severe foot drop, tendon transposition from the tibialis posterior muscle to a nonfunctional tibial anterior muscle can be performed. Most patients will no longer need ankle–foot orthoses after transposition.

Among the early onset distal myopathies, the slow, myosin heavy chain defect Laing myopathy may cause cardiomyopathy, although this occurs rarely in a minority of the mutations in the corresponding *MYH7* gene. In desminopathy cardiac and respiratory complications are very common and may even precede the distal weakness. These complications need regular monitoring.

Bibliography

Bolduc V, Marlow G, Boycott KM, et al. Recessive mutations in the putative calcium-activated chloride channel anoctamin 5 cause proximal LGMD2L and distal MMD3 muscular dystrophies. *Am J Hum Genet* 2010;**86**:213–21.

Gowers WR. Myopathy and a distal form. *BMJ* 1902;**ii**:89–92.

Griggs R, Vihola A, Hackman P, et al. Zaspopathy in a large classic late onset distal myopathy family. *Brain* 2007;**130**:1477–84.

Hackman P, Vihola A, Haravuori H, et al. Tibial muscular dystrophy is a titinopathy caused by mutations in TTN, the gene encoding the giant skeletal-muscle protein titin. *Am J Hum Genet* 2002;**71**:492–500.

Laing NG, Laing BA, Meredith C, et al. Autosomal dominant distal myopathy: linkage to chromosome 14. *Am J Hum Genet* 1995;**56**:422–7.

Liu J, Aoki M, Illa I, et al. Dysferlin, a novel skeletal muscle gene, is mutation in Miyoshi myopathy and limb girdle muscular dystrophy. *Nat Genet* 1998;**20**:31–6.

Miyoshi K, Kawai H, Iwasa M, Kusaka K, Nishino H. Autosomal recessive distal muscular dystrophy as a new type of progressive muscular dystrophy. *Brain* 1986;**109**:31–54.

Nonaka I, Sunohara N, Ishiura S, Satoyoshi E. Familial distal myopathy with rimmed vacuole and lamellar (myeloid) body formation. *J Neurol Sci* 1981;**51**:141–55.

Selcen D, Engel AG. Mutations in myotilin cause myofibrillar myopathy. *Neurology* 2004;**62**: 1363–71.

Senderek J, Garvey SM, Krieger M, et al. Autosomal-dominant distal myopathy associated with a recurrent missense mutation in the gene encoding the nuclear matrix protein, matrin 3. *Am J Hum Genet* 2009;**84**:511–18.

Sjöberg G, Saavedra-Matiz C, Rosen D, et al. A missense mutation in the desmin rod domain is associated with autosomal dominant distal myopathy, and exerts a dominant negative effect on filament formation. *Hum Mol Genet* 1999;**8**:2191–8.

Udd B. 165th ENMC International Workshop: Distal myopathies III. *Neuromusc Disord* 2009; **19**:429–38.

Udd B, Partanen J, Halonen P, et al. Tibial muscular dystrophy: late adult-onset distal myopathy in 66 Finnish patients. *Arch Neurol* 1993;**50**: 604–8.

Wallgren-Pettersson C, Lehtokari V-L, Kalimo H et al. Distal myopathy caused by homozygous missense mutations in the nebulin gene. *Brain* 2007;**130**:1465–76.

Welander L. Myopathia distalis tarda hereditaria. *Acta Med Scand* 1951;**141**:1–124.

Muscle Channelopathies

James Burge and Michael G. Hanna

UCL MRC Centre for Neuromuscular Diseases, and National Hospital for Neurology and Neurosurgery, UCLH FT, London, UK

The inherited muscle ion channel diseases (muscle channelopathies) are rare disorders of the skeletal muscle cell membrane with manifestations that range from muscle stiffness (sarcolemmal hyperexcitability) to flaccid weakness (sarcolemmal inexcitability). Primary periodic paralyses are autosomal dominant disorders with the major feature being attacks of weakness, although some patients additionally experience muscle stiffness. Nondystrophic myotonias (which are distinct from the myotonic dystrophies) may be recessive or dominant and are characterized by muscle stiffness, although some patients also experience attacks of weakness. Triggers to attacks or worsening of symptoms are frequently identifiable and include alterations in serum potassium, cooling, rest after strenuous exercise, carbohydrate loading, or emotional stress (Figure 13.1).

Presentations and diagnostic tests

Myotonia and paramyotonia

Myotonia is the phenomenon of delayed muscle relaxation after contraction. It is experienced by patients as stiffness, cramp, or locking of muscles. Stiffness may be mildly worse in the cold or after periods of rest, but diminishes with repeated muscle contractions (the warm-up phenomenon). The clinical findings are an inability to immediately relax muscles after forceful contraction and contraction induced by direct percussion (percussion myotonia). Lid-lag may be seen on rapid downgaze. These findings become less marked with repetition (the warm-up phenomenon) but reappear after rest. In paramyotonia muscle stiffness is precipitated by exercise. This is the opposite of the warm-up phenomenon in myotonia (hence *paradoxical* myotonia or *para*myotonia). Paramyotonia is much more temperature-sensitive than classic myotonia. Exposure to cold not only produces muscle stiffness in paramyotonia, but may also trigger muscle weakness.

> ★ **TIPS AND TRICKS**
>
> - Marked exacerbation by cold and exercise is useful clinically in distinguishing paramyotonia from myotonia. Ask about the effects of eating ice-cream and swimming in cold water.
> - Exposure to cold not only produces muscle stiffness in paramyotonia, but also often produces muscle weakness.

Weakness

The hallmark of the periodic paralyses is episodic weakness, which may affect all the limbs, one side, or be extremely focal. Bulbar and respiratory muscles are rarely affected. Attacks of weak-

Neuromuscular Disorders, First Edition. Edited by Rabi N. Tawil, Shannon Venance.
© 2011 John Wiley & Sons, Ltd. Published 2011 by John Wiley & Sons, Ltd.

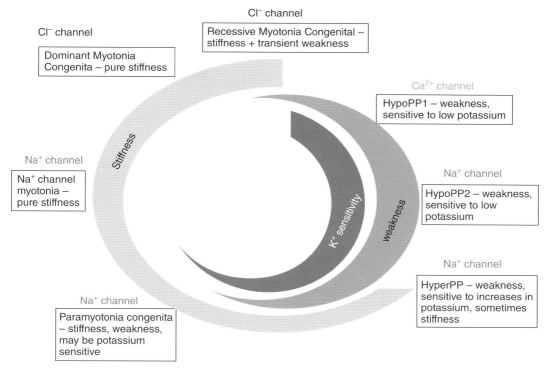

Figure 13.1. Triggers to attacks or worsening of muscle channelopathies. HyperPP, hyperkalemic periodic paralysis; HypoPP, hypokalemic periodic paralysis.

ness most commonly occur in the morning after waking from sleep. Triggers include stress, cold, fasting (hyperkalemic periodic paralysis or hyperPP), carbohydrate-rich meal (hypokalemic periodic paralysis or hypoPP), and exercise followed by rest. Tendon reflexes are depressed during an attack of periodic paralysis. Some patients with periodic paralysis develop a fixed myopathy, which can be disabling. Mild fixed weakness may develop in patients with myotonia congenita and paramyotonia congenita.

Muscle hypertrophy

Muscle hypertrophy is characteristic of the non-dystrophic myotonias and is a direct result of muscle overactivity. This is different from the pseudohypertrophy seen in some of the dystrophinopathies: the "true" hypertrophy of myotonic disorders results in increased muscle strength. Some individuals are able to participate in sports requiring strength rather than speed or endurance (e.g. Thomsen-type myotonia).

Clinical–genetic correlation

Skeletal muscle channelopathies produce a spectrum of clinical phenomena from pure muscle stiffness (myotonia) to pure muscle weakness (periodic paralysis), with overlap syndromes in between. Chloride channel mutations cause myotonia congenita, characterized by classic myotonia, warm-up phenomenon, and no periodic paralysis whatsoever. At the other end of the spectrum, calcium channel and potassium channel mutations both produce pure periodic paralysis without myotonia. Sodium channel disease sits in the central overlapping part of the spectrum and causes four syndromes: pure myotonia, paramyotonia, hyperPP, and hypoPP.

Genetic testing

The gold standard for the diagnosis of a skeletal muscle channelopathy is identification of the causative mutation from a blood sample. Sequencing ion channel genes is labor intensive and the clinician should suggest which gene to test first based on the clinical manifestations. The genetic laboratory will usually sequence regions of that gene where mutations are commonly found. If a mutation has been identified in another member of the patient's family, clearly indicating this to the genetics laboratory will enable a more focused search.

> ✋ CAUTION!
>
> A negative genetics test does not necessarily rule out a channelopathy because mutations may occur in regions of channel genes that have not been tested.

Electrodiagnosis

The roles of electrodiagnostic medicine are to indicate the presence of myotonia that is not detectable clinically or the presence of myopathy (e.g. where myotonic dystrophy is a possibility, or in longstanding periodic paralysis), or to exclude other causes of muscle weakness and stiffness (e.g. neuropathy causing cramp).

The long and short exercise tests, in which the compound motor action potential from a convenient muscle (e.g. abductor digiti minimi) is recorded before and after a period of exercise, can give additional information to guide genetic testing.

Muscle biopsy

Biopsy is generally not usually necessary for the diagnosis of muscle channelopathies. In patients with suspected periodic paralysis and where other diagnostic tests are inconclusive, finding characteristic vacuolar changes or tubular aggregates on muscle biopsy is helpful in establishing the diagnosis.

The nondystrophic myotonias

Myotonia congenita (MC), paramyotonia congenita (PMC), and potassium-aggravated myotonia (PAM) are known as "nondystrophic" to distinguish them from myotonic dystrophy, which is not a primary channelopathy. Myotonic dystrophy causes muscle wasting and weakness, whereas nondystrophic myotonia causes muscle hypertrophy.

> ⚛ SCIENCE REVISITED
>
> **ION CHANNELS**
> An ion channel is a transmembrane protein that controls the flow of a particular type of ion across a plasma membrane. The channels considered in this chapter are in surface and T-tubule membranes of skeletal muscle cells. An ion channel is formed by the association of several proteins, each protein being identified by a protein name and a gene name, e.g. the SCN4A gene encodes the NaV1.4 subunit of the voltage-gated skeletal muscle sodium channel. Four Nav1.4 proteins associate to form a sodium channel. A single gene can cause different syndromes depending on the mutation (e.g. paramyotonia congenita and periodic paralysis are caused by different mutations of SCN4A). Conversely a syndrome can be caused by mutation of different genes (e.g. myotonia can be caused by CLCN1 or SCN4A mutations). The channels discussed in this chapter are as follows:
>
> | Ion | Gene | Protein | Disease |
> | --- | --- | --- | --- |
> | Sodium | SCN4A | NaV1.4 | Sodium channel myotonia |
> | | | | Potassium aggravated myotonia |
> | | | | Paramyotonia congenita |
> | | | | Hyperkalemic periodic paralysis |
> | | | | Hypokalemic periodic paralysis (type 2) |
> | Calcium | CACNA1S | CaV1.1 | Hypokalemic periodic paralysis (type 1) |
> | Potassium | KCNJ2 | Kir2.1 | Andersen–Tawil syndrome |
> | Chloride | CLCN1 | ClC1 | Myotonia congenita |

Myotonia congenita – chloride channel

MC is caused by mutation of the voltage-gated chloride channel, ClC1, encoded by the *CLCN1* gene on chromosome 17. Recessive MC (Becker's disease) is more common and more severe than the dominant variant (Thomsen's disease). Muscle stiffness may be slightly worse in the cold, although never to the extent seen in paramyotonia, and improves with exercise. Onset is usually in the second decade and the condition progresses slowly over years. The legs are affected first, giving rise to a disproportionate figure with hypertrophic calf and gluteal muscle, but smaller neck and shoulder girdle muscles. Grip and percussion myotonia and the lid-lag phenomenon are easily elicited. Although later in onset, the recessive form is usually more disabling and may exhibit the following features:

(1) more severe myotonic stiffness
(2) transient weakness that accompanies the myotonic stiffness
(3) minor distal wasting and weakness.

Transient post-exercise weakness produces a characteristic pattern in the short exercise test.

Mutations occur throughout the *CLCN1* gene; some produce dominant disease whereas others give rise to recessive inheritance. A few mutations are reported to cause dominant disease in one family but recessive disease in another. Interestingly the abnormal RNA splicing underlying myotonic dystrophy, which is not a primary channelopathy, causes myotonia by reducing expression of ClC1.

★ TIP AND TRICKS

- Transient weakness can be tested by asking the patient to repeatedly abduct the shoulder strongly against the examiner's hand.
- The first abduction is usually strong but the second is weak, and with continued repetitions strength improves again (warm-up phenomenon)

Paramyotonia congenita – sodium channel

PMC is caused by mutation of the skeletal muscle voltage-gated sodium channel NaV1.4, encoded by the *SCN4A* gene. The hallmarks of PMC are autosomal dominant inheritance, myotonia that is exacerbated by exercise, and marked cold sensitivity. Symptoms of PMC start in infancy and, in contrast to MC, affect bulbar, facial, neck, and hand muscles more than lower limb muscles. Stiffness can be precipitated by exercise and is usually accompanied by weakness. Unlike the transient weakness of recessive MC, weakness in PMC may persist for hours. Cold sensitivity is typically much more extreme than in myotonia and can cause profound muscle weakness. Cold water presents a serious risk to children with PMC. Characteristic presentations include blepharospasm after prolonged crying and tongue stiffness after eating ice-cream. Symptoms of paramyotonia are usually static through life but attacks of weakness and hyperkalemia may appear during adolescence.

The diagnosis is often clear from the history and clinical examination, but needle electromyography (EMG) and the short exercise test before and after cooling of the muscle may be helpful where there is uncertainty.

Potassium-aggravated myotonia – sodium channel

Some individuals with mutation in the *SCN4A* sodium channel gene present with symptoms of myotonia which, unlike MC, are potassium sensitive. Several variants of PAM (also known as sodium channel myotonia) have been described. The myotonia can be painful and fluctuate, and may be induced by exercise but the variants share the characteristic of being worse after potassium ingestion (e.g. fruit juices). Unlike other sodium channelopathies, however, there is no weakness and symptoms are not usually worse in the cold. Distinguishing PAM from autosomal dominant MC is sometimes difficult.

Management of the nondystrophic myotonias

Management of nondystrophic myotonia comprises avoidance of precipitating factors such as cold or strenuous exercise, and drugs that reduce muscle excitability. However, in many cases myotonia is mild and no specific treatment is required. In others drug treatment can be ceased in the summer months.

Most muscle specialists consider mexiletine (a class Ib antiarrhythmic that acts on sodium channels) to be the most effective drug for myotonia but evidence is anecdotal. A randomized controlled trial is under way. Mexiletine is generally well tolerated but can prolong the Q–T interval and thereby predispose to arrhythmia. It should be avoided in patients who already have a long Q–T interval, and the Q–T interval should be checked regularly in those taking the drug. Other drugs that act on sodium channels are often effective, including phenytoin, carbamazepine, procainamide, propafenone, and flecanide. Acetazolamide, a carbonic anhydrase inhibitor, and quinine are generally considered to be second-line treatments.

> ✋ **CAUTION!**
>
> Mexiletine can prolong the Q–T interval and predispose to arrhythmia.

The periodic paralyses

> ✯ **TIPS AND TRICKS**
>
> The presence of clinical or EMG myotonia in a patient with periodic paralysis suggests a sodium channel disorder.

Hyperkalemic periodic paralysis – sodium channel

HyperPP is characterized by recurrent attacks of limb weakness (sometimes focal) lasting from minutes up to a few hours, with onset in the first decade of life. The term "hyperkalemic" is somewhat misleading because the potassium may be normal during an attack. The characteristic feature is precipitation of attacks by potassium-rich foods, e.g. fruit juice, but the serum potassium need not exceed normal. Attacks can occur on waking and can be precipitated by the cold, fasting, rest after exercise, and emotional stress. Tendon reflexes are depressed during an attack, but bulbar and respiratory muscles are usually spared. A large proportion of individuals with

hyperPP develop progressive proximal myopathy, similar to hypoPP, which is seen with increasing age.

HyperPP is distinguished from hypoPP by shorter, more focal attacks, potassium sensitivity, and the presence of myotonia. The last, however subtle, in a patient with periodic paralysis strongly suggests hyperPP. Interictally, lid lag and eyelid myotonia may be the only clinical signs. Electrical myotonia is found in 50–75% of affected individuals yet is clinically apparent in less than 20%.

Similar to PMC and PAM, hyperPP is caused by mutations in the skeletal muscle voltage-gated sodium channel gene, *SCN4A*. Sodium channel disorders span the middle of the spectrum between episodic weakness and muscle stiffness, and overlap syndromes exist with characteristics of both hyperPP and PMC or hyperPP and PAM.

Hypokalemic periodic paralysis – calcium or sodium channel

HypoPP is the most common form of primary periodic paralysis but is still a rare disorder with a prevalence of about 1 per 100 000. Paralytic attacks usually begin in the first or second decade, usually occurring early in the morning. Weakness may be focal or generalized, and tends to be more severe and prolonged than in hyperPP, lasting for hours (occasionally days) with gradual resolution. Tendon reflexes are depressed during an attack. Respiratory and facial muscles are usually spared. Attacks occur spontaneously or are provoked by prolonged rest after vigorous exercise or a carbohydrate-rich meal on the previous day, and serum potassium is invariably low during an attack.

> ✋ **CAUTION**
>
> Although cardiac muscle is not primarily affected by hypoPP, profound hypokalemia may cause arrhythmia during an attack.

Other triggers include emotional stress, intercurrent viral illness, lack of sleep, menstruation, and specific medications (e.g. β agonists, corticosteroids, and insulin). Attack frequency varies widely from patient to patient: some experience daily episodes of weakness, others have a few episodes in a lifetime. After the age of 40 attacks become less frequent and less distinct. With time, fixed proximal muscle weakness may develop.

Myotonia never occurs in hypoPP; the presence of myotonia in a patient with periodic paralysis strongly suggests hyperPP.

Patients without a family history or presenting after age 20 should be assessed for thyrotoxic periodic paralysis by checking for suppressed thyroid-stimulating hormone (TSH) and elevated free thyroxine (fT_4) or free triiodothyronine (fT_3) levels. The serum potassium is often profoundly low. Thyrotoxic periodic paralysis, which is otherwise indistinguishable from hypoPP, can be inherited and is more common in men and in particular individuals from east Asians.

Ninety percent of cases of hypoPP are caused by mutation of the *CACNA1S* gene which encodes the voltage-gated calcium channel, CaV1.1 (type I hypoPP). Mutations in *SCN4A*, encoding the voltage-gated sodium channel NaV1.4, account for only 10% of hypoPP families (type II hypoPP).

Andersen–Tawil syndrome – potassium channel

Andersen–Tawil syndrome (ATS) is caused by mutation of the inward rectifier potassium channel, Kir2.1, encoded by the *KCNJ2* gene. The prevalence is estimated at one-tenth that of hypoPP. Symptomatic onset typically is with episodic weakness in the first or second decade. This type of familial periodic paralysis is characterized by extramuscular features. The full clinical presentation in ATS is periodic paralysis (usually hypokalemic, although normo- or hyperkalemic attacks are reported), cardiac arrhythmia, and distinctive skeletal features. Intermittent weakness occurs spontaneously or may be triggered by prolonged rest or rest after exertion; permanent proximal weakness often develops. Attack frequency, duration, and severity are variable between and within affected individuals.

The cardiac manifestations are variable and may include prolongation of the Q°T interval (long-QT syndrome), prominent U waves, premature ventricular contractions, ventricular bigeminy, and polymorphic ventricular tachycardia. A subset of patients manifests bidirectional ventricular tachycardia, a unique form of ventricular tachycardia in which the QRS axis polarity alternates from one beat to the next. Although many patients with ventricular ectopy are asymptomatic, others present with palpitations, syncope, or rarely cardiac arrest.

ATS patients may remain asymptomatic despite frequent runs of tachycardia, and there appears to be a lower incidence of syncope and sudden death in ATS compared with other long QT (LQT) syndromes. Distinctive physical findings include: a small mandible, ocular hypertelorism, low-set ears, clinodactyly, syndactyly, and broad nasal root; short stature, unilateral hypoplastic kidney, vaginal atresia, and brachydactyly; and also learning difficulties and a neurocognitive phenotype. The penetrance of symptoms is highly variable in ATS and some affected members of the same family may have only cardiac arrhythmia or periodic paralysis, whereas others may have all three features.

A diagnosis of ATS can be made when at least two of the following are present: periodic paralysis; ventricular ectopy; and typical ATS physical features. However, the phenotypic variability in ATS may obscure the diagnosis so ATS should be considered in any individual presenting with isolated periodic paralysis or polymorphic ventricular ectopy. A prolonged Q–U interval or large-amplitude U wave may be more sensitive than the Q–Tc interval, which overlaps with the upper limit of normal.

Management of periodic paralysis

The management of periodic paralysis comprises prevention of attacks and giving patients a contingency plan for the emergency treatment of an attack. Prevention is achieved by avoidance of the precipitants outlined above, and by drug treatment with a carbonic anhydrase inhibitor (either acetazolamide 125–1000 mg/day or dichlorphenamide 50–400 mg/day in divided doses). Carbonic anhydrase inhibitors are effective in both hypoPP and hyperPP, and are thought to exert their effect by producing metabolic acidosis. If hypoPP attacks persist on a carbonic anhydrase inhibitor, oral potassium should be added. In hyperPP, potassium-sensitivity symptoms are helped by lowering serum potassium, e.g. with an oral carbohydrate load, exercise, or inhaled β agonists.

Attacks of paralysis are rarely acutely life threatening but may render the patient incapable of self-care, sometimes for more than 24 hours, and the associated shifts in serum potassium can lead to cardiac arrhythmia. In an acute hypoPP attack, oral potassium 0.2–0.4 mmol/kg improves strength. Intravenous potassium is rarely necessary unless the patient cannot swallow. In the rare case that bulbar and respiratory muscles are affected by an attack, respiratory support and measures to prevent aspiration may be necessary. As the disease is rare, emergency physicians are unlikely to be familiar with its management, and giving the patient a letter explaining the condition and its treatment and a telephone contact for the patient's specialist is helpful.

Bibliography

Cannon S. Pathomechanisms in channelopathies of skeletal muscle and brain. *Annu Rev Neurosci* 2006;**29**:387–415.

Cannon SC. Voltage-sensor mutations in channelopathies of skeletal muscle. *J Physiol* 2010;**588**(Pt 11):1887–95.

Colding-Jorgensen E. Phenotypic variability in myotonia congenita. *Muscle Nerve* 2005;**32**: 19–34.

Davies N, Hanna M. The skeletal muscle channelopathies: distinct entities and overlapping syndromes. *Curr Opin Neurol* 2003;**16**:559–68.

Fournier E, Arzel M, Sternberg D, et al. Electromyography guides toward subgroups of mutations in muscle channelopathies. *Ann Neurol* 2004;**56**:650–61.

Fournier E, Viala K, Gervais H, et al. Cold extends electromyography distinction between ion channel mutations causing myotonia. *Ann Neurol* 2006;**60**:356–65.

Matthews E, Hanna MG. Muscle channelopathies: does the predicted channel gating pore offer new treatment insights for hypokalaemic periodic paralysis? *J Physiol* 2010;**588**(Pt 11): 1879–86.

Matthews E, Tan S, Fialho D, et al. What causes paramyotonia in the United Kingdom?: Common and new SCN4A mutations revealed. *Neurology* 2008;**70**:50–3.

Miller T. Differential diagnosis of myotonic disorders. *Muscle Nerve* 2008;**37**:293–9.

Rakowicz W, Hanna M. Muscle ion channel diseases. *Adv Clin Neurosci Rehabil* 2003;**3**: 14–17.

Trip J, Drost G, van Engelen, BG, Faber, CG. Drug treatment for myotonia (Review). *Cochrane Database System Rev* 2006;(**1**):CD004762.

Venance S, Cannon S, Fialho D, et al. The primary periodic paralyses: diagnosis, pathogenesis and treatment. *Brain* 2006;**129**:8–17.

Congenital Myopathies

Nigel Clarke and Kathryn North

Institute for Neuroscience and Muscle Research, The Children's Hospital at Westmead, Sydney, NSW, Australia

An overview of diagnosis and management of the congenital myopathies

The classification of congenital myopathies is based on histopathological features

The congenital myopathies are a group of genetic muscle disorders that are defined by the presence of distinct structural abnormalities seen on muscle biopsy and that share a common pattern of clinical features. As a group they probably account for around 2% of all patients with genetic muscle conditions. There are four broad pathological patterns: protein inclusion myopathies (e.g. nemaline myopathy, myosin storage myopathy), core myopathies (e.g. central core disease, multi-minicore disease), myopathies with internalized nuclei (e.g. myotubular and centronuclear myopathies), and myopathies associated with abnormal fiber size (e.g. congenital fiber size disproportion). These abnormalities reflect chronic relatively stable changes in the architecture of muscle fibers although pathological features can evolve over time.

Common clinical features in congenital myopathies

The congenital myopathies share common clinical features and the absence of these should alert the clinician to other diagnoses. The most common presentation is at birth or soon after with generalized hypotonia and weakness, difficulty with sucking, and often a need for temporary respiratory support. Mildly affected patients may be diagnosed during childhood or later. Many children have a long face, dolichocephy, and a high arched palate together with facial weakness (*myopathic facies*; Plate 14.1). Weakness is usually generalized or more prominent in axial and/or proximal limb muscles and of variable severity. Except for weakness of ankle dorsiflexion, prominent distal limb weakness is atypical. The facial, extraocular, swallowing, and respiratory muscles are often involved. This can lead to difficulties in feeding, susceptibility to chest infections and respiratory failure in more severely affected children. Hypotonia and reduced or absent deep tendon reflexes are almost universally present. The most severe patients present *in utero* with reduced fetal movements and polyhydramnios, and may never achieve independent respiration.

Congenital dislocation of the hips can be seen in all forms of congenital myopathies but is especially common in myopathies due to the ryanodine receptor (*RYR1*). Progressive scoliosis in childhood or adolescence and proximal or distal joint contractures are common when there is moderate or severe weakness. Usually the clinical course is static or only slowly progressive. Some children with severe neonatal weakness, most notably those with nemaline myopathy or

Neuromuscular Disorders, First Edition. Edited by Rabi N. Tawil, Shannon Venance.

DNM2-related centronuclear myopathy, often become more robust with age if they survive the first year or two. Intellectual function is usually normal and, in contrast to some of the muscular dystrophies, primary cardiac involvement is rare.

The diagnostic approach

Excluding other diagnoses

The first task in the diagnosis of a congenital myopathy is to exclude other causes of muscle weakness that can be diagnosed without the need for a muscle biopsy. A detailed history and clinical examination, with attention to the pattern of muscle weakness and clinical features may suggest alternative diagnoses. Most congenital myopathy patients have a normal creatine kinase (CK) level after the first week of life. CK levels more than five times normal makes a muscular dystrophy or metabolic myopathy much more likely. Electrophysiological tests are most useful to exclude other disorders such as neuropathies and anterior horn cell disorders. Common alternative diagnoses to consider include: congenital myotonic dystrophy, spinal muscular atrophy (SMA), and Prader–Willi syndrome, all of which are best diagnosed by genetic testing. A much rarer and more challenging group of disorders with clinical features that can overlap congenital myopathies are the congenital myasthenic syndromes (Box 14.1).

The role of muscle biopsy

A genetic diagnosis can be made in around two-thirds of patients with congenital myopathy (Table 14.1). Muscle biopsy findings provide the strongest clues as to the underlying genetic cause. It is also useful to exclude congenital muscular dystrophies, which can be difficult to differentiate clinically. Many structural abnormalities become more prominent with age, and pathological changes can be patchy so that a second biopsy may need to be performed to establish a specific diagnosis. Muscle biopsies are best performed in a center with experience in handling muscle.

Muscle imaging

Magnetic resonance imaging (MRI) of the thigh and lower leg muscles is proving a useful adjunct

---

Box 14.1. Tests to consider in the diagnosis of congenital myopathies

1. **Tests to exclude other causes of muscle weakness**
   Plasma creatine kinase (CK) and lactate
   EMG, nerve conduction studies,
      ±repetitive nerve stimulation
   In neonates or infants also consider
   Urine metabolic screen
   Genetic testing for spinal muscular
      atrophy, myotonic dystrophy, Prader–
      Willi syndrome
2. **If a congenital myopathy is suspected**
   Muscle biopsy for frozen sections,
      paraffin-embedded sections, electron
      microscopy
   Consider muscle MRI in children aged 4
      years or older

---

in diagnosis because many congenital myopathies have consistent distinct patterns of muscle involvement, in particular those due to *RYR1*, *DNM2*, and *SEPN1* (see Box 14.1).

Gene testing

Definition of the gene causing a congenital myopathy should be a goal for all families because this informs genetic counseling, gives important information about prognosis, often guides management, and in the future will be essential to prescribe specific therapies.

Common approaches to management

Not unexpectedly, health complications from congenital myopathies largely arise from weakness of various muscle groups.

Orthopedic issues

Patients with mild generalized weakness may develop contractures of the Achilles tendon but other joint contractures are unusual if patients remain ambulant. Scoliosis is a common complication and often seen in myopathies due to *RYR1* and *SEPN1*. Surgical fixation is recommended for moderate progressive curves, to prevent major deformity for comfort and to preserve respiratory

Table 14.1. The genetic causes of congenital myopathies

Congenital myopathy	Protein (gene)	Inheritance pattern
Nemaline myopathy	Nebulin (*NEB*)	AR
	Skeletal α-actin (*ACTA1*)	AD, uncommonly AR
	α-Tropomyosin$_{slow}$ (*TPM3*)	AD, AR
	β-Tropomyosin (*TPM2*)	AD, uncommonly AR
	Troponin T$_{slow}$ (*TNNT1*)	AR
	Cofilin (*CLF2*)[a]	AR
Myosin storage myopathy	Slow/β-cardiac myosin heavy chain (*MYH7*)	AD, rarely AR
Central core disease	Ryanodine receptor (*RYR1*)	AD > AR
Multi-minicore disease	Selenoprotein N (*SEPN1*)	AR
	Ryanodine receptor (*RYR1*)	AR > AD
	Skeletal α-actin (*ACTA1*)[a]	AD
Centronuclear myopathy	Myotubularin (*MTM1*)	X-linked
	Dynamin 2 (*DNM2*)	AD
	Ryanodine receptor (*RYR1*)	AR
	Amphiphysin 2 (*BIN1*)	AR
Congenital fiber type disproportion	α-Tropomyosin$_{slow}$ (*TPM3*)	AD
	Ryanodine receptor (*RYR1*)	AR
	Skeletal α-actin (*ACTA1*)	AD
	β-Tropomyosin (*TPM2*)[a]	AD

Genetic causes are shown in rough order of population frequency.
[a]Indicates when two or fewer families are reported.
AD, autosomal dominant; AR, autosomal recessive.

function. Mild or moderately affected patients may benefit from regular low-impact moderate-intensity aerobic exercise, such as swimming or cycling, to improve stamina and motor abilities.

Feeding and nutrition issues

Pharyngeal muscle weakness is common in patients with moderate or severe weakness and is associated with feeding and swallowing difficulties, difficulties with managing secretions, and increased risk of aspiration. In severe congenital myopathies, establishing oral feeding after birth may take weeks or months. Some patients require tube feeds to maintain adequate nutrition. Bulbar function often improves during childhood and gastrostomy tubes may be required only temporarily.

Respiratory issues

Respiratory muscle weakness that requires continuous ventilation from birth for more than a month generally predicts a poor prognosis. If the degree of weakness is sufficient to significantly impair gait, functionally significant respiratory muscle weakness is often present. All patients with moderate or severe weakness require regular sleep studies and a forced vital capacity (FVC) below 60% indicates a possible need for nocturnal ventilatory support. Nocturnal bilevel positive airway pressure (BiPAP) can enable patients with FVC measures as low as 15% of predicted to manage without a tracheostomy, so long as daytime respiratory function is adequate. Annual influenza immunization and early aggressive treatment of respiratory tract infections can reduce the risk of severe lower respiratory tract infections. General strength and respiratory function may slowly deteriorate from mid-adulthood and late scoliosis can develop.

> ✋ **CAUTION!**
>
> Patients with mutations in *SEPN1* and *TPM3* may develop nocturnal hypoventilation while fully ambulant and monitoring of respiratory function from early ages is advised in proven or suspected cases.

The different types of congenital myopathy

Nemaline myopathy

Nemaline myopathy (NM) is one of the most common forms of congenital myopathy and is defined by the presence of numerous dense rod-like protein inclusions in skeletal muscles (nemaline rods or nemaline bodies). Rods tend to increase with age and vary in number between muscles and sometimes re-biopsy is required to establish the diagnosis. Rods are best seen on Gomori trichrome stain as dark red/purple dense bodies. The spectrum of muscle weakness in NM extends from children who never establish independent respiration to patients with mild weakness that has little impact on daily life into adulthood. A clinical categorization based on early disease severity is useful to predict prognosis and genetic cause (see Ryan et al. in the Bibliography at the end of the chapter).

There are six known genetic causes that overlap in clinical phenotype. A diagnostic difficulty is the expense of genetic testing for *NEB*, an enormous gene encoding nebulin which likely accounts for over half of NM families worldwide. All *NEB* families to date have autosomal recessive inheritance. *ACTA1* encodes α-skeletal actin and is the second most common cause, accounting for around 25% of NM patients, but around 50% of those with severe congenital weakness. Over 90% of *ACTA1* mutations are autosomal dominant and many are new mutations; however, 10% of families have recessive disease. Two tropomyosin genes (*TPM2* and *TPM3*) each account for around 5% of NM and may be either dominant

or recessive. The *NEB*, *TPM3*, and *TPM2* genes cause a very similar range of clinical phenotypes, with prominent neck and ankle dorsiflexor weakness in mild or moderately affected patients. At present muscle MRI appears less useful in NM than in other congenital myopathies.

Currently, genetic testing for NM usually begins with *ACTA1*, particularly in patients with severe weakness, numerous nemaline rods, or if there is a dominant family history. When rods are confined to slow muscle fibers, a mutation in *TPM3* is likely because α-tropomyosin$_{slow}$ is expressed only in slow fibers. Mutation analysis of *TPM3* and *TPM2* is often undertaken before *NEB* because testing is less expensive despite their relative rarity. *TNNT1* and *CFL2* also cause NM but these forms are so rare that these genes are not usually tested for.

The core myopathies

There are two main forms of core myopathy, central core disease (CCD) and multi-minicore disease (MmD). Although there is overlap between these entities, the distinction remains useful because the genetic basis differs. The "cores" in all core myopathies are regions within muscle fibers that lack staining on the oxidative stains (SDH and NADH) due to marked reduction or absence of mitochondria in those areas. In CCD, the cores are often single, large, and central with well-defined borders that extend along the fiber a considerable distance (best appreciated on longitudinal muscle sections). In contrast, in MmD, the cores are usually smaller, multiple, often have less well defined boundaries, and involve only a few adjacent sarcomeres. Electron microscopy (EM) is particularly helpful to confirm the diagnosis in MmD because poorly defined cores can be difficult to distinguish from staining artifacts.

Classic CCD is usually due to mutations in *RYR1* and there is a strong co-association with malignant hyperthermia (MH). Most CCD mutations are dominant (heterozygous) changes that cluster in three CCD/MH hotspot regions. Most patients with CCD present in infancy or childhood with delayed gross motor skills, mild or moderate proximal limb weakness, and facial weakness, and remain ambulant in adulthood. Most patients do not have ophthalmoplegia, difficulty swallowing, or significant respiratory muscle involvement, but scoliosis and congenital hip dislocation are common. A few patients with CCD have severe weakness and resemble patients with MmD due to *RYR1* (see below).

Multi-minicore disease

This has two common genetic causes identified to date. Up to half of MmD patients have autosomal recessive disease due to mutations in *SEPN1*, which encodes the protein selenoprotein N. Mutations in *SEPN1* result in variable histological abnormalities that include mild dystrophic changes, as well as multiple cores. The clinical phenotype is more consistent and recognizable, particularly in older children; the clinical features and muscle MRI offer the best clues for diagnosis. Children with *SEPN1*-related myopathy are usually well at birth and walk and sit at normal ages, but may present with hypotonia and axial weakness in infancy (a dropped-head phenotype). They usually have slight builds and mild limb weakness during childhood. Facial and eye movements are normal but spinal rigidity and neck weakness may be marked. CK levels can be mildly elevated or normal. Most children require surgical stabilization of scoliosis in adolescence and, even though they remain fully ambulant, most require nocturnal respiratory support from late childhood to late adolescence.

The second common cause of MmD is the *RYR1* gene. In contrast to CCD, MmD due to *RYR1* is most often autosomal recessive and more severe, although the range of disease severity is wide. Patients may present from birth with generalized hypotonia and weakness, poor head control, and difficulty swallowing. Axial weakness is usually prominent and scoliosis common. The presence of facial weakness, ptosis, and ophthalmoplegia (which may develop only during childhood) is helpful in discriminating MmD due to *RYR1* from that due to *SEPN1*. Muscle MRI also shows a relatively consistent pattern. All patients with possible, suspected, or known mutations in *RYR1* have a high risk of MH during general anesthesia and precautions are required.

The *RYR1* gene is large and contains many harmless sequence variants in the general population (polymorphisms), and both dominant and recessive patterns are common. This complicates the interpretation of genetic testing results. It is prudent to ask the advice of a specialist laboratory or neuromuscular service if there is any uncertainty.

☡ CAUTION!

All patients with possible, suspected, or proven mutations in *RYR1* are at high risk of malignant hyperthermia and precautions must be taken during general anesthesia.

Centronuclear myopathies

After 17 weeks' gestation, nuclei in skeletal muscle usually have peripheral positions, just under the plasma membrane. Internal nuclei may be seen after muscle repair but in normal individuals are present in less than 3% of fibers. Increased internalization of nuclei is the main abnormality on muscle histology in centronuclear myopathy (CNM). However, increased internal nuclei are also a common feature of muscular dystrophies and the distinction can be difficult. There are two common (*MTM1*, *DNM2*) and one rare (*BIN1*) established genetic cause, and they are best differentiated using a combination of clinical and histological features and muscle MRI. Recently, recessive *RYR1* mutations have been reported in some CNM-like patients as well.

X-linked myotubular myopathy

This is a severe form of CNM that is classified apart from other forms of CNM because of the distinct clinical features and inheritance pattern. It is caused by mutations in the *MTM1* gene, which encodes the protein myotubularin, and affects mainly boys due to the X-linked inheritance. Most mutations cause severe generalized weakness, facial weakness, feeding difficulties, and respiratory failure in the newborn period in affected males. Ophthalmoplegia, prematurity, and increased body length at birth are common. Most die before age 1 year even with aggressive treatment, and most survivors are ventilator dependent. Muscle biopsy in the neonatal period or infancy shows numerous large nuclei in central positions in muscle fibers and, when present with typical clinical features, a relatively firm clinical diagnosis can be made. Mutation analysis of the *MTM1* gene is recommended to confirm the diagnosis, so that genetic counseling is accurate and carrier testing in female relatives and prenatal diagnosis for families possible. Usually females with *MTM1* mutations are asymptomatic, but uncommonly they can present with proximal limb weakness in childhood or adulthood.

DNM2–related centronuclear myopathy

Mutations in *DNM2*, which encodes dynamin II, are the most common cause of autosomal dominant CNM. Mutations in *DNM2* also cause Charcot–Marie–Tooth disease (CMTDIB) and combined phenotypes are reported. Most patients with CNM due to *DNM2* present in infancy or childhood with weakness of limb–girdle, trunk, and neck muscles. Ptosis and ophthalmoparesis are also common. Often there is a family history. A few patients have more severe disease and present in the neonatal period with generalized hypotonia and weakness, and ptosis, and with early swallowing and respiratory difficulties that improve. These patients are more likely to have new *DNM2* mutations. Common complications are nocturnal hypoventilation, swallowing difficulties, loss of ambulation, and contractures of the Achilles tendon and long finger flexors. Radial sarcoplasmic strands (seen on NADH stains) and an abundance of geographically central nuclei are hallmarks of CNM due to *DNM2* but are not always present. Muscle MRI shows a distinctive pattern.

Myosin storage myopathy

The hallmark histological abnormality in myosin storage myopathy (MSM; previously also called hyaline body myopathy) is the presence of hyaline bodies beneath the plasma membrane in type 1 (slow twitch) muscle fibers that stain intensely for slow myosin. Most families have dominant mutations in the *MYH7* gene which encodes the myosin isoform in both type 1 (slow twitch) muscle fibers and cardiac muscle. The most common clinical pattern is childhood onset of slowly progressive generalized weakness, but the most severely affected patients have congenital weakness, scoliosis and contractures, lose ambulation, and need ventilatory support in early adulthood. An unusual aspect of the condition is the variability in severity, clinical course, and phenotype even within the same family. Common clinical features include scapuloperoneal or limb–girdle weakness, foot drop, calf hypertrophy, scoliosis, and respiratory failure. Some MSM patients also have cardiomyopathy and arrhythmias.

Congenital fiber-type disproportion

Finally, patients may present with typical clinical features of a congenital myopathy (Figure 14.1) who do not have cores, rods, or internalized nuclei but have abnormalities in fiber sizes or ratios as the main abnormality. Such changes are common in all congenital myopathies and are therefore regarded as relatively nonspecific. However, when the main histological abnormality is type 1 fibers consistently smaller than type 2 fibers, this is termed "congenital fiber-type disproportion" (CFTD). A range of other congenital myopathies, and neurological and metabolic conditions should be considered and excluded before making the diagnosis. The most common causes identified to date are mutations in the *TPM3* (approximately 25–40%), *RYR1* (approximately 10–25%) and *ACTA1* (approximately 5%) genes. Some CFTD patients will reveal features of another congenital myopathy if biopsied at an older age or from a different muscle, but often the genetic basis can be identified from the initial biopsy and clinical features. Early respiratory failure is a common feature in many patients with CFTD, particularly those with mutations in *TPM3*, and vigilance for nocturnal hypoventilation is advised, even in ambulant patients.

Future perspectives

Even the best clinical services are unable to identify the genetic cause in around a third of congenital myopathy families. The clinical and histological patterns arising from the known congenital myopathy genes continue to expand. The large genes remain difficult to analyze and there is good evidence that more genes remain to be identified. Whole genome sequencing is likely to simplify the task of discovering new congenital

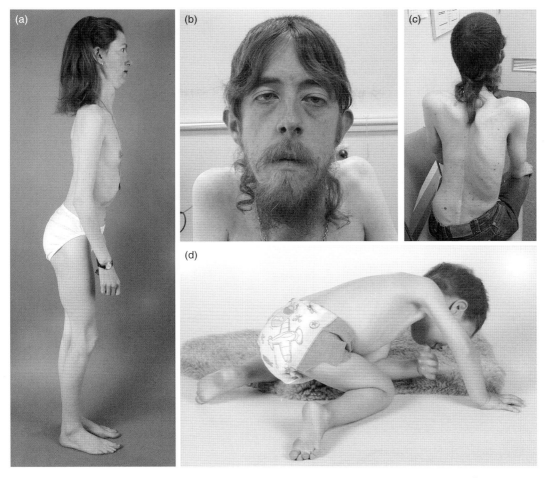

Figure 14.1. Clinical photographs of patients with different forms of congenital myopathy. (a) *SEPN1*-related myopathy: this woman requires nocturnal bilevel positive airway pressure (BiPAP) and has had scoliosis fixation. (b,c) *RYR1*-related congenital fiber-type disproportion (CFTD) due to recessive mutations. Note the long face, ptosis, strabismus (associated with ophthalmoparesis), generalized muscle wasting, and scoliosis post-fixation. (d) *TPM3*-related CFTD patient mid-way through rising from a supine position showing generalized mild-to -moderate muscle weakness and reduced muscle bulk.

myopathy genes. Advances in genetic technology are also likely to simplify diagnosis once afford-able, large-scale gene sequencing becomes rou-tinely available.

Acknowledgments

The authors were supported by the National Health and Medical Research Council (NC by grants 206529 and 571287, and KN by grant 403941).

Bibliography

Bitoun M, Bevilacqua JA, Prudhon B, et al. Dynamin 2 mutations cause sporadic centro-nuclear myopathy with neonatal onset. *Ann Neurol* 2007;**62**:666–70.

Clarke NF, North KN. Congenital fiber type dis-proportion – 30 years on. *J Neuropathol Exp Neurol* 2003;**62**:977–89.

Clarke NF, Kolski H, Dye DE, et al. Mutations in TPM3 are a common cause of congenital fiber type disproportion. *Ann Neurol* 2008;**63**: 329–37.

Ferreiro A, Quijano-Roy S, Pichereau C, et al. Mutations of the selenoprotein N gene, which is implicated in rigid spine muscular dystrophy, cause the classical phenotype of multiminicore disease: reassessing the nosology of early-onset myopathies. *Am J Hum Genet* 2002; **71**:739–49.

Goebel HH, Laing NG. Actinopathies and myosinopathies. *Brain Pathol* 2009;**19**:516–22.

Jungbluth H, Zhou H, Hartley L, et al. Minicore myopathy with ophthalmoplegia caused by mutations in the ryanodine receptor type 1 gene. *Neurology* 2005;**65**:1930–5.

Mercuri E, Pichiecchio A, Counsell S, et al. A short protocol for muscle MRI in children with muscular dystrophies. *Eur J Paediatr Neurol* 2002; **6**:305–7.

Norwood FL, Harling C, Chinnery PF, Eagle M, Bushby K, Straub V. Prevalence of genetic muscle disease in Northern England: in-depth analysis of a muscle clinic population. *Brain* 2009;**132**:3175–86.

Quinlivan RM, Muller CR, Davis M, et al. Central core disease: clinical, pathological, and genetic features. *Arch Dis Child* 2003;**88**:1051–5.

Ryan MM, Schnell C, Strickland CD, et al. Nemaline myopathy: a clinical study of 143 cases. *Ann Neurol* 2001;**50**:312–20.

Susman RD, Quijano-Roy S, Yang N, et al. Expanding the clinical, pathological and MRI phenotype of DNM2-related centronuclear myopathy. *Neuromusc Disord* 2010;**20**:229–37.

Wallgren-Pettersson C, Clarke A, Samson F, et al. The myotubular myopathies: differential diagnosis of the X linked recessive, autosomal dominant, and autosomal recessive forms and present state of DNA studies. *J Med Genet* 1995; **32**:673–9.

Part II

Disorders of the Neuromuscular Junction

Approach to Diseases of the Neuromuscular Junction

Donald B. Sanders

Duke University Medical Center, Durham, NC, USA

The first admonition has stayed with me ever since I heard it from a senior physician more than 40 years ago. The second quotation reflects the reality of contemporary medicine. As Groopman points out, physicians make diagnoses based on their experience and the rules of thumb (heuristics) from that experience. Myasthenia gravis (MG), the most common neuromuscular junction (NMJ) disease, is far from common, and the Lambert–Eaton syndrome (LES) is even rarer, thus most physicians have seen too few examples to develop their own sense of how these patients present. The first, and most important, step in diagnosing NMJ disorders is to think of them. However, MG was included in the differential by the first evaluating physician in less than half the patients with MG ultimately referred to the author's clinic (Table 15.1). The characteristic clinical presentations of MG and LES are described in this chapter. Once these distinctive patterns of weakness are recognized from the history and examination, confirmation by appropriate diagnostic tests is usually straightforward.

The clinical presentation of MG

Patients with MG (and LES) seek medical attention because of specific muscle dysfunction. Although they frequently also have excessive fatigue, that is not usually their major complaint. Weakness of ocular or eyelid muscles brings most MG patients to the doctor – in the author's clinic, 70% of MG patients had eyelid ptosis, diplopia, or blurred vision at onset, and these were the only initial symptoms in 60% (Figure 15.1). Bulbar symptoms – slurred, nasal, or garbled speech, or difficulty chewing or swallowing – are the next most common presenting symptoms. When prompted, patients may recall previous transient episodes of ocular or bulbar muscle weakness – a drooping eyelid or double vision – that resolved spontaneously after several days, frequent changes in spectacles to improve blurred vision, trouble reading or watching TV in the evening, not driving in bright daylight because of double vision, giving up singing because of voice changes, avoiding foods that have become difficult to chew or swallow, coughing after eating because of aspiration, and nasal regurgitation of liquids.

Neuromuscular Disorders, First Edition. Edited by Rabi N. Tawil, Shannon Venance.

© 2011 John Wiley & Sons, Ltd. Published 2011 by John Wiley & Sons, Ltd.

Patients with a recently described subset of MG associated with antibodies to muscle-specific tyrosine kinase (MuSK) frequently have findings atypical for MG. As many do not have ocular muscle weakness and weak muscles may be atrophic, the clinical findings may be more suggestive of motor neuron disease or a myopathy than of MG. Suspect MuSK-MG if there is facial or tongue weakness and atrophy, or weakness that predominates in neck or shoulder muscles.

Table 15.1. Initial diagnosis in 700 patients with definite acquired myasthenia gravis (MG)

Initial diagnosis	Number (%)
MG	329 (47)
Eye disease	96 (14)
Cerebrovascular accident	84 (12)
Psychological	20 (3)
Myopathy	15 (2)
Bell's palsy	13 (2)
Thyroid disease	10 (1.4)
Brain lesion	8 (1.1)
Multiple sclerosis	8 (1.1)
Allergy	8 (1.1)
Blepharospasm	3 (0.4)
Other	106 (15)

From Sanders DB, Massey JM – unpublished data.

☝ CAUTION!

- Patients with MG associated with MuSK antibodies may have clinical findings suggestive of motor neuron disease or a myopathy, rather than of MG.
- Suspect MuSK-MG if there is facial or tongue weakness and atrophy, or weakness that predominates in neck or shoulder muscles.

Examination of the patient with suspected MG

★ TIPS AND TRICKS

- In MG, the weakness on examination is frequently worse than the symptoms would suggest.

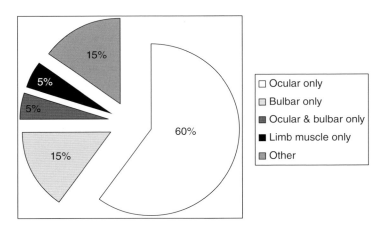

Figure 15.1. Initial symptoms in 919 patients with myasthenia gravis seen at the Duke University myasthenia gravis clinic (Sanders DB and Massey JM, unpublished data). Seventy percent had ocular symptoms (ptosis, diplopia, or blurred vision) at onset, and these were the only initial symptoms in 60%. Twenty-two percent had bulbar symptoms (dysarthria, dysphagia, or facial weakness), and these were the only symptoms in 15%; 5% had ocular and bulbar symptoms, and these were the only initial symptoms in 4%; and 5% had isolated weakness of limb or axial muscles alone. Twelve percent had initial symptoms of generalized weakness or fatigue, with or without other symptoms.

- Demonstrating mild or even moderate weakness requires exertion of more physician effort than is used during the typical physical exam.
- Weakness that varies during the examination, becoming worse after activity and improving after rest, should always raise the question of MG.

✋ CAUTION

The weakness in MG typically comes and goes, and may not be present during the examination, confusing the physician when physical findings do not confirm the symptoms.

The alert physician can frequently detect dysfunction by observing patients in action – how they walk and talk, and their facial appearance. At rest, the corners of the mouth often droop downward, giving a depressed appearance. Attempts to smile often produce contraction of the medial portion of the upper lip and a horizontal contraction of the corners of the mouth without the natural upward curling, resembling a sneer. The patient may support a weak jaw (and neck) with the thumb under the chin, the middle finger curled under the nose or lower lip, and the index finger extended up the cheek, producing a studious or attentive appearance. To compensate for eyelid ptosis, the frontalis muscle contracts, producing a worried or surprised look – unilateral frontalis contraction is a clue that the lid elevators are weak on that side. The voice may be nasal or slurred, especially after prolonged talking.

Asymmetric weakness of several muscles in both eyes is typical of MG, in patterns that cannot be localized to lesions of one or more nerves, and the pupillary responses are normal. When mild, ocular weakness may not be obvious on routine examination and appears only upon provocative testing. The medial rectus is particularly likely to be weak in MG – this can be seen as limited medial deviation or lateral drift of the affected eye during sustained gaze to the opposite side, or as an inability to maintain conjugate fixation on sustained

upgaze. If there is weakness in any eye muscle, fatigability may be convincingly demonstrated by examining the patient again after a few minutes of rest or after applying an icepack to the eye.

Almost all MG patients have weakness of eyelid closure, which is usually asymptomatic. With moderate weakness of these muscles, the patient cannot "bury" the eyelashes during forced eye closure. More severe weakness may result in involuntary opening of the eyes during sustained forced eye closure, the so-called peek sign. Do not mistake blepharospasm or voluntary eye closure for lid ptosis – with the former, the lower lid rises as the upper lid descends.

✋ CAUTION!

Do not mistake blepharospasm or voluntary eye closure for lid ptosis – with the former, the lower lid rises as the upper lid descends.

★ TIPS AND TRICKS

- A history of eyelid ptosis that shifts from one eye to the other is virtually diagnostic of MG.
- Almost all patients with MG have weakness of eyelid closure.

Muscle strength should be assessed by manual muscle testing during maximum effort and again after rest so as to detect variable weakness – most physicians do not exert sufficient effort during manual muscle testing to detect mild or moderate weakness. However, keep in mind that performance may also fluctuate if effort varies or testing causes pain.

Any trunk or limb muscle may be weak in MG, but some are more often affected than others. Neck flexors are usually weaker than neck extensors, and the deltoids, triceps, and extensors of the wrist and fingers, and ankle dorsiflexors are frequently weaker than other limb muscles. Rarely, MG presents with focal weakness in single muscle groups, such as a "dropped head syndrome" due to severe neck extensor weakness or isolated vocal fold or respiratory muscle weakness.

The edrophonium test

This has fallen out of favor in most clinics, unfortunately so, in the author's opinion. Serious complications (bradyarrhythmia or syncope) have been reported in only 0.16% of edrophonium tests, and these symptoms generally resolve with rest in the supine position. The author can recall only one such adverse reaction, many years ago, when he injected the entire 10 mg dose in one bolus in an elderly man, who promptly fainted, fortunately without sequelae. I never did that again, and learned that the diagnostic response is usually seen after injecting only 2 or 5 mg.

Serological testing

This confirms the diagnosis of MG in most patients – 80% of patients with generalized MG and 50% with ocular MG have serum antibodies to the acetylcholine receptor (AChR). Antibodies to MuSK are found in about 50% of generalized MG and occasional ocular MG patients who lack the AChR antibodies. The presence of either of these antibodies assures the diagnosis.

If the edrophonium test is positive or MG antibodies are found, the patient can be referred to a neuromuscular disease expert for confirmation of the diagnosis and management (Sanders and Howard 2008). No dangerous or sustained treatment should be used until the diagnosis is certain, particularly thymectomy.

Electrodiagnostic testing

The most efficient approach to diagnosing MG (or LES) is to perform electrodiagnostic testing early to demonstrate that neuromuscular transmission (NMT) is abnormal. In the author's clinic, the patient with suspected NMJ disease usually goes directly from the exam room to the electromyography (EMG) lab. Repetitive nerve stimulation (RNS) testing demonstrates abnormal NMT in about 80% of patients with generalized MG, but in only about 50% of those with ocular MG. If RNS is normal, single-fiber EMG virtually always demonstrates abnormal NMT.

The clinical presentation of LES

★ TIPS AND TRICKS

- Lambert–Eaton syndrome is characterized by the triad of weakness, dry mouth, and reduced or absent tendon reflexes.
- In LES, the weakness on examination is frequently less than the symptoms would suggest.

LES usually presents with symptoms that suggest a myopathy – gradually progressive lower extremity weakness, sometimes with muscle tenderness – but, unlike most myopathies, tendon reflexes are almost always absent or diminished. Ocular and bulbar symptoms are generally not prominent. Most patients have a dry mouth, and many have other autonomic symptoms: erectile dysfunction in males, postural hypotension, constipation, and dry eyes. Respiratory failure is uncommon unless there is also primary pulmonary disease. Approximately half of LES patients have an underlying malignancy – in 80% this is small cell lung cancer (SCLC), which may be discovered before or years after the onset of symptoms. The weakness in LES is frequently attributed to cachexia, polymyositis, or, in patients with known cancer, a paraneoplastic neuromuscular syndrome.

Antibodies to voltage-gated calcium channels are found in almost all patients with LES who have an underlying malignancy, and in more than 90% without cancer.

Electrodiagnostic testing

Simple nerve stimulation tests demonstrate characteristic abnormalities in almost all LES patients. The amplitude of the muscle responses to nerve stimulation is low, and increases markedly after the muscle is activated, either by brief maximum voluntary contraction or by high-frequency stimulation of the nerve.

✋ CAUTION!

- Many medications are known to exacerbate the weakness in patients with MG or LES, sometimes with fatal outcome.
- Aminoglycoside, fluoroquinolone, or macrolide antibiotics are the drugs most frequently involved, as are magnesium salts, especially intravenous Mg^{2+}

replacement. Telithromycin should never be used in myasthenic patients. Many other drugs may exacerbate the weakness in some patients with MG. All MG and LES patients should be observed for increased weakness whenever any new medication is started.

Bibliography

Groopman J. *How Doctors Think*. Boston, MA: Houghton Mifflin Harcourt, 2007.

Guptill JT, Sanders DB. Update on MuSK antibody positive myasthenia gravis. *Curr Opin Neurol* 2010;**23**:530–5.

Harper CM, Lennon VA. The Lambert–Eaton myasthenic syndrome. In: Kaminski HJ (ed.), *Current Clinical Neurology: Myasthenia gravis and related disorders*. Totowa, NJ: Humana Press, 2002: 269–91.

Ing EB, Ing SY, Ing T, Ramocki JA. The complication rate of edrophonium testing for suspected myasthenia gravis. *Can J Ophthalmol* 2005; **35**:141–4.

Pascuzzi RM. The edrophonium test. *Semin Neurol* 2003;**23**:83–8.

Sanders DB, Howard JF Jr. Disorders of neuromuscular transmission. In: Bradley WG, Daroff RB, Fenichel GM, Jancovic J (eds), *Neurology in Clinical Practice*. Philadelphia, PA: Butterworths Heinemann Elsevier, 2008: 2383–402.

Sanders DB, Juel VC. Lambert–Eaton myasthenic syndrome. In: Engel AG (ed.), *Neuromuscular Junction Disorders*. Amsterdam: Elsevier, 2008: 274–83.

Stålberg EV, Trontelj JV, Sanders DB. Myasthenia gravis and other disorders of neuromuscular transmission. In: *Single Fiber EMG*. Fiskebåckskil, Sweden: Edshagen Publishing House, 2010: 218–66.

Myasthenia Gravis

Michael K. Hehir and Emma Ciafaloni

Department of Neurology, University of Rochester, Rochester, NY, USA

Myasthenia gravis (MG) is an autoimmune disease of the peripheral nervous system caused by antibody-mediated alteration of the postsynaptic acetylcholine (ACh) receptors at the neuromuscular junction. This results in a reduced ability to depolarize the muscle and the classic fluctuating, fatigable weakness. There is selective vulnerability of the extraocular, bulbar, and proximal limb muscles. All age groups are affected.

Epidemiology

MG is a rare disease. The prevalence rate is approximately 20 in 100 000 and the incidence ranges from 10 cases to 20 cases/million per year. The incidence is higher in men after the age of 50 and in women younger than 40. Before puberty the incidence is equal among the sexes.

Clinical presentation

Classic MG is marked by fluctuating, fatigable weakness either isolated to ocular muscles (ocular MG) or generalized to ocular, bulbar, and limb muscles (generalized MG).

The ocular symptoms of ptosis and diplopia are the presenting feature in 85% of cases; approximately 80% of cases will go on to generalize by 2 years from initial presentation. In patients with restricted ocular symptoms at 2 years, there is a 90% likelihood that they will not generalize.

The typical ptosis of MG is frequently asymmetric and always without pupillary changes.

Patients report blurred vision or double vision that is worse at the end of the day, and improves with rest and when the patient covers one eye. Diplopia and ptosis are elicited by having the patient look upwards or to the side for 2–3 min. The curtain sign is demonstrated when the examiner lifts the more affected eyelid, which results in worsened ptosis on the contralateral, less affected side. Eye closure weakness (e.g. the inability to fully bury the eyelashes) is also frequently observed.

> **SCIENCE REVISITED**
>
> - Of those with MG 85% present with ocular symptoms.
> - The likelihood of progression to generalized MG is low if a patient does not generalize within 2 years of developing ocular symptoms.

Bulbar symptoms are the presenting feature in about 15% of cases. Dysarthria is described as breathy, nasal speech due to palatal weakness, in contrast to the spastic dysarthria of amyotrophic lateral sclerosis (ALS). Patients report liquids escaping through the nose when drinking due to palatal weakness and fatigue with chewing. Weakness of the orbicularis oris muscle causes the classic myasthenic snarl caused by the inabil-

Neuromuscular Disorders, First Edition. Edited by Rabi N. Tawil, Shannon Venance.
© 2011 John Wiley & Sons, Ltd. Published 2011 by John Wiley & Sons, Ltd.

ity to raise the corners of the mouth when attempting to smile.

Neck flexion is typically more affected than neck extension but rare patients can present with a dropped head syndrome. Proximal limb weakness is usually symmetric. Respiratory weakness is not uncommon in severe generalized MG. Myasthenic crisis is due to severe respiratory weakness and/or severe dysphagia and can be potentially fatal without mechanical ventilation and intensive care support.

Pathophysiology

The weakness observed in MG is due to alteration of neuromuscular transmission at the neuromuscular junction, and reduced ability to depolarize muscle caused by elevated serum antibodies against the postsynaptic ACh receptors (seropositive MG). A subset of patients without ACh receptor antibodies has elevated titers of muscle-specific kinase (MuSK) antibodies. MuSK is believed to help cluster ACh receptors at the postsynaptic neuromuscular junction. The development of ACh receptor antibodies is both T- and B-cell dependent. Alteration in neuromuscular transmission in MG is multifactorial and ultimately leads to loss of the normal folded pattern of the postsynaptic membrane.

Thymic pathology is often observed in MG; 65% of individuals with MG have thymic hyperplasia and 10% have a thymoma. Patients with thymoma typically have more severe phenotypes of generalized MG. Most thymomas are encapsulated and amenable to complete resection; occasional highly invasive malignant thymomas are observed.

Diagnosis

The diagnosis of MG requires a combination of clinical history, physical examination, and confirmatory tests. The authors recommend a stepwise approach to diagnosis (Figure 16.1). The differential diagnosis of MG is short (Box 16.1).

History and bedside examination

Obtaining a quality clinical history in suspected MG is imperative because the degree of MG

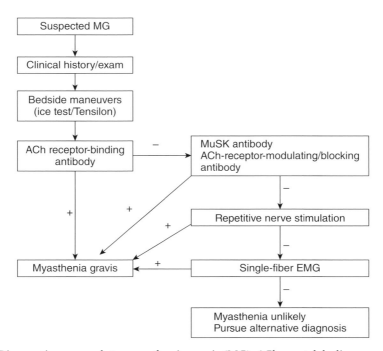

Figure 16.1. Diagnostic approach to myasthenia gravis (MG). ACh, acetylcholine.

Box 16.1. Differential diagnosis of myasthenia gravis

Neuromuscular junction disease
Lambert–Eaton myasthenic syndrome
Botulism
Tick paralysis

Anterior horn cell disease
Amyotrophic lateral sclerosis

Peripheral nerve
Acute inflammatory demyelinating
  polyneuropathy
Chronic inflammatory demyelinating
  polyneuropathy

Myopathy
Ocular pharyngeal muscular dystrophy
Progressive external ophthalmoplegia

weakness fluctuates; an affected patient may have a normal bedside exam in early or partially treated disease. All patients should be asked if they are experiencing the following: diplopia, blurred vision, chewing fatigue, choking, loss of liquids from nose, dysarthria, shortness of breath, and difficulty with repetitive proximal limb tasks (e.g. brushing hair, standing from a chair).

Ice test

The application of an ice bag to the eyelids for 2–5 min can partially or fully resolve ptosis but does not impact other signs of MG, including dysconjugate gaze. The sensitivity ranges from 84% to 92% and specificity from 97% to 98%.

Edrophonium chloride test

Edrophonium chloride (Tensilon) is a short-acting acetylcholinesterase inhibitor that can be administered at the bedside. The medication achieves effect in about 30 s and its duration of action is about 10 min. An initial test dose of 2 mg is injected intravenously. If the patient tolerates the dose, an additional injection of 8 mg is given. A positive result is defined as unequivocal improvement in strength in an involved muscle in 2–5 min. The sensitivity of the test ranges from 60% to 95% in ocular MG and from 71% to 95% in generalized MG.

✋ CAUTION!

Atropine (1–2 mg) should be available during a Tensilon test in case the patient develops the rare complication of severe bradycardia and hypotension.

Laboratory testing

ACh-receptor antibodies

Approximately 70–80% of patients with generalized MG have positive antibodies directed against the ACh receptor. Only about 50% of ocular MG patients have positive ACh-receptor antibodies. The presence of ACh-receptor antibodies is reported to be about 97–98% specific for MG. Occasional false-positive results are reported in patients with asymptomatic thymoma and other autoimmune diseases. In patients with typical symptoms of ocular or generalized MG, positive ACh-receptor antibodies should be considered diagnostic.

★ TIPS AND TRICKS

- ACh-receptor antibodies are 97–98% specific for MG.
- Positive ACh-receptor antibodies are diagnostic in patients with typical symptoms of MG.

MuSK antibodies

Approximately a third of patients with seronegative MG have antibodies directed against MuSK. This is approximately 7% of the total cases of MG and raises the probability of detectable antibodies in generalized MG to 87–90%. Most MuSK-positive patients are females, and MuSK antibodies should be checked only in cases where ACh-receptor antibodies are negative.

Seronegative MG

Antibodies are not detected in 10–13% of generalized MG cases and diagnosis must be confirmed by electrodiagnostic testing.

★ TIPS AND TRICKS

- 10–13% of generalized MG cases have no detectable antibodies.

Electrodiagnostic evaluation

Routine electromyographic (EMG)/nerve conduction studies are useful to exclude non-neuromuscular junction causes of weakness (e.g. ALS, myopathy, chronic inflammatory demyelinating polyneuropathy [CIDP]) and presynaptic neuromuscular junction disease (e.g. Lambert–Eaton myasthenic syndrome and botulism).

Slow repetitive motor nerve stimulation

During repetitive motor nerve stimulation (RNS), a motor nerve is stimulated at 2–5 Hz in trains of six stimulations at rest and then after a period of exercise. This results in depletion of ACh stores at the neuromuscular junction and reduces successful competition of ACh for the limited ACh receptors in MG. It is imperative to test clinically affected muscles to improve the likelihood of a positive result. The sensitivity of RNS ranges from 53% to 100% in generalized MG and 10% to 20% in ocular MG.

Single-fiber EMG

Single-fiber EMG (SFEMG) is the most sensitive test to detect pathology at the neuromuscular junction. Increased variability in the time two muscle fibers of the same motor unit depolarize in relation to each other is observed in MG (jitter).

When facial and limb muscles are examined, SFEMG is reported to be 97% sensitive. A normal SFEMG of a weak muscle performed by an experienced electromyographer essentially excludes the diagnosis of MG.

★ TIPS AND TRICKS

SFEMG has high sensitivity but low specificity for MG, and must be combined with a clinical history and physical exam to establish a diagnosis.

Chest imaging

All patients with seropositive MG should undergo chest computed tomography (CT) or magnetic resonance imaging (MRI) to rule out thymoma. MRI can be substituted in patients in whom CT is contraindicated but does not add to the diagnostic sensitivity.

Treatment

A two-tiered approach is typically employed in the treatment of MG (Table 16.1). Acetylcholinesterase inhibitors, which do not alter disease course, are used to reduce the symptoms of fatigable weakness. Immunosuppressants and thymectomy are employed to modulate the immune system and alter disease course in more severe cases.

Acetylcholinesterase inhibitors

Acetylcholinesterase inhibitors increase the amount of ACh at the neuromuscular junction and increase the likelihood of successful competition with ACh-receptor antibodies for the limited number of ACh receptors in MG. This results in increased strength for short periods of time. Patients with mild disease and purely ocular disease can occasionally be managed with acetylcholinesterase inhibitors alone. Patients with moderate-to-severe disease require immunosuppression. Pyridostigmine is the most common acetylcholinesterase inhibitor (see Table 16.1). The dose and dosing frequency are adjusted to maximize benefit and limit side effects.

Side effects are usually mild and related to excess cholinergic effect (see Table 16.1). Cholinergic crises manifested by muscle weakness are rarely observed in patients taking more than 450 mg daily and can mimic MG exacerbation. Crises are typically accompanied by other cholinergic side effects but are occasionally observed alone.

★ TIPS AND TRICKS

Oral pyridostigmine 60 mg is equivalent to 1.5 mg intramuscular or 0.5 mg intravenous neostigmine.

Corticosteroids

Prednisone and prednisolone (see Table 16.1) are considered first-line immunosuppressant therapy. Improvement in strength usually begins about 2–3 weeks after initiating steroid therapy; full improvement is not observed until after about 3 months of therapy. Patients with severe

Table 16.1. Treatment of myasthenia gravis

Medication	Indication	Dose	Side effects	Monitoring	Prophylaxis
Pyridostimine	Symptomatic management	30 mg three times a day increase to 30–60 mg four to five times a day orally	GI upset Cholinergic effects Cholinergic crisis	None	None
Prednisone	Maintenance immunosuppression	60 mg/day oral Slow taper with improvement	Bone loss, gastric ulcers, weight gain, hyperglycemia, cataracts, hypertension Exacerbation at initiation of treatment	DXA pre-treatment Blood pressure/Glucose monitoring	Vitamin D/Calcium Bisphosphonate (consider) Proton pump inhibitor or H_2-receptor blocker Low-fat diet
Azathioprine	Maintenance immunosuppression	50 mg/day increase to 2.5 mg/kg per day	Myelosuppression Hepatitis Idiosyncratic reaction Nausea/Vomiting	CBC with differential monthly Hepatic enzymes monthly	None
Mycophenolate mofetil	Maintenance immunosuppression	1000–1500 mg every 12 h	Myelosuppression Diarrhea/Abdominal pain	CBC with differential monthly for 1 year then every 3 months	None
Cyclosporine	Maintenance immunosuppression	25 mg/kg every 12 h	Nephrotoxicity Hypertension Drug interactions	Creatinine/GFR monthly Blood pressure	None
IVIG	Immunosuppression with exacerbation or refractory disease	1–2 g/kg i.v. divided over 2–5 days	Renal failure Thrombosis/Stroke Aseptic meningitis Volume overload Fever Headache	1. Allergic reaction during first infusion	Pre-treatment diphenhydramine/ acetaminophen
Plasma exchange	Immunosuppression with exacerbation or refractory disease	1–2 plasma volumes every other day for 4–6 treatments	Volume overload Intravenous line infection/thrombosis	1. Infusion center 2. Blood pressure	1. Meticulous line care

CBC, complete blood count; DXA, dual energy X-ray absorptiometry; GFR, glomerular filtration rate; GI, gastrointestinal; IVIG, intravenous weakness, especially of bulbar muscles often require intravenous immunoglobulin (IVIG) or plasma exchange before starting prednisone because initiation of corticosteroid therapy can initially increase myasthenic weakness in up to 15% of patients. The most common strategy of corticosteroid therapy involves the use of high-dose prednisone until the patient achieves significant improvement, followed by a slow taper to the lowest possible dose without return of symptoms. Treatment is limited by long-term side effects (see Table 16.1).

Azathioprine

Azathioprine (AZA; see Table 16.1) is converted to the active metabolite, 6-mercaptopurine, which blocks nucleotide synthesis and reduces T-cell proliferation. AZA was primarily studied as an adjunctive therapy with corticosteroids and was shown to reduce both relapses during steroid taper and the dose of steroid needed to maintain remission. Some clinicians use AZA as monotherapy, especially in patients in whom steroids are contraindicated. The primary limiting factor to AZA monotherapy is the long duration (about 9 months) needed before seeing an effect of the medication; maximal benefit is not observed until after about 18 months.

Potential side effects (see Table 16.1) require monitoring of a monthly comprehensive blood count and hepatic profile. An allergic idiosyncratic reaction, manifest by flu-like symptoms while taking AZA ,is observed in 15% of patients within 3 weeks of starting treatment. AZA should be discontinued and not restarted if this reaction is observed because it recurs in all patients with re-challenge.

Mycophenolate mofetil

Mycophenolate mofetil (MMF; see Table 16.1) selectively blocks purine synthesis in B and T cells by inhibiting the action of inosine-5-monophosphate dehydrogenase. Similar to AZA, MMF is typically employed as an adjunctive therapy to prednisone. However, some clinicians use MMF as monotherapy in selected patients.

Two randomized controlled trials did not demonstrate additional benefits of adjunctive MMF over prednisone alone as initial immunosuppression in generalized MG or a steroid-sparing effect over a period of 9 months. A subsequent, nonconflicting, long-duration, retrospective analysis suggests that MMF may be an effective therapy in MG as an adjunctive agent to prednisone, and as monotherapy after the second and third year of therapy. Based on these results, other retrospective analyses, and clinical experience, the authors continue to use MMF in the treatment of their MG patients.

Potential side effects (see Table 16.1) require following routine monthly blood counts for 1 year and then every 3 months for subsequent years.

Cyclosporine

Cyclosporine (see Table 16.1) blocks interleukin-2 and inhibits CD4 helper-T cell proliferation. It is an effective adjunctive therapy to prednisone in MG. Its use is limited by its unfavorable side-effect profile (see Table 16.1) and interaction with other medications. Clinical benefit is usually observed after 6 months with maximal benefit observed in the second and third years of treatment.

Pooled intravenous immunoglobulin

The mechanism of IVIG (see Table 16.1) in autoimmune disease is unknown. It is believed to reduce circulating pathological antibodies. Due to cost and the need for intravenous infusion, IVIG is employed in patients experiencing increased weakness while on other immunosuppressive agents or in those who have developed a myasthenic exacerbation or crisis. Maximal benefit is typically observed over 1–2 weeks. The duration of effect is variable but likely persists at least 1 month. The typical dose is 1–2 g/kg in divided doses over 2–5 days. Severe side effects (see Table 16.1) require close patient monitoring and education before instituting therapy.

Plasma exchange

Plasma exchange (PLEX; see Table 16.1) removes patient plasma containing pathological antibodies and exchanges it with antibody-free fresh frozen plasma or albumin. Rapid improvement in MG weakness occurs over days and lasts for several weeks. PLEX is reserved for treatment of severe myasthenic exacerbation and crisis. A randomized trial of MG exacerbation found PLEX and IVIG to be equally effective. The decision to choose one over the other revolves around side-effect profiles and availability. Again, side effects (see Table 16.1) require close patient monitoring.

Thymectomy

Thymectomy is indicated in all patients with MG-associated thymoma. Thymectomy may also be of benefit in patients with associated thymic hyperplasia. Benefit may be delayed for years and timing of surgery is debated. Thymectomy is not usually recommended in patients over age 60. Many clinicians pre-treat patients scheduled for thymectomy with a course of PLEX; this is especially important in patients with active bulbar and respiratory involvement.

☟ CAUTION!

DRUGS THAT MAY CAUSE MG EXACERBATION:

- Aminoglycoside antibiotics
- Other antibiotics: erythromycin, ciprofloxacin, azithromycin
- β-Blocking agents
- Botulinum toxin
- Interferon-α
- Calcium channel blockers
- Magnesium, magnesium salts contained in some laxatives and antacids
- Quinine, quinidine, procainamide
- Neuromuscular blocking agents such as succinylcholine, vecuronium, curare-like agents
- Iodinated contrast agents
- Penicillamine
- Eyedrops used in the management of glaucoma: timolol, betaxolol hydrochloride, echothiopate

Special circumstances

Myasthenic crisis/exacerbation

The goal of therapy during acute exacerbations of MG is to rapidly improve weakness and to avoid progression to respiratory failure (e.g. myasthenic crisis). Clinicians can follow serial measurements of forced vital capacity, negative inspiratory force, and maximal numbers able to be counted in a single breath to help establish a trend in the respiratory status and guide the decision to pursue intubation.

Patients are typically treated with a course of either PLEX or IVIG. A long-term immunosuppressant should be added if a patient is not already on one. Management of the acute MG patient may require transfer to a center with experience managing these patients and with available intensive care.

Ocular MG

Treatment of purely ocular MG (isolated ptosis/diplopia) is evolving. Retrospective data suggest that patients treated with prednisone show greater improvement than those treated with acetylcholinesterase inhibitors alone, and that early use of prednisone may delay or prevent progression to generalized MG. The choice to employ immunosuppression in these patients varies among clinicians.

MuSK-positive MG

MuSK-positive MG patients have a unique response to treatment. Acetylcholinesterase inhibitors are less effective and may be associated with acute worsening and generalized fasciculations. The best response is observed with prednisone and PLEX therapies. Indication for thymectomy in this subgroup is unclear.

Pregnancy

The peak incidence of MG in women occurs during childbearing years (mean age of onset 28). New-onset MG has been observed in the partum and postpartum periods. MG exacerbation is observed in a third of pregnant patients and is most common in the first trimester. Management of MG must be adjusted during pregnancy to account for changes in maternal physiology as well as the health of the fetus. We recommend that all pregnant MG patients deliver at a major medical center with a neonatal intensive care unit due to the risks of transient neonatal MG and arthrogryposis from passive transfer of ACh-receptor antibodies.

Prognosis

Approximately 20% of patients with MG experience spontaneous remission without need for immunosuppression. It is difficult to predict which patients will enter remission. Some clinicians attempt to wean immunosuppression if patients remain asymptomatic for 1 year.

Bibliography

AAEM Quality Assurance Committee. Literature review of the usefulness of repetitive nerve stimulation and single fiber EMD in the electrodiagnostic evaluation of patients with suspected myasthenia gravis or Lambert Eaton myasthenic syndrome. *Muscle Nerve* 2001;**24**: 1239–47.

Bhanushali MJ, Wuu J, Benatar M. Treatment of ocular symptoms in myasthenia gravis. *Neurology* 2008;**71**:1335–41.

Ciafaloni E, Massey JM. Myasthenia gravis and pregnancy. *Neurol Clin* 2004;**22**:771–82.

Gajdos P, Chevret S, Clair B, Tranchant C, Chastang C, for the Myasthenia Gravis Study Group. Clinical trial of plasma exchange and high-dose intravenous immunoglobulin in myasthenia gravis. *Ann Neurol* 1997;**41**:789–96.

Grob D, Brunner N, Namba T, Pagala M. Lifetime course of myasthenia gravis. *Muscle and Nerve* 2008;**37**:141–9.

Hehir MK, Burns TM, Alpers J, Conaway MR, Sawa M, Sanders DB. Mycophenolate mofetil in AChR-antibody-positive myasthenia gravis: outcomes in 102 patients. *Muscle Nerve* 2010; **41**:593–8.

Juel VC, Massey JM. Myasthenia gravis. *Orphanet J Rare Dis* 2007;**2**:44.

Meriggioli MN, Sanders DB. Autoimmune myasthenia gravis: emerging clinical and biological heterogeneity. *Lancet Neurol* 2009;**8**: 475–90.

The Muscle Study Group. A trial of mycophenolate mofetil with prednisone as initial immunotherapy in myasthenia gravis. *Neurology* 2008;**71**:394–9.

Palace J, Newsom-Davis J, Lecky B, for Myasthenia Study Group. A randomized double-blind trial of prednisolone alone or with azathioprine in myasthenia gravis. *Neurology* 1998;**50**: 1778–83.

Pascuzzi, RM, Coslett HB. Johns Long-term corticosteroid treatment of myasthenia gravis: Report of 116 patients. *Ann Neurol* TR. 1984;**15**: 291–8.

Pasnoor M, Wolfe GI, Nations S, et al. Clinical findings in MuSK- antibody positive myasthenia gravis: a U.S. experience. *Muscle Nerve* 2010;**41**:370–4.

Phillips LH. The epidemiology of myasthenia gravis. *Ann NY Acad Sci* 2003;**998**:407–12.

Sanders DB, Hart IK, Mantegazza R, et al. An international, phase III, randomized trial of mycophenolate mofetil in myasthenia gravis. *Neurology* 2008;**71**:400–6.

Tindall RS, Phillips JT, Rollins JA, Wells L, Hall K. A clinical therapeutic trial of cyclosporine in myasthenia gravis. *Ann NY Acad Sci* 1993l;**681**: 539–51.

Botulism

Nikhil Balakrishnan[1] and Matthew N. Meriggioli[2]

[1]Wake Forest University Baptist Medical Center, Winston Salem, NC, USA
[2]Division of Neuromuscular Medicine, University of Illinois College of Medicine, Chicago, IL, USA

Botulism is a paralytic illness caused by neurotoxins secreted by anaerobic spore-forming bacilli of the genus *Clostridium*. *Clostridium botulinum* is responsible for the vast majority of human infections, with rare cases being caused by *Clostridium baratii* (type F toxin) and *Clostridium butyricum* (type E toxin). Botulinum toxins are among the most potent toxins known to humans, with the lethal dose of the type A toxin estimated to be 1 ng/kg,

Pathogenesis of botulism

The clinical effects of *Clostridium botulinum* infection are mediated entirely by the toxin, the actions of which are limited to blockade of the peripheral cholinergic nerve terminals (Figure 17.1). The sites of action of the toxin are located not only at the axon terminals of the neuromuscular junction, but also at autonomic ganglia and parasympathetic nerve terminals.

The toxin is initially synthesized as a single-chain polypeptide and is subsequently cleaved to yield a heavy chain linked by a disulfide bond to a light chain. After endocytosis, the disulfide bond is cleaved separating the chains. The N terminus of the light chain is the active proteolytic site responsible for cleavage of SNARE (SNAP (**s**oluble **N**SF **a**ttachment **p**rotein) **re**ceptor) proteins and the resultant permanent inhibition of acetylcholine (ACh) release. Recovery occurs only when the axon sprouts another nerve terminal to re-establish synaptic transmission.

Clinical features of botulism

Exposure to botulinum toxin occurs through the following mechanisms:

1. Ingestion of pre-formed toxin (food-borne botulism)
2. Local production of toxin by *C. botulinum* organisms at the site of a penetrating wound (wound botulism)
3. Local production of toxin by *C. botulinum* in the gastrointestinal tract (infant botulism and adult intestinal botulism)
4. Inhalation of pre-formed toxin (inhalational botulism)
5. Inadvertent systemic exposure to the toxin during injection for therapeutic or cosmetic reasons (iatrogenic botulism).

The classic clinical presentation for botulism is an acutely evolving symmetrical, descending motor paralysis with autonomic symptoms in an alert patient, with no sensory deficits.

Classic botulism (food-borne botulism)

Almost all human cases of food-borne botulism are caused by A, B, and E strains. The geographical distribution parallels the distribution of

Neuromuscular Disorders, First Edition. Edited by Rabi N. Tawil, Shannon Venance.

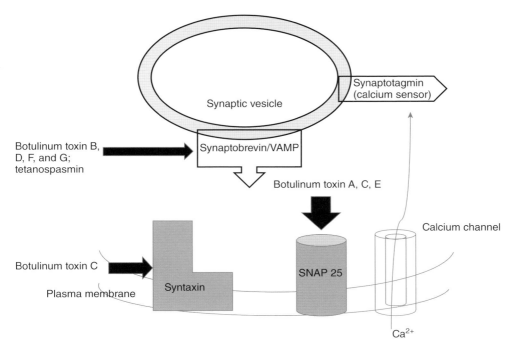

Figure 17.1. SNARE proteins involved in the docking of synaptic vesicles and the release of acetylcholine (ACh). The increase in free Ca^{2+} triggers the interaction between vesicle-bound synaptotagmin which acts as a Ca^{2+} sensor and presynaptic membrane-bound syntaxin, thus clamping the vesicle to the presynaptic membrane. SNAP-25 is cleaved by types A, C, and E toxin. Syntaxin is cleaved by type E toxin and synaptobrevin is the target of types B, D, F, and G toxins. VAMP, vehicle-associated membrane protein.

spores with type A predominating in western USA and type B predominating in north-eastern and central USA. Marine food products account for 91% of type E outbreaks. Type A infections cause more severe illness. The most common sources of infection are home-canned (preserved) vegetables, fruit, and fish. Prevention of food-borne botulism requires killing the bacterium with heating to at least 120°C for 5 min, preferably in a high pressure setting. In contrast to the spores, the toxins are heat labile and inactivated by heating to 85°C for a minimum of 5 min.

The incubation period typically ranges from 12 h to 72 h. The illness may sometimes be so mild that no medical attention is sought, and not all people who ingest the contaminated food become symptomatic. The initial symptoms are typically gastrointestinal with nausea, vomiting, diarrhea, and abdominal cramping. Presenting neurological signs and symptoms are referable to extraocular and bulbar weakness and include blurring of vision, ptosis, diplopia, ophthalmoplegia, dysarthria, and dysphagia. This is followed by a characteristic bilateral, symmetric, descending paralysis with weakness of the upper limbs followed by truncal and lower extremity weakness and autonomic dysfunction. Respiratory compromise may occur due to upper airway obstruction and/or to diaphragmatic weakness. There are typically no sensory symptoms.

★ **TIPS AND TRICKS**

- Botulism differs from other flaccid paralyses in that it always manifests initially with prominent cranial paralysis, it invariably has a descending progression,

and there is an absence of sensory symptoms or signs.
- Prominent oculobulbar and facial weakness are early manifestations with pupillary abnormalities in 50%.
- Patients are afebrile unless a concurrent infection is present.
- Nausea, vomiting, and diarrhea often precede or accompany neurological manifestations in food-borne botulism.

Wound botulism

Wound botulism is caused by infection of a contaminated wound with *C. botulinum* (a natural contaminant of soil throughout the USA), with subsequent absorption of locally produced toxin into the circulation. First reported almost exclusively in patients with traumatic and surgical wounds, it is more recently associated with injection drug users, and in particular with subcutaneous injection of heroin in a method called "skin popping," designed to slowly release the drug. Infection is believed to result from *C. botulinum* spores contaminating the heroin. After injection, the spores germinate in an anaerobic tissue environment and release toxin. The presence of skin abscesses may suggest the diagnosis, but the clinical diagnosis is often challenging. Maxillary sinusitis associated with intranasal cocaine use has rarely been the source of wound botulism. The clinical syndrome of wound botulism closely resembles classic botulism, save for the absence of gastrointestinal symptoms. The diagnosis is established by detection of the organism in the wound or toxin from the circulation.

Infant botulism

Infant botulism is caused by ingestion of *C. botulinum* spores, which colonize the gastrointestinal tract and produce toxin that is absorbed into the circulation. The source of spores in most cases is unknown, although the more common sources of infection for infants appear to be honey and environmental exposure. The age of onset is between 3 weeks and 8 months, with most cases occurring before the age of 6 years. The disease characteristically begins with lethargy and poor feeding, usually accompanied by constipation. This is typically followed by weakness of bulbar and limb muscles, hypotonia, loss of head control, poor sucking ability, and decreased movements. Autonomic involvement is common with constipation, tachycardia, hypotension, neurogenic bladder, and dry mouth.

Adult intestinal botulism

The pathogenesis of adult intestinal botulism is similar to that of infant botulism. Only a few cases have been recognized, and most have occurred postoperatively, or in adults with underlying pathology of the gastrointestinal tract causing an alteration of the normal gut flora, including prior antimicrobial therapy, achlorhydria, Crohn's disease, or surgery. Diagnosis is established by isolation of the organism or toxin from fecal samples.

Inhalational botulism

This form of botulism is caused by inhalation of aerosolized, pre-formed toxin which is absorbed into the circulation through the lungs. The use of aerosolized toxin as an agent of bioterrorism has the potential to lead to high numbers of casualties.

Iatrogenic botulism

This refers to generalized weakness or autonomic dysfunction related to the use of botulinum toxin as a therapeutic agent.

Differential diagnosis

The diagnosis should be suspected in an alert patient presenting with an acute onset of descending, painless paralysis without sensory involvement. Clinical suspicion may be increased in the case of an outbreak where there is a history of a common source of food exposure. The differential diagnosis for botulism may be systematically broken down into central, peripheral nerve, neuromuscular junction, and muscular causes as shown in Table 17.1.

Given the widespread pure motor dysfunction, three broad categories of disorders should be considered: myopathy, motor neuropathy/neuronopathy, and neuromuscular junction disease. Few myopathies produce rapidly pro-

Table 17.1. Diagnostic considerations in a patient presenting with acute weakness with prominent ocular/bulbar involvement

Etiology	Distinguishing features/Ancillary tests
Central nervous system Brain-stem strokes Demyelination Rhombencephalitis/Infections Thiamin deficiency	Altered sensorium, long tract signs, upgoing toes, abnormalities of hearing, facial sensory loss; nystagmus and ataxia if present would be incompatible with botulism and suggest CNS/alternate etiology. Test: MRI of the brain, lumbar puncture
Anterior horn hell Poliomyelitis West Nile virus	Fever, meningeal signs. Classically asymmetric flaccid paralysis. CSF pleocytosis. West Nile serology

Peripheral nerve
a. Guillian–Barré syndrome (GBS)[a]
b. Miller-Fisher syndrome[a]
c. Heavy metal poisoning[a]
d. Lyme disease
e. Tick paralysis
f. Diphtheria
g. Porphyria
h. Critical illness neuropathy/myopathy
i. Sarcoidosis
j. Marine poisoning:
  saxitoxin
  tetrodotoxin
  ciguatera toxin
	a. GBS is usually associated with sensory symptoms at onset. NCS/EMG shows demyelination. LP: albuminocytological dissociation
	b. Ataxia, anti-GQ1b antibodies in Miller-Fisher syndrome
	c. Urine, blood heavy metal screen
	d. Lyme serology, CSF Lyme PCR, CSF studies
	e. Usually children. Search skin for tick exposure
	f. Check for tonsillar exudates, culture
	g. Porphyria screen
	h. Neuropathic/myopathic findings in light of severe systemic illness, steroid use
	i. Radicular pattern, sensory involvement. Chest radiograph/imaging, serum ACE levels, MRI of the brain and spine as indicated. CSF studies
	j. Prominent sensory symptoms, pure motor presentation is very unusual

Neuromuscular junction a. Myasthenia gravis[a] b. Lambert–Eaton syndrome[a] c. Aminoglycosides, neuromuscular blocking agents (drugs, venoms, Mg^{2+}) d. Organophosphate poisoning	a, b. Subacute/chronic onset. Areflexia may be seen in LES but not in MG. NCS/EMG may show a decrement with repetitive nerve stimulation in MG and LEMS. Low baseline CMAPs with prominent facilitation seen with the latter. Serological studies: anti-AChR, anti-MuSK, anti-voltage-gated calcium channel antibodies maybe helpful. Organophosphate poisoning shows prominent oral/respiratory secretions, pinpoint pupils
Muscle disease a. Polymyositis[a] b. Dermatomyositis[a] c. Periodic paralysis d. Muscular dystrophy (oculopharyngeal muscular dystrophy, mitochondrial disorders)	Elevated serum creatine kinase in (a, b). NCS/EMG shows prominent spontaneous activity and myopathic features on EMG (c) Serum hypokalemia/hyperkalemia. History of repeated episodes with recovery in between. Respiratory, autonomic, extraocular involvement extremely rare Muscular dystrophies have normal pupillary reflexes, diplopia is rare

[a]More common etiologies.
ACE, angiotensin-converting enzyme; AChR, acetylcholine receptor; CMAP, compound muscle action potential; CNS, central nervous system; CSF, cerebrospinal fluid; EMG, electromyography; LEMS, Lambert–Eaton myasthenic syndrome; LES, Lambert–Eaton syndrome; LP, lumbar puncture; MG, myasthenia gravis; MRI, magnetic resonance imaging; NCS, nerve conduction studies; PCR, polymerase chain reaction.

gressive weakness and early bulbar/respiratory signs. Although the periodic paralyses may cause acute paralysis, involvement of ocular and facial muscles is rare.

The presence of sensory symptoms, prodromal viral or diarrheal illness, and an ascending pattern of weakness suggests Guillain–Barré syndrome (GBS). However, early in the course, it may be difficult to differentiate some GBS variants, such as the Miller-Fisher syndrome (MFS) or the cervical–pharyngeal–brachial variant, from botulism. Anti-GQ1b antibodies may be helpful in this clinical scenario, but results of testing may be delayed. Electrophysiological testing (showing the typical findings of demyelination) is required to rule out GBS or MFS. Tick paralysis classically has an ascending pattern resembling GBS and a careful search of the skin, especially the scalp, for tick exposure helps make the diagnosis. Poliomyelitis and West Nile infections usually cause asymmetric weakness, in association with a febrile onset and signs of meningeal irritation.

The neuromuscular junction transmission disorders – myasthenia gravis (MG) and Lambert–Eaton syndrome (LES) – resemble botulism in that they result in weakness caused by abnormal neuromuscular transmission. In addition to weakness, areflexia and autonomic involvement are common to both LES and botulism, but, in LES, cranial nerve involvement is typically not conspicuous and respiratory failure is rare. The facilitation/potentiation of muscle stretch reflexes, reported in LES, has not been observed in botulism. In MG, reflexes are typically preserved unless there is severe limb weakness. Serological studies for MG, and for LES, if positive, help make the distinction. The major distinguishing feature is that MG and LES present in a subacute to chronic manner while botulism is acute and progresses precipitously. Hypermagnesemia or the administration of other drugs adversely affecting neuromuscular transmission may cause rapid neuromuscular blockade, but is ruled out by the history.

Diagnosis of botulism

The clinical diagnosis of botulism is supported by electrophysiological and microbiological studies. Important investigations that should be normal in botulism include: complete blood count (CBC), imaging of the brain and spinal cord, and cerebrospinal fluid (CSF) glucose, protein, and cell count.

Electrophysiological findings in botulism

A low-amplitude compound muscle action potential (CMAP) in a clinically weak muscle is seen in up to 85% of botulism cases. However, the sensitivity of this finding may be as low as 50% when testing is limited to distal muscles routinely performed in the electromyography (EMG) laboratory. A decremental response (>10% reduction in amplitude or area) on slow repetitive nerve stimulation (2–5 Hz) is seen in both presynaptic and postsynaptic disorders of the neuromuscular junction, including botulism (Figure 17.2). Post-tetanic facilitation, after 10 s of maximal isometric exercise or with high-frequency repetitive stimulation at 30–50 Hz is seen in up to 62% of botulism cases. The degree of facilitation is modest, typically ranging from 20% to 60%, whereas facilitation in LES is typically 100–300%.

Needle EMG shows motor units with myopathic features or mixed myopathic–neuropathic features in more severe cases. Single-fiber EMG shows evidence of increased jitter and blocking in virtually all cases of botulism, but increased jitter is not specific for botulism. The finding of normal jitter in a clinically weak muscle effectively excludes a disorder of neuromuscular transmission.

Microbiological diagnosis of botulism

Establishing a microbiological diagnosis involves detection of the toxin in samples from serum, stool, gastric aspirate, and wound aspirate. The gold standard for laboratory diagnosis remains the mouse lethality assay. The test is expensive, restricted to a few specialized centers, and results are delayed. False-positive and false-negative results are reported and a negative test does not exclude the diagnosis. Alternate immunological methods remain investigational. Polymerase chain reaction (PCR) assays are used for the detection of *C. botulinum* toxin genes in food and fecal samples.

Detection of toxin in the stool, serum, or wound, and isolation of *C. botulinum* using anaerobic culture methods from relevant samples, are methods for making the diagnosis of infant, wound, and adult intestinal botulism.

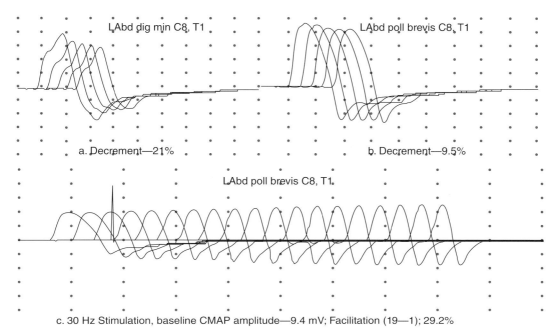

Figure 17.2. Top: repetitive nerve stimulation at 3 Hz of the left abductor digiti minimi (Abd Dig Min) and left abductor pollicis brevis (Abd Poll Brevis) muscles. Bottom: high-frequency repetitive nerve stimulation showing modest pseudofacilitation in the abductor pollicis brevis muscle.

In suspected inhalational cases the toxin is believed to be present for up to 24 hours in upper airway secretions; however, the utility of nasopharyngeal secretions in establishing the diagnosis is unknown.

Treatment of botulism

Botulism is a reportable disease. Clinicians should be familiar with state, provincial, or country reporting requirements, emergency contact numbers, and, if indicated, the process for release of antitoxin.

The cornerstones of treatment remain supportive care and early administration of antitoxin. The case fatality rate is approximately 15% for wound botulism, approaches 5% for food-borne cases, and is less than 5% for infant botulism. Death usually occurs from respiratory failure or from complications such as pneumonia.

Supportive care

All patients should be admitted to the intensive care unit (ICU) for monitoring of upper airway patency and respiratory function. The decision to intubate and institute mechanical ventilation should be made on an individual basis by monitoring of upper airway patency and deterioration of respiratory flow volumes and pressures. Arterial hypoxemia and hypercapnia occur late in impending respiratory failure and are insensitive for guiding decisions about intubation. Supportive management of blood pressure, urinary retention, and constipation is needed with autonomic failure. In food-borne cases, purgatives and activated charcoal may be administered if there is concern for residual unabsorbed toxin in the gastrointestinal tract.

Administration of antitoxin

The decision to administer antitoxin should be made early (within first 24 h) in suspected cases without waiting for laboratory confirmation, because the antitoxin neutralizes circulating toxin but has no effect on internalized and bound toxin. Antitoxin use does not ameliorate established weakness, but may help prevent progression. In the USA, antitoxin is made available by the Centers for Disease Control (CDC) through the state and local public health departments. In the USA, licensed bivalent equine antiserum against types A, B, and an investigational monovalent type E antiserum are available through the CDC. In cases where the type of toxin is unknown, it is recommended that all three types be administered. The bivalent A and B antitoxin or monovalent E antitoxin can be administered in cases where the type has been identified.

✋ CAUTION!

During administration of antitoxin, the following reactions may occur:

- Anaphylaxis
- Thermal reactions (usually occurring 20 min to 1 h after administration and characterized by chills, dyspnea, and a rapid rise in temperature)
- Serum sickness (occurring within 14 days after administration and characterized by fever, urticaria or a maculopapular rash, arthritis, or arthralgias, and lymphadenopathy).

Skin testing for hypersensitivity should be performed on all patients before they receive antitoxin. If skin testing is positive, the patient can be desensitized over several hours before the full dose of antitoxin is administered.

Diphenhydramine and epinephrine should be available during administration of antitoxin, and the patient should be kept under careful observation for 1–2 h after administration (then under close surveillance for a full 24 h).

Hypersensitivity reactions including urticaria, serum sickness, febrile reactions, and anaphylaxis are reported in 9% of cases. Diphenhydramine and epinephrine should be available during administration. Botulism immune globulin (BIG-IV) is a bivalent human antiserum approved by the Food and Drug Administration (FDA) in 2003 for the treatment of infant botulism. BIG-IV is available through the California Department of Health Services. A 5-year, randomized, double-blind, placebo-controlled trial of BIG-IV demonstrated reduced duration of hospital stay, ICU stay, duration of mechanical ventilation, and duration of tube/intravenous feeding.

Additional aspects of treatment

Antibiotics are not indicated in classic and infant botulism, and may worsen illness in infants not treated with BIG-IV due to systemic absorption of toxins released into the gut from bacterial lysis. In all cases, aminoglycosides and macrolides should be avoided in treatment of secondary infections to prevent further deleterious effects on neuromuscular transmission. Wound debridement should be performed in all cases of wound botulism and antibiotics should be given after administration of antitoxin to prevent worsening of symptoms from toxins released from antibiotic-induced bacterial lysis. Acetylcholinesterase inhibitors are not usually beneficial although 3,4-diaminopyridine may improve strength but not respiratory function.

Conclusion

Botulism is a life-threatening infection caused by neurotoxins secreted by *Clostridium botulinum*. Diagnosis is based on the clinical history and physical examination, with supporting evidence from electrophysiological and laboratory studies. Close coordination with regulatory health authorities is necessary to establish the diagnosis and to initiate prompt administration of antitoxin. Effective treatment involves not only early administration of antitoxin, but high-quality supportive treatment in an intensive care setting. Depending on the initial severity of illness, recovery may be quite prolonged, with many patients continuing to have symptoms a year or longer after the onset of illness.

Bibliography

Arnon SS, Schechter R, Maslanka SE, Jewell NP, Hatheway CL. Human botulism immune globulin for the treatment of infant botulism. *N Engl J Med* 2006;**354**:445–7.

Bleck TP. *Clostridium botulinum* (botulism). In: Mandell GL, Bennett JE, Dolin R (eds), *Principles and Practice of Infectious Diseases*, 5th edn. Philadelphia, PA: Churchill Livingstone, 2000: 2443–548.

Cherrington M. Clinical spectrum of botulism. *Muscle Nerve* 1998;**21**:701–10.

Centers for Disease Control and Prevention. *Botulism: Treatment overview for clinicians.* Online. Available at: www.bt.cdc.gov/agent/Botulism/clinicians/treatment.asp (accessed July 26, 2010).

Center for Infectious Disease Research and Policy (CIDRAP). *Botulism: Current, comprehensive information on pathogenesis, microbiology, epidemiology, diagnosis, and treatment*, 2009. Online. Available at: www.cidrap.umn.edu/cidrap/content/bt/botulism/index.html (accessed July 31, 2010).

Davis LE, King MK. Wound botulism from heroin skin popping. *Curr Neurol Neurosci Rep* 2008;**8**: 462–8.

Gupta A, Sumner CJ, Castor M, et al. Adult botulism type F in the United States, 1981–2002. *Neurology* 2005;**65**:1694–700.

Juel VC, Bleck TP. Botulism. In: Fink MP, Abraham E, Vincent J-L, Kochanek PM (eds), *Textbook of Critical Care*, 5th edn. Philadelphia, PA: Elsevier Saunders, 2005: 1405–10.

Kongsaengdao S, Samintarapanya K, Rusmeechan S, et al. Electrophysiological diagnosis and patterns of response to treatment of botulism with neuromuscular respiratory failure. *Muscle Nerve* 2009;**40**:271–8.

Lindstrom M, Korkeala H. Laboratory diagnosis of botulism. *Clin Microbiol Rev* 2006;**19**: 298–314.

Maselli RA. Pathogenesis of human botulism. *Ann N Y Acad Sci* 1998;**841**:122–39.

Maselli RA, Bakshi N. Botulism. *Muscle Nerve* 2000;**23**:1137–44.

Padua L, Aprile I, Monaco ML, et al. Neurophysiological assessment in the diagnosis of botulism: usefulness of single fiber EMG. *Muscle Nerve* 1999;**22**:1388–92.

Souyah N, Karim H, Kamin SS *et al.* (2006) Severe botulism after focal injection of botulinum toxin. *Neurology.* **67**(10), 1855–1856.

Department of Public Health, California. Botulism, 2005. Online. Available at: www.sfcdcp.org/botulism.html#providers (accessed July 26, 2010).

Lambert–Eaton Myasthenic Syndrome

Michael W. Nicolle

Department of Clinical Neurological Sciences, University of Western Ontario, and Myasthenia Gravis Clinic, University Hospital, London, ON, Canada

Pathophysiology

To understand the diagnosis and treatment of Lambert–Eaton myasthenic syndrome (LEMS), it is helpful to understand neuromuscular transmission (NMT). Voltage-gated calcium channel (VGCC) antibodies reduce Ca^{2+} influx into the presynaptic nerve terminal, resulting in NMT failure at muscle fibers and cholinergic transmission failure at autonomic synapses. The effects of VGCC antibodies are transiently overcome by increasing presynaptic nerve terminal Ca^{2+} content after high-frequency nerve depolarization, which increases acetylcholine (ACh) release. Thus, a maximal voluntary contraction (MVC) of muscle or high-frequency stimulation (HFS) of nerves in the electromyography (EMG) lab explains the clinical phenomenon of a transient increase in deep tendon reflexes and perhaps strength after an MVC, and the characteristic electrophysiological findings in LEMS (see below). In approximately half of LEMS cases, an underlying malignancy is found, with a small cell lung cancer (SCLC) in most paraneoplastic LEMS (P-LEMS). Non-paraneoplastic LEMS (NP-LEMS) is a primary autoimmune disease.

> ### 🔬 SCIENCE REVISITED
>
> **NEUROMUSCULAR TRANSMISSION**
> The steps involved in neuromuscular transmission are:
>
> - Motor nerve depolarization produces action potentials
> - **Sodium** enters the nerve through voltage-gated sodium channels
> - Repolarization of motor nerves, stopping action potential propagation
> - **Potassium** leaves the nerve through voltage-gated potassium channels
> - Opening of presynaptic nerve terminal VGCCs in response to nerve terminal depolarization, allowing calcium to enter the nerve terminal
> - Migration and exocytosis of ACh-containing vesicles
> - Binding of released ACh to ACh receptors (AChR) on the muscle surface
> - ACh binds transiently to the AChR before being released and metabolized by acetylcholinesterase (AChE), or diffusing away

Neuromuscular Disorders, First Edition. Edited by Rabi N. Tawil, Shannon Venance.
© 2011 John Wiley & Sons, Ltd. Published 2011 by John Wiley & Sons, Ltd.

- Opening of AChRs, cation influx (mainly sodium) and muscle membrane depolarization
- Nerve depolarization produces the release of about 100 vesicles which is measured on the muscle surface as an end-plate potential (EPP)
- If the EPP is of sufficient amplitude an all-or-none muscle fiber action potential is generated
- Excitation–contraction coupling and muscle contraction

OTHER IMPORTANT PHENOMENA

- The generation of a muscle fiber action potential depends on the product of pre- and postsynaptic events:

[ACh released] × [Available muscle surface AChRs].

- An excess of released ACh and available AChRs constitutes the "safety factor" of neuromuscular transmission.
- A reduction in either of these may result in neuromuscular transmission failure at a muscle fiber.
- If NMT fails at sufficient numbers of muscle fibers, the compound muscle action potential (CMAP) amplitude will be reduced and the muscle will be weak.
- High-frequency nerve depolarization (during a maximal voluntary contraction or with high-frequency [20–50 Hz] repetitive nerve stimulation [RNS]) increases nerve terminal calcium. This increases ACh release if this is a limiting factor.
- With low-frequency nerve depolarization (e.g. 3 Hz RNS), ACh release is gradually reduced, reaching its nadir at the fourth or fifth stimulation. Other ACh stores are then mobilized and ACh release increases again. If the reduction in released ACh causes the product of [released ACh available × AChRs] to fall below the safety factor – neuromuscular transmission fails at that muscle fiber.

Clinical features

Although overlapping somewhat with myasthenia gravis (MG), LEMS has distinctive symptoms and signs (Table 18.1) with gradual onset over months or even years. P-LEMS may have a more rapid progression and be associated with recent weight loss. However, P-LEMS and NP-LEMS are otherwise indistinguishable clinically. The cardinal features of LEMS are weakness, usually predominantly affecting the proximal legs and producing gait problems, areflexia or hyporeflexia, and autonomic dysfunction. Subjective gait problems and leg weakness are often more than the objective weakness of individual muscle groups would suggest, underlying the "3 As" of LEMS: gait apraxia, areflexia, and autonomic involvement.

Weakness

Present in at least two-thirds of patients initially, almost all LEMS patients eventually develop proximal leg, and to a lesser degree arm, weakness. A history of fluctuation and fatigue suggests a disorder of NMT. Extraocular or bulbar weakness, especially if early or prominent, is unusual in LEMS. Ptosis is more common than diplopia. Severe ptosis or external ophthalmoplegia suggests MG. Said to be characteristic in LEMS is an initial improvement in strength during muscle contraction, before strength fatigues again. This author is not impressed with the sensitivity or specificity of this finding in a blinded assessment.

Hypo- or areflexia

Deep tendon reflexes (DTRs) are reduced or absent in over 90% of LEMS patients. DTRs of 2+ or more virtually exclude the diagnosis of LEMS. The DTRs may also increase or return after an MVC.

Autonomic

Up to 75% of LEMS patients eventually develop autonomic manifestations. Cholinergic dysfunction produces parasympathetic, or less frequently sympathetic, involvement. A dry mouth is the most common symptom, along with postural hypotension, constipation, or erectile dysfunction. Sluggish pupillary reflexes and abnormal sweating also occur.

Table 18.1. Myasthenia gravis (MG) versus Lambert–Eaton myasthenic syndrome (LEMS)

	LEMS	MG
Pathophysiology and target antigen	Presynaptic disorder of NMT with antibodies against VGCC	Postsynaptic disorder of NMT with antibodies against AChR or MuSK
Clinical	"Legs first" with leg weakness earlier and more severe and EOM or bulbar involvement later and milder	"Head first" with early and more striking EOM and bulbar involvement and legs involved later, if at all
	DTRs reduced or absent	DTRs normal
	Autonomic (PNS > SNS) involvement	No autonomic involvement
Associations	50% P-LEMS with SCLC in >90% of these	Thymoma in 15% generalized AChR antibody positive MG
	50% NP-LEMS with increased rate of other autoimmune diseases and HLA-B8, -DR3, and -DQ2	Hyperplastic thymus in early onset MG with increased rate of other autoimmune diseases and HLA-B8, -DR3, and- DQ2
Electrophysiology	Reduced CMAP amplitudes	Normal CMAP amplitudes
	Decrement with low frequency (2–5 Hz) RNS	Decrement with low frequency (2–5 Hz) RNS
	Increment (>60–100%) with high frequency (20–50 Hz) RNS or after MVC	Significant increment rare
	+++ jitter and blocking on SFEMG	++ jitter and blocking on SFEMG
Serology	Anti-VGCC antibodies in > 90%	Anti-AChR antibodies in 85% generalized MG and 50% ocular MG
		Anti-MuSK abs in 5% generalized MG
Treatment	3,4-DAP most useful symptomatic	Pyridostigmine most useful symptomatic
	Immunomodulation with IVIG ≥ Plex (?)	Immunomodulation with Plex = IVIG
	Immunosuppression	Immunosuppression
	±removal of SCLC	±removal of hyperplastic thymus

3,4-DAP, 3,4-diaminopyridine; AChR, acetylcholine receptor; CMAP, compound muscle action potential; DTR, deep tendon reflexes; EOM, extraocular muscles; IVIG, intravenous immunoglobulin; LEMS, Lambert–Eaton myasthenic syndrome; MG, myasthenia gravis; MuSK, muscle-specific kinase; MVC, maximal voluntary contraction; NMT, neuromuscular transmission; Plex, plasma exchange; RNS, repetitive nerve stimulation; SCLC, small cell lung cancer; SFEMG, single-fiber EMG; VGCC, voltage-gated calcium channel.

Other

Less common manifestations include respiratory involvement, rarely the presenting feature. Given its association with smoking and SCLC, dyspnea from LEMS must be differentiated from underlying pulmonary disease. Myalgia, especially of the proximal legs, occurs in a fifth patients initially and a third eventually. Prominent sensory symptoms with an underlying SCLC suggest a coexistent paraneoplastic sensory neuronopathy. Similarly, ataxia occurs in up to 10% of LEMS cases, and may represent a cerebellar paraneoplastic disorder with antibodies against Hu or even VGCC.

Epidemiology

LEMS is uncommon, with an incidence of approximately 0.4 in 10^6, 15 times less than MG. The prevalence, even more reduced because of the poor survival of P-LEMS, is about 30–45 times less than MG at 2.5 in 10^6. However, when specifically looked for, approximately 3% (range 0–6%) of SCLC cases have LEMS, suggesting that it is underdiagnosed. In the author's experience P-LEMS is more common in newly diagnosed patients than NP-LEMS. Although LEMS occurs from childhood through to being elderly, its association with SCLC means that most individuals are diagnosed in the fifth decade or later. Both genders are equally represented.

Paraneoplastic LEMS

Of LEMS patients 50–60% have an underlying malignancy – SCLC in >90%. SCLC is rare when LEMS starts before the age of 40. Malignancies other than SCLC may simply be incidental findings in P-LEMS, with an as yet undetected SCLC, or in NP-LEMS. In most patients, a SCLC is discovered within 2 years of diagnosing LEMS, rarely as long as 5 years. SCLC may be less extensive in the presence of LEMS, so that investigations looking for a SCLC may initially be negative.

Non-paraneoplastic LEMS

In 40–50% of LEMS patients no malignancy is found. Other autoimmune diseases and organ-specific autoantibodies are found in up to 30% of patients with NP-LEMS, more than in P-LEMS. NP-LEMS, is associated with the "autoimmune" human leukocyte antigen (HLA) haplotype -B8, -DR3, -DQ2. Thus, NP-LEMS is likely a primary autoimmune disorder such as myasthenia gravis, pernicious anemia, or Graves' disease.

Diagnosis

The diagnosis of LEMS is often delayed because it is uncommon and may be confused with the more common MG. Presumably because of its association with SCLC, P-LEMS tends to be diagnosed more rapidly than NP-LEMS.

Clinical

The biggest obstacle to diagnosing LEMS is to consider it in the differential of patients presenting with leg weakness. In a patient with what looks like MG, but where extraocular and bulbar manifestations are minimal and DTRs reduced, especially if there is autonomic involvement, LEMS should be considered and the appropriate electrodiagnostic studies and VGCC antibodies performed.

Electrophysiological

The electrophysiological triad in LEMS consists of:

- reduced CMAP amplitudes
- decrement >10% with low-frequency repetitive nerve stimulation (LFS)
- increment with high-frequency stimulation (HFS) or after an MVC.

Motor conduction velocities and sensory studies are normal, unless there is an associated neuropathy.

CMAP amplitudes are reduced, often less than 10% of the lower limit of normal, in over 90% of LEMS patients, especially in studies of distal hand muscles such as abductor digiti minimi (ADM), the most sensitive muscle for studies in LEMS (a paradox given the prominent proximal leg weakness clinically). If normal and LEMS is still suspected, studies to abductor pollicis brevis (ABP), anconeus, or extensor digitorum brevis (EDB) can be performed. Normal amplitudes in all of these muscles virtually exclude LEMS.

Decrement with LFS is found in over 95% of LEMS patients, although this can be difficult to detect if initial CMAP amplitudes are significantly reduced.

Once LEMS is suspected, this should lead to studies looking for *increment* (also described as facilitation or potentiation) – an increase in CMAP amplitude within seconds of a brief (10–15 s) MVC or during high-frequency (20–50 Hz) RNS. The former is as sensitive as and much less painful than HFS. HFS is still useful in patients too weak to maximally contract or when cooperation is suboptimal, such as in the intensive

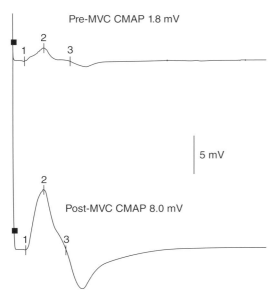

Figure 18.1. Post-maximal voluntary contraction (MVC) studies of the ulnar nerve to abductor digiti minimi in a patient with Lambert–Eaton myasthenic syndrome. A supramaximal compound muscle action potential (CMAP) was obtained at rest (top) and after 10 s of MVC (bottom). A 340% increment in the CMAP amplitude is demonstrated.

care unit (ICU). Studies of distal muscles are also more sensitive to detect increment in LEMS. The degree of increment needed to diagnose LEMS is controversial. Although most LEMS patients have increment of more than 2 standard deviations (SDs) above control values, this cut-off would also include a number of MG patients, where increment is occasionally seen. Various authors have used increments of 60%, 100%, or even more as a cut-off for LEMS. Depending on the cut-off, increment is eventually found in over 95% of LEMS patients in at least one of the above target muscles. An increment of more than 100% is seldom found in MG, although rare patients with MG have increments of 300% or more (Figure 18.1).

The electrophysiological abnormalities in LEMS may not be striking early on, and if suspicious, the studies should be repeated in a few months. A common but unexplained observation in LEMS is that the electrophysiological abnormalities are more severe than one would predict for the degree of weakness, the opposite situation from MG. Needle EMG may show unstable or even "myopathic" motor unit potentials, but these are not specific to LEMS. Single-fiber EMG is often markedly abnormal in LEMS, but again is not specific for LEMS.

Serological

Antibodies against P-/Q-type VGCCs are found in almost all cases of P-LEMS and >90% of cases of NP-LEMS. Given their high sensitivity and the electrophysiological overlap with MG, when VGCC antibodies are negative, MG should be considered. Anti-VGCC antibodies are also found in patients with SCLC without LEMS, and can be independently associated with a paraneoplastic cerebellar disorder. These antibodies, through VGCC blockade, are directly pathogenic in LEMS. There is no relationship between antibody titer and disease severity among LEMS patients. Within a single patient there is only a rough correlation between longitudinal changes in antibody levels and the clinical course, so, once positive, it is preferable to follow the clinical and perhaps electrophysiological response to treatment rather than antibody titers.

Other investigations

The injection of edrophonium (the "Tensilon test") may transiently improve weakness, but is not specific for LEMS and less sensitive than in MG. Patients at risk for SCLC (arguably any LEMS patient with disease onset at age >50, especially if a current or ex-smoker) should be investigated with computed tomography (CT) of the chest, and if negative with bronchoscopy. The role of positron electron tomography (PET) remains uncertain. If negative, scans should be repeated every 3–6 months for 2 years and then yearly for the next 3–4 years. SCLC is highly unlikely in patients aged <40 years who are non-smokers.

★ **TIPS AND TRICKS**

LEMS should be considered in patients who present with:

- Prominent proximal leg weakness, which may fluctuate and fatigue over the course of the day

- Reduced or absent deep tendon reflexes
- Autonomic involvement (dry mouth, constipation, postural hypotension, erectile dysfunction)
- History of smoking and/or an underlying SCLC
- Electrodiagnostic results of reduced CMAP amplitudes, decrement at low frequency stimulation of distal hand muscles and an increment of >100% with high-frequency RNS or after maximal voluntary contraction.

LEMS is highly unlikely if:

- The initial symptoms are mainly ocular or bulbar
- The DTRs are 2+ or better
- Electrodiagnostic studies show that CMAP amplitudes are normal, there is no decrement, and there is no increment in several different muscles (ADM, APB, EDB).

Differential diagnosis

The main differential diagnosis of LEMS is MG. A careful history and exam will usually allow a distinction between the two (see Table 18.1). There are rare overlap cases in which both AChR and VGCC antibodies are positive. Some reported VGCC antibody-negative "overlap" cases may simply be MG with atypical electrophysiological results. Given this potential overlap, clinical and serological criteria should be used to distinguish LEMS from MG and not solely electrophysiological ones. The combination of proximal leg weakness and reduced reflexes might also suggest a myopathy or inflammatory neuropathy in which sensory involvement is minimal. In the ICU a critical illness neuromyopathy may have diffusely reduced CMAP amplitudes with normal sensory studies. Given the available treatments, HFS should be done in all such cases to rule out LEMS. The weakness of P-LEMS may be mistaken for the systemic effects of SCLC or adverse effects of chemotherapy.

Management

The treatment of LEMS is individualized and partially depends on the presence of an underlying malignancy. Although similar to the treatment options for MG, significant differences mandate a definitive diagnosis of LEMS. Available treatment options include the symptomatic improvement of NMT, modulation or suppression of the autoimmune response, and, if present, treatment of the underlying malignancy, usually SCLC.

Symptomatic: 3,4-diaminopyridine

Given that ACh release is reduced in LEMS, it is not surprising that pyridostigmine has minimal benefit in LEMS, even in combination with 3,4-diaminopyridine (3,4-DAP). Pyridostigmine may be useful to treat the dry mouth commonly seen in LEMS. The mainstay of symptomatic treatment in LEMS is with 3,4-DAP, which inhibits nerve voltage-gated potassium channels, prolonging nerve depolarization and increasing ACh release (see "Science revisited"). 3,4-DAP increases muscle strength and may increase CMAP amplitudes. The dosing regimen is individualized. Starting doses are 5–10 mg orally four times a day. Based on the clinical response the dose is increased by 5- to 10-mg increments every 1–2 weeks to a maximum of 100 mg/day (20–25 mg four times daily). Optimal doses are usually between 20 and 60 mg/day. Benefit starts within 30–60 min of each dose, is optimal at 1–2 h. but may last only 3–4 h. so that sometimes the total daily dose must be divided as five to six doses per day. Proximal leg weakness is usually the yardstick by which efficacy is judged, although improvement in autonomic dysfunction also occurs. Once stable clinical improvement happens, each dose is reduced by 5-mg decrements to a maintenance dose. 3,4-DAP is removed during plasma exchange, so that the timing of administration may need to be adjusted.

Doses below 60 mg/day have minimal toxicity. Common adverse effects are transient perioral or acral paraesthesias, usually beginning with minutes of a dose and resolving within 15 min or so. Nausea, increased sweating, salivation, anxiety, and insomnia may also occur. The last dose should be at least 4 h before bedtime to avoid the latter. Doses over 100 mg/day increase the risk of seizures, which may occur at lower doses when brain metastases or the use of other drugs such as theophyllines increase the risk of seizures. 3,4-DAP is contraindicated in patients with known seizures.

Immunomodulation

Either intravenous immunoglobulin (IVIG) or plasma exchange (Plex) is useful for the treatment of severe weakness in LEMS. The doses and regimens are similar to those used in MG. Given their transient benefit and considerable expense, their use should be limited to adjuvant and not maintenance treatment.

Immunosuppression

In patients with a suboptimal response to 3,4-DAP immunosuppression is useful. The drugs and doses used are similar to MG, including prednisone and azathioprine. Other immunosuppressives including cyclosporine, tacrolimus, and mycophenolate might work, although there is little published evidence of their use in LEMS.

In P-LEMS, there are concerns that immunosuppression may reduce immunosurveillance and promote tumor growth, although the poor prognosis from SCLC may mean that this is an acceptable risk in order to improve the remaining quality of life.

Treatment of underlying malignancy

Although widely reported, there is little evidence that the treatment of the underlying SCLC improves LEMS beyond the immunosuppressive effects of chemotherapy and radiotherapy used. Nevertheless, in P-LEMS, this seems a reasonable management strategy.

Prognosis

The prognosis in LEMS is not predicted by the initial anti-VGCC antibody titer or electrophysiological results. In P-LEMS, the underlying SCLC determines the prognosis. P-LEMS is associated with less extensive SCLC, and the presence of LEMS, not just VGCC antibodies without clinical LEMS, doubles the survival from approximately 8 months with extensive SCLC. This may reflect earlier diagnosis as well as improved immunosurveillance conferred by functional anti-VGCC antibodies. NP-LEMS has an excellent prognosis, although it is perhaps not as treatable as MG. Many patients have persistent mild weakness despite optimal medical management.

Bibliography

Elrington G, Murray N, Spiro S, et al. Neurological paraneoplastic syndromes in patients with small cell lung cancer. A prospective survey of 150 patients. *J Neurol Neurosurg Psychiatry* 1991;**54**:764–7.

Engel A, Fukuoka T, Lang B, et al. Lambert–Eaton myasthenic syndrome IgG: early morphologic effects and immunolocalization at the motor endplate. *Ann N Y Acad Sci* 1987; **505**:333–45.

Keesey JC. AAEE Minimonograph #33: electrodiagnostic approach to defects of neuromuscular transmission. *Muscle Nerve* 1989;**12**:613–26.

Maddison P, Lang B. Paraneoplastic neurological autoimmunity and survival in small-cell lung cancer. *J Neuroimmunol* 2008;**201–202**: 159–62.

Maddison P, Newsom-Davis J. Treatment for Lambert–Eaton myasthenic syndrome. *Cochrane Database System Rev* 2005;(2): CD003279.

Maddison P, Lang B, Mills K, et al. Long term outcome in Lambert-Eaton myasthenic syndrome without lung cancer. *J Neurol Neurosurg Psychiatry* 2001;**70**:212–17.

O'Neill JH, Murray N, Newsom-Davis J. The Lambert–Eaton myasthenic syndrome. A review of 50 cases. *Brain* 1988;**111**:577–96.

Oh SJ, Kurokawa K, Claussen G, et al. Electrophysiological diagnostic criteria of Lambert-Eaton myasthenic syndrome. *Muscle Nerve* 2005;**32**:515–20.

Payne M, Bradbury P, Lang B, et al. Prospective study into the incidence of Lambert Eaton myasthenic syndrome in small cell lung cancer. *J Thorac Oncol* 2010;**5**:34–8.

Sher E, Carbone E, Clementi F. Neuronal calcium channels as target for Lambert–Eaton myasthenic syndrome autoantibodies. *Ann N Y Acad Sci* 1993;**681**:373–81.

Tim R, Massey J, Sanders D. Lambert–Eaton myasthenic syndrome: electrodiagnostic findings and response to treatment. *Neurology* 2000;**54**:2176–8.

Titulaer M, Wirtz P, Kuks J, et al. The Lambert–Eaton myasthenic syndrome 1988–2008: a clinical picture in 97 patients. *J Neuroimmunol* 2008;**201–202**:153–8.

Wirtz P, Lang B, Graus F, et al. P/Q-type calcium channel antibodies, Lambert–Eaton myasthenic syndrome and survival in small cell lung cancer. *J Neuroimmunol* 2005;**164**:161–5.

Wirtz P, Nijnuis M, Sotodeh M, et al. The epidemiology of myasthenia gravis, Lambert–Eaton myasthenic syndrome and their associated tumours in the northern part of the province of South Holland. *J Neurol* 2003;**250**:698–701.

Wirtz P, Sotodeh M, Nijnuis M, et al. Difference in distribution of muscle weakness between myasthenia gravis and the Lambert–Eaton myasthenic syndrome. *J Neurol Neurosurg Psychiatry* 2002;**73**:766–8.

Congenital Myasthenic Syndromes

Andrew G. Engel

Department of Neurology, Mayo Clinic, Rochester, MN, USA

Definitions and basic principles

The congenital myasthenic syndromes (CMSs) represent a heterogeneous group of disorders in which the safety margin of neuromuscular transmission is compromised by one or more specific mechanisms.

During neuromuscular transmission, synaptic vesicles in the nerve terminal exocytose acetylcholine (ACh) quanta into the synaptic space. The released quanta open postsynaptic acetylcholine receptor (AChR) channels to evoke an endplate potential (EPP) that activates the $Na_v1.4$ voltage-dependent sodium channels to trigger a propagated action potential. The muscle AChR is a heteropentamer. After birth, it is composed of two α units, and one each of β, δ, and ε subunits. AChR in fetal muscle harbors a γ instead of an ε subunit. A high concentration of AChRs on the terminal expansions of the junctional folds and of $Na_v1.4$ in the depth of the folds ensures that excitation is propagated beyond the endplate. The safety margin of neuromuscular transmission is a function of the difference between the depolarization caused by the EPP and the depolarization required to activate $Na_v1.4$.

The safety margin of neuromuscular transmission can be resolved into the following major categories: factors that affect the number of ACh molecules per synaptic vesicle, factors that affect quantal release mechanisms reflected by the quantal content of EPP, and factors that affect the efficacy of individual quanta. Quantal efficacy is determined by the endplate geometry, the density of acetylcholinesterase (AChE) in the synaptic space, the density and distribution of AChRs on the junctional folds, and the kinetic properties of the AChR and $Na_v1.4$ channels.

Electrophysiological and morphological studies can probe the involvement of these different mechanisms in CMSs. If the clinical data, alone or in combination with results of special tests, point to a candidate gene, then molecular genetic analysis becomes feasible. If a mutation is discovered in a candidate gene, expression studies with the genetically engineered mutant protein can be used to confirm pathogenicity and to analyze the properties of the abnormal protein. To date, the candidate gene approach has led to discovery of pathogenic mutations in genes encoding subunits of AChR, the ColQ subunit of AChE, rapsyn, Dok-7, choline acetyltransferase (ChAT), β_2-laminin, muscle-specific kinase (MuSK), agrin, $Na_v1.4$, and plectin as causes of CMSs. Close to 80% of CMS patients have postsynaptic defects and most postsynaptic defects reside in the AChR ε subunit (Figure 19.1 and Table 19.1).

The slow-channel CMSs and sodium-channel myasthenia are transmitted by dominant inheritance. All other CMSs identified to date are transmitted by recessive inheritance.

Neuromuscular Disorders, First Edition. Edited by Rabi N. Tawil, Shannon Venance.
© 2011 John Wiley & Sons, Ltd. Published 2011 by John Wiley & Sons, Ltd.

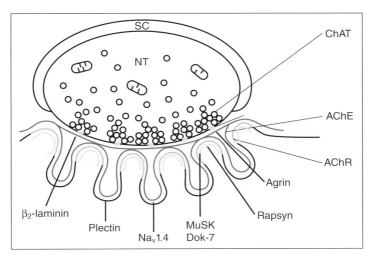

Figure 19.1. Schematic representation of an endplate region showing locations of congenital myasthenic syndrome disease proteins. AChE, acetylcholinesterase; AChR, acetylcholine receptor; ChAT, choline acetyltransferase; SC, Schwann cell; NT, nerve terminal.

Phenotypic features and pathological mechanisms in the different CMSs

This section considers the more frequently encountered CMSs before those identified in only a few kinships.

Choline acetyltransferase deficiency

Mutations in ChAT either reduce the expression or decrease the catalytic efficiency of the enzyme. This decreases the rate of ACh resynthesis and the ACh content of the synaptic vesicles during physiological activity. Consequently the amplitude of the synaptic response, reflected by the amplitude of the miniature EPP (MEPP) and EPP, also decrease. This disorder leaves no anatomic footprint.

Endplate AChE deficiency

The endplate species of AChE is composed of catalytic subunits encoded by *ACHET* and a structural subunit encoded by *COLQ*. No spontaneous mutations have been observed in *ACHET*. ColQ anchors the enzyme complex in the synaptic basal lamina. Different mutations in different ColQ domains prevent its association with the catalytic subunits, reduce ColQ expression, or prevent ColQ from anchoring the enzyme in the synaptic basal lamina. Absence of AChE from the endplate prolongs the lifetime of ACh in the synaptic space so that each ACh can bind to a series of AChRs before leaving the synaptic space by diffusion, and this prolongs the decay phase of the MEPP and EPP. When the EPP outlasts the absolute refractory period of the muscle fiber, it generates a second or repetitive compound muscle action potential (CMAP). Cholinergic overactivity at the endplate results in cationic overloading of the postsynaptic region; this causes degeneration of the junctional folds with loss of AChR.

Perhaps to protect the endplate from overexposure to ACh, the nerve terminals are abnormally small; this reduces the number of readily releasable quanta and hence the quantal content of the EPP. Thus, the safety margin of neuromuscular transmission is compromised by the decreased quantal content of the EPP, loss of AChR from degenerating junctional folds, altered endplate geometry, and desensitization of AChR from overexposure to ACh.

Pathogenic mutations in AChR

These can either decrease the expression of AChR at the endplate or alter the kinetic properties of the receptor, so as to shift the thermodynamic equilibrium to favor the open channel state and result in slowly decaying EPPs (slow-channel

Table 19.1. Classification and frequency of the congenital myasthenic syndromes (CMSs)

CMS	Index cases identified at Mayo Clinic
Presynaptic (7%)	
• ChAT deficiency[a]	17
• Paucity of synaptic vesicles and reduced quantal release	1
• Congenital Lambert–Eaton -like	2
• Other presynaptic defects	2
Synaptic space (14%)	
• Endplate AChE deficiency due to defects in ColQ[a]	43
• β_2-Laminin deficiency[a,b]	0
Postsynaptic (79%)	
• Primary kinetic defect ± AChR deficiency[a]	53
• Primary AChR deficiency ± minor kinetic defect[a]	109
• Rapsyn deficiency[a]	48
• Dok-7 myasthenia[a]	30
• Na^+ channel myasthenia[a]	1
• Plectin deficiency[a]	2
• MuSK deficiency[a,b]	0
• Agrin deficiency[a,b]	0
Total	308

[a]Gene defects identified.
[b]Gene defects in single kinships were identified at other medical centers (see text).
AChE, acetylcholinesterase; AChR, acetylcholine receptor; ChAT, choline acetyltransferase; MuSk, muscle-specific kinase.

syndromes) or to favor the closed channel state and result in fast decaying EPPs (fast-channel syndromes).

Primary endplate AChR deficiency

Endplate AChR deficiency results from mutations in the α, β, δ, or ε subunits of the receptor. The types of identified mutations include frameshift, splice-site, or nonsense mutations, chromosomal microdeletions, or missense mutations in the promoter or signal peptide region, or in residues essential for assembly of the pentameric AChR. Morphological studies show an increased number of small endplate regions distributed over an increased span of the muscle fiber, and the distribution of AChRs on the junctional folds is patchy and attenuated. The structural integrity of the junctional folds is preserved but the postsynaptic region is simplified due to the decreased height and number of the folds. The safety margin is compromised by the AChR deficiency and the postsynaptic simplification that reduces the input resistance of the postsynaptic region. Both factors reduce the amplitude of the MEPPs and EPPs. Low-expressor or null mutations in the ε subunit are partially compensated for by expression of small amounts of AChR harboring the fetal γ subunit and this likely rescues the phenotype. Low-expressor or null mutations in non-ε subunits either are embryonic lethal or generate severe phenotypes with high mortality in early life. Consequently, most identified low-expressor or null mutations of AChR reside in the ε subunit.

Slow-channel syndrome

Pathogenic mutations occurring in different AChR subunits prolong the opening events of the AChR channel by increasing the rate at which the channel opens, decrease the rate at which it closes, or increase its affinity for ACh, resulting in repeated channel reopenings during the prolonged sojourn of ACh at the receptor-binding site. The prolonged channel-opening events prolong the duration of the EPP so that it outlasts the refractory period of the muscle fiber, and thereby eliciting a repetitive CMAP. The prolonged synaptic response also causes cationic overloading of the postsynaptic region and degeneration of the junctional folds with loss of AChR from the folds. The safety margin is compromised by loss of AChR, altered endplate geometry, and progressive depolarization block of the endplate at physiological rates of stimulation, as a result of each consecutive EPP arising in the wake of the preceding EPP before the postsynaptic membrane has repolarized.

Fast-channel syndrome

Pathogenic mutations residing in different subunits of the AChR curtail the duration of the channel-opening events by decreasing the rate at which the AChR channel opens, increasing the rate at which it closes, decreasing the affinity for ACh, or altering the fidelity of channel openings, which typically become briefer than normal. The kinetic mutations are generally accompanied by a null mutation in the second allele so that the kinetic mutation dominates the phenotype. Endplate structure is normal. The safety margin of neuromuscular transmission is compromised by a decreased probability of channel openings, which decreases the synaptic response to ACh and accelerates its decay.

Rapsyn deficiency

Rapsyn, under the influence of agrin and MuSK, concentrates AChR on the terminal expansions of the junctional folds. Mutations in different domains of rapsyn cause endplate AChR deficiency. Nearly all white patients carry a common *N88K* mutation. The morphological features of the endplate and the factors that impair the safety margin are like those in primary AChR deficiency.

Dok-7 myasthenia

Dok-7 is a muscle intrinsic activator of MuSK required for normal development and maintenance of the neuromuscular junction. The clinical hallmarks are limb–girdle weakness with lesser face, jaw, and neck muscle weakness. Mild ptosis is common but the ocular ductions are usually spared. The neuromuscular junctions are composed of single or multiple small regions. The postsynaptic membrane is less folded than normal and there is ongoing destruction of endplates and attempts to form new endplates. Different parameters of neuromuscular transmission (MEPP amplitude, quantal release, AChR content) are reduced to a different extent in different patients. The safety margin of neuromuscular transmission is likely impaired by a combination of factors that operate to a different extent in different patients.

Paucity of synaptic vesicles and reduced quantal release

In a single investigated patient, the number of quanta released by nerve impulse was decreased due to a decreased number of readily releasable quanta. Electron microscopy revealed that the decrease in quantal content of the EPP was due to a decrease in the number of readily releasable quanta, and this was proportionate to a decreased density of synaptic vesicles in the nerve terminals.

Congenital Lambert–Eaton-like syndrome

A CMS in which the EMG features resembled those in the acquired autoimmune form of the disease was reported in a single patient. In another patient, the number of quanta released by nerve impulse was decreased due to a decreased probability of quantal release. Electron microscopy revealed no structural abnormality of the endplate.

β_2-Laminin myasthenia

β_2-Laminin, encoded by *LAMB2*, is a component of the basal lamina of different tissues and is highly expressed in the kidney, eye, and neuromuscular junction. In vitro microelectrode studies revealed decreased quantal release by nerve impulse and decreased MEPP amplitude. The nerve terminals were abnormally small and often encased by Schwann cells, the synaptic space was widened, and the junctional folds were simplified.

CMSs due to defect in agrin

Agrin, encoded by *AGRN*, is a multidomain proteoglycan secreted into the synaptic basal lamina by the nerve terminal. The muscle isoform of agrin harbors A and B regions near its C terminus. Agrin phosphorylates and thereby activates MuSK by way of its receptor, LRP4. Two siblings with eyelid ptosis but normal ocular ductions and only mild weakness of the facial and hip–girdle muscles carried a homozygous missense mutation in the agrin A region. Light microscopic preparations showed newly formed, partially denervated, and remodeled endplates. Electron microscopy revealed some abandoned and partially occupied postsynaptic regions. The aggregation of AChR at the endplates was not affected. The number of AChRs per endplate was not determined.

CMSs due to defects in MuSK

MuSK under the influence of agrin and LRP4 plays a role in maturation and maintenance of the synapse and in directing rapsyn to concentrate AChR in the postsynaptic membrane. In one kinship there was decreased expression and stability of the mutant protein, decreased AChR aggregation, and reduced AChR expression at simplified endplates. The safety margin is likely compromised by the AChR deficiency. Endplate fine structure was not examined.

Sodium-channel myasthenia

In the single patient observed to date, quantal release by nerve impulse and the amplitude of the EPPs were normal, but suprathreshold EPPs failed to generate muscle action potentials. This disease was traced to a p.V1442E mutation in an S4/S5 linker in domain IV of Nav1.4. This mutation enhances fast inactivation of Nav1.4 at a resting membrane potential, rendering a large fraction of the channels inexcitable at rest, and also enhances use-dependent inactivation of the channel. The endplates show no structural abnormality.

CMSs, muscular dystrophy, and epidermolysis bullosa simplex caused by plectin deficiency

Plectin is an intermediate filament-associated protein that orchestrates the internal cytoskeleton in a variety of cells and tissues in an isoform-dependent manner. Plectin deficiency in muscle results in impaired anchoring and defective function of the muscle fiber organelles, breaks in the sarcolemma, and degeneration of the junctional folds. Plectin deficiency in skin causes dermoepidermal disjunction and epidermolysis bullosa simplex. The safety margin of neuromuscular transmission is likely impaired by the abnormal endplate geometry and by loss of AChR and Nav1.4 from the postsynaptic membrane.

Prenatal CMS with fetal akinesia and deformities

Fetal hypomotility can result in intrauterine growth retardation, multiple joint contractures, subcutaneous edema, pterygia (webbing of the neck, axilla, elbows, fingers, or popliteal fossa), lung hypoplasia, and other congenital malformations. The syndrome is often lethal; the nonlethal form is referred to as Escobar's syndrome. Fetal akinesia has many causes. Those due to defects in neuromuscular transmission include transplacental transfer from mother to fetus of anti-AChR antibodies that contain a high titer of complement-fixing anti-γ subunit specificities. Mutations in the AChR gamma subunit and severe or null mutations in non-epsilon AChR subunits, *RAPSN*, and *DOK7* can also cause fetal akinesia and congenital deformities.

Diagnosis of the CMSS

A generic diagnosis of a CMS can be made on the basis of fatigable weakness since birth or early childhood involving oculobulbar, axial, and limb muscles, similarly affected relatives, a decremental electromyographic (EMG) response of the evoked CMAP at 2- to 3-Hz stimulation, and negative tests for antibodies directed against AChR, MuSK, and P-/Q-type of calcium channels. There are exceptions, however. In some CMSs the onset is delayed, the weakness may not involve the oculobulbar muscles, often there are no similarly affected relatives, and the symptoms can be episodic. Further, the EMG abnormalities may not be present in all muscles, are present only intermittently, or are elicited only after a prolonged train of subtetanic stimuli. Box 19.1 summarizes the clinical clues pointing to the diagnosis of specific types of CMSs.

When neither clinical nor EMG clues point to a specific diagnosis, specialized studies that investigate neuromuscular transmission in vitro by microelectrode methods may still point to the correct diagnosis. However, such studies are available in only a few medical centers in North America or elsewhere. A molecular diagnosis may still be feasible but can be expensive and desultory because there are now no fewer than 13 CMS disease genes to analyze. A practical guide to this approach is as follows:

1. Sequence genes in order of the frequency that they are associated with CMSs. In the Mayo cohort of patients these frequencies were as follows: *CHRNE*, 34%; *CHRNA1*, *CHRNB*, and

Box 19.1. Clinical clues pointing to specific types of congenital myasthenic syndromes

Low-expressor or null mutations in the AChR subunit
  Early fixed ophthalmoparesis refractory to therapy
  Mutations in non-ε subunits carry worse prognosis than mutations in ε subunit
  Respond to cholinergic agonists
Slow-channel congenital myasthenic syndrome
  Dominant inheritance
  Repetitive CMAP
  Selective involvement of cervical and wrist and finger extensor muscles in most cases
  Refractory to or worsened by cholinergic agonists; responds to fluoxetine
Endplate acetylcholinesterase deficiency
  Repetitive CMAP
  Refractory to or worsened by cholinergic agonists
  Delayed pupillary light reflexes in some cases
  Ocular ductions spared in some patients
  Improved by ephedrine or albuterol
Endplate ChAT deficiency
  Recurrent apneic episodes, spontaneous or with fever, vomiting, or excitement
  Variable or no myasthenic symptoms between acute episodes
  Subtetanic stimulation at 10 Hz for 5 min causes marked decrease of CMAP followed by slow recovery over 6–10 min
  Responds to pyridostigmine
Rapsyn deficiency
  Multiple congenital joint contractures in a quarter of patients
  Increased weakness and respiratory insufficiency precipitated by intercurrent infections
  Ocular ductions usually spared; limb–girdle pattern of weakness
  Responds to cholinergic agonists; ephedrine or albuterol can be beneficial

Dok-7 myasthenia
  Ocular ductions usually spared; limb–girdle pattern of weakness in most cases
  Significant bulbar muscle involvement in some patients
  Worsened by cholinergic agonists; improved by ephedrine or albuterol
β_2-Laminin myasthenia
  Nephrotic syndrome, ocular abnormalities (Pierson's syndrome)
  Refractory to pyridostigmine
Plectin-related myasthenia
  Association with epidermolysis bullosa simplex and muscular dystrophy
  Refractory to cholinergic agonists

AChR, acetylcholine receptor; ChAT, choline acetyltransferase; CMAP, compound muscle action potential.

Box 19.2. Treatment of the congenital myasthenic syndromes (CMSs)

The currently available therapeutic agents include 3,4-diaminopyridine (3,4-DAP), pyridostigmine, ephedrine, albuterol, fluoxetine, and quinidine. 3,4-DAP increases the number of quanta released from the nerve terminal. The acetylcholinesterase (AChE) inhibitor pyridostigmine increases the lifetime of acetylcholine (ACh) in the synaptic space so that each released quantum can activate a larger number of ACh receptors (AChRs). These two cholinergic agonists act synergistically. The cholinergic antagonists quinidine and fluoxetine are long-lived open-channel blockers of AChR that shorten the duration of the synaptic current. The mechanisms of action of albuterol and ephedrine are not known. In the USA, 3,4-DAP is available for compassionate use with an investigational new drug (IND) number obtained from the Food and Drug Administration. The list below indicates the medications used in the different types of CMSs.

Simple AChR deficiency
Pyridostigmine; 3,4-DAP also helps in
30–50%.
Avoid fluoxetine or quinidine.
Slow-channel CMSs
Fluoxetine and quinidine are beneficial.
Avoid pyridostigmine and 3,4-DAP
Fast-channel CMSs
Pyridostigmine and 3,4-DAP
AChE deficiency
Avoid cholinergic agonists; ephedrine or
albuterol can be beneficial
Rapsyn deficiency
Pyridostigmine, 3,4-DAP; ephedrine or
albuterol can also be beneficial
Choline acetyltransferase deficiency
Pyridostigmine; neostigmine methyl sulfate
intramuscularly for apneic attacks
Na⁺ channel myasthenia
Pyridostigmine and acetazolamide
Muscle-specific kinase deficiency
Pyridostigmine and 3,4-DAP
Agrin deficiency
Ephedrine or albuterol
β₂-Laminin deficiency
Ephedrine or albuterol

CHRND combined 19%; *RPSN*, 15%; *COLQ*,
16%; *DOK7*, 10%; and *CHAT*, 6%.
2. Search for common mutations in *RPSN*
(p.N88K) and *DOK7* (c.1124_1127dupTGCC).
3. Search for common mutations in ethnic
groups (e.g. c.1267delG in *CHRNE* in gypsies).

Treatment of CMSs

Appropriate therapy of CMSs must be based on
an accurate diagnosis. It is important to note that
some agents effective in one type of CMS can be
ineffective or harmful in another type. As a rough
guide, one can use the edrophonium test to
determine whether a patient will respond to
cholinergic agonists. However, slow-channel
syndrome and Dok-7 myasthenia patients may
transiently respond to edrophonium but are
worsened by long-term exposure to pyridostigmine. Box 19.2 provides guidelines for the treatment of different types of CMSs.

Acknowledgment

Work done in the author's laboratory was sup-
ported by NIH Research Grant NS6277 and a
Research Grant from the Muscular Dystrophy
Association.

Bibliography

Beeson D, Higuchi O, Palace J, et al. Dok-7 mutations underlie a neuromuscular junction syn-
aptopathy. *Science* 2006;**313**:1975–78.

Chevessier F, Faraut B, Ravel-Chapuis A, et al.
MUSK, a new target for mutations causing
congenital myasthenic syndrome. *Hum Mol
Genet* 2004;**13**:3229–40.

Engel AG, Ohno K, Milone M, et al. New mutations in acetylcholine receptor subunit genes
reveal heterogeneity in the slow-channel congenital myasthenic syndrome. *Hum Mol Genet*
1997;**6**:753–66.

Engel AG, Ohno K, Sine SM. Sleuthing molecular
targets for neurological diseases at the neuromuscular junction. *Nat Rev Neurosci* 2003;**4**:
339–52.

Engel AG, Ohno K, Sine SM. Congenital
myasthenic syndromes. In: Engel AG, Franzini-
Armstrong C (eds), *Myology*, 3rd edn. New
York: McGraw-Hill, 2004: 1755–90.

Harper CM, Fukudome T, Engel AG. Treatment of
slow channel congenital myasthenic syndrome
with fluoxetine. *Neurology* 2003;**60**:170–3.

Huze C, Bauche S, Richard P, et al. Identification
of an agrin mutation that causes congenital
myasthenia and affects synapse function. *Am J
Hum Genet* 2009;**85**:155–67.

Maselli RA, Ng JJ, Andreson JA, et al. Mutations
in *LAMB2* causing a severe form of synaptic
congenital myasthenic syndrome. *J Med Genet*
2009;**46**:203–8.

Milone M, Shen XM, Selcen D, et al. Myasthenic
syndrome due to defects in rapsyn: Clinical
and molecular findings in 39 patients.
Neurology 2009;**73**:228–35.

Ohno K, Brengman JM, Tsujino A, et al. Human
endplate acetylcholinesterase deficiency caused
by mutations in the collagen-like tail subunit
(ColQ) of the asymmetric enzyme. *Proc Natl
Acad Sci USA* 1998;**95**:9654–9.

Ohno K, Tsujino A, Brengman JM, et al. Choline
acetyltransferase mutations cause myasthenic

syndrome associated with episodic apnea in humans. *Proc Natl Acad Sci USA* 2001;**98**: 2017–22.

Reimann J, Jacobson L, Vincent A, et al. Endplate destruction due to maternal antibodies in arthrogryposis multiplex congenita. *Neurology* 2009;**73**:1806–8.

Selcen D, Milone M, Shen X-M, et al. Dok-7 myasthenia: phenotypic and molecular genetic studies in 16 patients. *Ann Neurol* 2008;**64**: 71–87.

Sine SM, Engel AG. Recent advances in Cys-loop receptor structure and function. *Nature* 2006; **440**:448–55.

Tsujino A, Maertens C, Ohno K, et al. Myasthenic syndrome caused by mutation of the *SCN4A* sodium channel. *Proc Natl Acad Sci USA* 2003; **100**:7377–82.

Wood SJ, Slater CP. Safety factor at the neuromuscular junction. *Prog Neurobiol* 2001;**64**: 393–29.

Part III

Disorders of Peripheral Nerve

Approach to Diagnosis of Peripheral Nerve Disease

James C. Cleland[1] and Eric L. Logigian[2]

[1]Auckland City Hospital and University of Auckland School of Medicine, Auckland, New Zealand
[2]University of Rochester Medical Center, Rochester, NY, USA

Anatomy

Peripheral nerves convey information to and from the central nervous system via afferent (sensory), efferent (motor), and autonomic ("vasomotor" and "sudomotor") fibers. Most nerves are "mixed" containing all three components, but exceptions include cutaneous afferents that contain sensory and autonomic fibers only.

Sensory fibers conduct information from peripheral receptor organs via myelinated and unmyelinated fibers. Pain and temperature sensibility are conveyed from nociceptors and bare nerve endings in skin via "small" thinly myelinated or unmyelinated axons (Aδ- and C-fibers respectively), whereas conscious and unconscious proprioception is conveyed from muscle spindles, mechanoreceptors (e.g. pacinian corpuscles), joint capsule receptors, and Golgi tendon bodies via "large", heavily myelinated axons (Aα- and Aβ-fibers). Disease of sensory neurons or axons results in "positive" symptoms of pain, and tingling, along with "negative" symptoms such as numbness, balance difficulty, and trouble performing fine motor tasks out of proportion to weakness. Signs include "small fiber" sensory loss to pin and temperature, painless foot ulcers, or Charcot's arthropathy, and "large fiber" loss to joint position and vibration with hyporeflexia, Rombergism, and limb or gait ataxia.

Motor axons arise from anterior horn cells in the ventral horn of the spinal cord and exit via the ventral roots. Dorsal and ventral roots combine to form a spinal root that then divides into anterior and posterior rami. The posterior ramus innervates parapsinal musculature and adjacent skin, and the anterior ramus supplies cutaneous innervation referable to that spinal level ("dermatome") and innervates all limb musculature referable to that spinal level ("myotome"). Unlike sensory fibers, all motor axons under voluntary control are myelinated. The motor axon terminates in the neuromuscular junction, where the neurotransmitter acetylcholine mediates neuromuscular transmission. Disease of motor neurons or axons results in "positive" symptoms, such as fasciculations or muscle cramps, along with "negative" symptoms, such as weakness and resulting functional disability (e.g. distal weakness: foot drop and falling, hand weakness, and trouble opening jars; proximal weakness: arising from chairs, going upstairs, reaching overhead;respiratory failure). Signs include muscle atrophy, fasciculations, skeletal deformities (e.g. pes cavus, kyphoscoliosis), hypotonia, and weakness.

The autonomic nervous system is composed of the parasympathetic and sympathetic systems.

Neuromuscular Disorders, First Edition. Edited by Rabi N. Tawil, Shannon Venance.

The "craniosacral" parasympathetic system comprises fibers of the tenth cranial nerve (vagus) and fibers originating in the intermediolateral zone of segments S2–4 of the sacral spinal cord. The sympathetic system comprises fibers originating from cells in the intermediolateral cell column of spinal segments T1–L2. Both systems use exclusively thinly myelinated or unmyelinated axons, and innervate endorgans including sweat glands ("sudomotor" fibers), blood vessels ("vasomotor" fibers), as well as cardiac tissue and other endocrine organs (e.g. adrenal glands). Disease of autonomic neurons or axons result in "positive" symptoms of hyperhidrosis or gustatory sweating, along with "negative" symptoms such as orthostasis, sicca symptoms, anhidrosis, heat and exercise intolerance, impotence, and bladder or bowel disturbance. Bedside signs include postural hypotension (without compensatory tachycardia), poorly reactive pupils, and dry skin.

★ TIPS AND TRICKS

When symptoms and signs indicate involvement of only one of the three fiber types the differential diagnosis is narrowed, e.g. severe sensory neuropathies associated with sensory limb or gait ataxia are caused by only a few conditions (mainly paraneoplastic, Sjögren's syndrome, a few toxins, and rare hereditary neuropathies). Peripheral causes of isolated muscle weakness are limited and include motor neuronopathy, multifocal motor neuropathy, or some forms of acute and chronic inflammatory demyelinating polyneuropathy (AIDP and CIDP). Pure autonomic dysfunction is seen in acute panautonomic neuropathy (sometimes post-infectious), pure autonomic failure, or as an immune mediated syndrome.

Case 1

A 65-year-old woman with asthma presents with a progressive right foot drop along with numbness and pain in the lateral calf and dorsum of the right foot; 14 days later, she develops weakness of the left hand with numbness and pain of the ulnar border. There is low-grade fever, weight loss of 10 kg, and a nonproductive cough. Examination confirms a right peroneal and a left ulnar neuropathy, both of moderate clinical severity. Her complete blood count is normal other than eosinophilia, and the erythrocyte sedimentation rate is elevated at 90 mm/h. A chest radiograph demonstrates a hazy interstitial infiltrate. Electrodiagnostic examination confirms a multifocal axonal polyneuropathy with low-amplitude right peroneal and left ulnar motor and sensory responses, normal conduction velocities, without motor conduction block.

Discussion

The diagnostic algorithm in peripheral nerve disorders follows a logical and stepwise approach in which the following questions are addressed:

1. What is the localization for the patient's symptoms (e.g. central, peripheral, or both)?
2. Is the onset acute, subacute, or chronic, and is the course relapsing–remitting, progressive, or static?
3. What is the pattern and clinical severity of deficits (e.g. sensory, motor, or autonomic)?
4. What is the pattern of involvement (e.g. symmetric or asymmetric; proximal, distal, or mixed)?
5. Are there associated systemic features (e.g. weight loss, rash, joint swelling, fever)?
6. Are there clues to a hereditary cause in the family history?
7. Is there exposure to neurotoxins (drugs, occupational toxins, alcohol), or inadequate nutrition?
8. Is the past medical history notable for diseases associated with neuropathy (diabetes, cancer, connective tissue disease, etc)?

Involvement of individual named nerve territories with both motor and sensory involvement is due to a peripheral neuropathy, not a central disorder. The onset is subacute, stepwise in nature, and clearly asymmetric. Such a presentation is typical of *mononeuropathy multiplex,* in which motor and sensory fibers of individual peripheral nerves are affected in sequential fashion. Although this is a typical presentation of a vasculitic illness, other causes are listed in Table 20.1. This patient's asthmatic symptoms,

Table 20.1. Causes of neuropathy

Neuropathy type	Acute	Subacute or chronic
Demyelinating		
Symmetric	Immune-mediated, AIDP, SLE, HIV-associated AIDP, Lyme disease-associated AIDP Infectious, e.g. diphtheria Toxic, hexacarbons (*n*-hexane)	Immune-mediated, CIDP, anti-MAG, POEMS/Castleman's syndrome Hereditary, CMT type 1A, 1B (childhood), CMT3, CMT4, CMTX Drugs, e.g. amiodarone, perhexilene Toxic, e.g. *n*-hexane, gold, arsenic Leukodystophies, e.g. Krabbe's, metachromatic, adrenomyelopathy Mitochondrial
Asymmetric/ Multifocal	Immune-mediated, AIDP (rarely) Hereditary, e.g. HNPP Inflammatory, vasculitis[a]	Immune-mediated, e.g. MADSAM, MMNCB, CIDP (upper extremity variant) Hereditary, e.g. HNPP
Axonal		
Symmetric	Immune-mediated, e.g. AMAN, AMSAN Hereditary, porphyria Toxic, e.g. alcohol, arsenic, thallium, hexacarbon, pyrinuron Drugs, e.g. vincristine, cisplatin, high-dose pyridoxine Critical illness Inflammatory, vasculitis (rarely), cryoglobulinemia	Metabolic, e.g. diabetes, renal failure, hypothyroidism Toxic, e.g. alcohol, arsenic, thallium, acrylamide, organophosphates, hexacarbon Hereditary, e.g. CMT type II ("axonal" CMT) Infectious, e.g. Lyme, HIV Paraneoplastic Infiltrative, e.g. amyloidosis Drugs, e.g. vincristine, cisplatin, thalidomide, dapsone, nucleoside analogs Inflammatory, e.g. connective-tissue disease, Sjögren's syndrome, cryoglobulinemia, celiac disease
Asymmetric/ Multifocal	Inflammatory, vasculitis, perineuritis Infectious, e.g. leprosy, Lyme disease Toxic, e.g. lead Paraneoplastic (sensory only) Metabolic, e.g. diabetes	Inflammatory, e.g. vasculitis, sarcoidosis Infectious, e.g. leprosy, Lyme disease Infiltrative disorders, e.g. amyloidosis, neurolymphomatosis Inflammatory, Sjögren's syndrome, cryoglobulinemia

[a]May be associated with acute motor conduction block, but axon loss then predominates.
AIDP/CIDP, acute/chronic inflammatory demyelinating polyradiculoneuropathy; AMAN/AMSAN, acute motor/sensorimotor axonal neuropathy; CMT, Charcot–Marie–Tooth disease; HNPP, hereditary neuropathy with pressure palsies; MADSAM, multifocal acquired demyelinating sensorimotor polyneuropathy; MMNCB, multifocal motor neuropathy with conduction block; POEMS, **p**eripheral neuropathy, **o**rganomegaly, **e**ndocrinopathy, **M**-protein, **s**kin changes.

peripheral eosinophilia, and pulmonary infil-trates all suggest a new diagnosis of Churg–Strauss syndrome. See Table 20.2 for examples of other systemic manifestations of diseases known to cause neuropathy. Nerve conduction studies disclosed axon loss physiology; biopsy of super-ficial peroneal nerve and adjacent peroneus brevis muscle confirmed a necrotizing vasculitis, and laboratory studies confirmed markedly ele-vated p-ANCA (perinuclear anti-neutrophil cyto-plasmic antibodies) titers (anti-myeloperoxidase or anti-MPO positive).

Patterns of involvement: length dependency

Most peripheral nerve diseases affect nerves in a "length-dependent" fashion, i.e. the longer the nerve fiber, the more severely it is affected. The result is a symmetric pattern of sensory, motor, and reflex symptoms and signs beginning in the feet, and "ascending" to the knees, fingers, etc. as the disease progresses. However, there are notable exceptions to this pattern dependent on the site of pathology; in diseases of the vasa nervorum (e.g. vasculitis), the deficits are asymmetric or multifocal as in the case above. In addition, in disease affecting proximal neural elements such as nerve roots (e.g. AIDP and CIDP), anterior horn cells (e.g. motor neuron diseases), or dorsal root ganglia cells (e.g. paraneoplastic sensory neuron-opathies), proximal weakness or sensory loss may be prominent. Identification of non-length dependency is an important clinical clue limiting the broad range of differential diagnoses in peripheral nerve disorders (see Table 20.1).

Case 2

A 45-year-old man presents with slowly progres-sive distal weakness and wasting in his hands and feet with increasing clumsiness and several falls. He noted foot weakness as far back as he can remember, and, on focused questioning, recalls that a former schoolteacher commented on his clumsiness during childhood. He has no positive sensory symptoms or autonomic symptoms. There is no clear family history, although he recalls that many family members have high arches. Examination reveals pes cavus foot deformity, a distal–predominant pattern of weak-ness and wasting, and generalized areflexia. Nerve conduction studies disclose uniform slowing of motor conduction velocities (median

conduction velocity or CV = 22 m/s) with reduc-tion in motor and sensory response amplitudes in the legs more than arms.

Diagnosis: Charcot–Marie–Tooth (CMT) disease type 1A due to PMP22 duplication.

This patient exhibits many of the typical features of a hereditary neuropathy phenotype: long history with slow progression, lack of positive sensory symptoms, and skeletal deformity (pes cavus). A carefully taken history may identify subtle neuropathic symptoms before the devel-opment of frank weakness (e.g. childhood clum-siness). Weakness follows a length-dependent pattern, and may be quite severe, but only comes to medical attention when functional limitation or disability develops (e.g. falls). An exception to the length-dependent pattern of most hereditary polyneuropathy syndromes that deserves special mention is hereditary neuropathy with pressure palsies (HNPP), due to *PMP22* deletions (see Chapter 21).

☙ CAUTION: SKELETAL DEFORMITIES

Although common in hereditary neuropathy, foot deformities may also be seen in central nervous system (CNS) diseases such as Friedreich's ataxia or hereditary spastic paraparesis, among others. Spinal abnormalities such as kyphosis or scoliosis, although non-specific, are clues to a hereditary neuropathy, and should be sought. Foot deformity may be in the form of "pes cavus" (high arch) or "pes planus" (fallen arch); both have similar diagnostic significance and typically reflect weakness of the intrinsic foot musculature with relative preservation of the extrinsic foot inverters and toe flexors and extensors. Finally, foot deformities may rarely be seen in chronic acquired neuropathies (e.g. longstanding CIDP).

Case 3

A 75-year-old man presents with progressive dif-ficulty climbing stairs and clumsiness of his right hand over 9 months, associated with muscle wasting of the hands. He has intermittent dys-phagia, and his weight has dropped 5 kg in 6

Table 20.2. Systemic manifestations of diseases associated with neuropathy

Systemic manifestation	Disease
Rheumatological	
Arthritis	Lyme disease, lupus, rheumatoid arthritis, sarcoidosis
Destructive arthropathy	Diabetes, leprosy, hereditary neuropathy
Hematological	
Hepatosplenomegaly	POEMS, myeloma, amyloidosis
Lymphadenopathy	POEMS, Castleman's disease, lymphoma, HIV, sarcoidosis
Macrocytosis – with or without anemia	Arsenic poisoning, vitamin B_{12} deficiency
Renal	HIV disease
	Fabry's disease
	Hepatitis B and C
	Diabetes
	Systemic vasculitis
	Lupus
	Amyloid
Gastrointestinal	Celiac disease
	Arsenic, thallium, or lead poisoning
	Porphyria
	Vitamin deficiency associated with malabsorption (e.g. thiamin, vitamin B_{12}, copper)
Dermatological	
Purpura	Systemic vasculitis, cryoglobulinemia
Hypopigmentation	Leprosy
Hyperpigmentation	Adrenomyeloneuropathy, POEMS
Ichthyosis	Refsum's disease
Angiokeratoma	Fabry's disease
Mees' lines	Arsenic, thallium poisoning
Alopecia	Thallium poisoning
Erythema nodosum	Sarcoidosis, connective tissue disease
Macroglossia	Amyloidosis, vitamin B_{12} deficiency
Thickened nerves	Hereditary neuropathy, leprosy
Raynaud's phenomenon	Cryoglobulinemia, connective tissue disease
Nodules	Rheumatoid arthritis
Kaposi's sarcoma	HIV
Cardiovascular	
Cardiac failure	Amyloidosis
Hypertrophic cardiomyopathy	Freidreich's ataxia
Pericarditis/pericardial effusion	Lupus, paraneoplastic syndrome

(*Continued*)

Table 20.2. (*Continued*)

Systemic manifestation	Disease
Cardiac conduction defects	Mitochondrial diseases
Respiratory	
Digital clubbing	Paraneoplastic syndrome, sarcoidosis, inflammatory bowel disease
Interstitial lung disease	Connective tissue diseases
Hilar adenopathy	Sarcoidosis
Endocrine	
Gynecomastia	Kennedy's disease
Hypothyroidism	POEMS
Diabetes	Mitochondrial diseases
Multiple system involvement	Critical illness polyneuropathy

months. He has no sensory symptoms. Examination shows atrophy of the intrinsic muscles of both hands, scattered fasciculations over the arms, legs, and trunk, and asymmetric moderate-to-severe proximal and distal limb weakness. Reflexes are normal to brisk, and the right plantar response is extensor. The speech has a nasal quality, and the cough is weak. The patient is dyspneic in the supine position, where there is paradoxical abdominal movement with respiration. The sensory examination is normal.

Diagnosis: amyotrophic lateral sclerosis
This is a typical presentation of moderately advanced motor neuron disease with gradual progression of proximal and distal weakness and wasting, bulbar and respiratory dysfunction, and weight loss. Although diagnostic confusion is unlikely in this case, the diagnosis may be delayed, particularly in patients who exhibit more subtle features early in the course of the disease. In addition to motor neuronopathy, the absence of sensory symptoms in patients with progressive limb or bulbar weakness should suggest a myopathy, neuromuscular junction disorder, or motor neuropathy with conduction block (MNCB). In such patients, the presence of preserved or brisk reflexes in wasted muscles is a strong clue to combined upper and lower motor neuron lesions as in amyotrophic lateral sclerosis (ALS). By contrast, marked muscle weakness without wasting or hyperreflexia should bring to

mind MNCB. Patients with neuromuscular junction disease (e.g. myasthenia gravis) often describe a fluctuating rather than a progressive course, do not have upper motor neuron signs, and typically show oculomotor signs that are not observed in ALS. With some exceptions (e.g. inclusion body myopathy), myopathies typically present with proximally predominant, symmetric muscle weakness, with wasting commensurate to the degree of weakness, and preservation of reflexes until weakness is advanced.

> ✋ **CAUTION!**
>
> **NORMAL AGING**
> A relatively common diagnostic error is to inappropriately attribute changes in peripheral nervous system physiology associated with normal aging to a peripheral neuropathic process, e.g. ankle jerks are commonly reduced or absent in 5% of otherwise healthy individuals over age 50 and up to 30% of those over age 70. In addition, both large-fiber (e.g. vibration thresholds) and small-fiber (e.g. warming/cooling thresholds) functions may be reduced in older patients to the extent that quantitative sensory testing may not be reliable in individuals over the age of 70. At the bedside, a useful guide to vibratory threshold testing is that 3 s or more of sensation from a 128 Hz

tuning fork at maximal intensity is typically considered normal in those aged over 70. Although vibratory sensation is physiologically reduced with normal aging, joint position sensation should be relatively preserved. Furthermore, such individuals should be not report symptoms otherwise suggestive of a neuropathic disorder (e.g. numbness, paraesthesias, weakness, or allodynia).

Case 4

A 65-year-old man with colonic adenocarcinoma is treated with adjuvant chemotherapy (5-fluorouracil, oxaloplatin, and folinic acid). Intermittent paraesthesias began in the feet within hours of each chemotherapy infusion. Following the completion of 6 months of chemotherapy, the symptoms progressed over the next 6 months to frank numbness that ascended symmetrically from the feet to the mid-calf, and to the fingertips of both hands. Examination revealed reduced pinprick to the mid-calf and wrist-crease bilaterally, reduced vibratory sensation to the level of the pelvis, severely diminished joint position sensation in the feet, but only slight weakness of hallux extension in both feet. Reflexes were absent at the knees and ankles, and reduced but present at the biceps and triceps. Electrodiagnostic testing confirmed a length-dependent axonal sensorimotor polyneuropathy with absent sural and reduced distal lower extremity motor response amplitudes.

Diagnosis: toxic polyneuropathy due to oxaloplatin chemotherapy
This case demonstrates a classic cause–effect relationship typical of a toxic polyneuropathy syndrome, in this case due to platinum-based chemotherapy. The temporal link between toxin exposure and symptom onset is less evident in cases where the exposure is chronic and low level, so specific inquiry into possible exposures is crucial. The onset of symptoms is remarkably symmetric, length dependent, and sensory predominant, and is typical of most toxic neuropathies. In addition, the neuropathy may progress after the termination of toxic exposure ("coast-

ing" phenomenon). In axonal polyneuropathies, reflexes are lost in a distal–proximal fashion, with preservation of proximal upper extremity reflexes until extremely advanced, whereas in demyelinating polyneuropathy syndromes early and diffuse hypo- or areflexia is the rule. With rare exception, almost all toxic neuropathies are axonal in nature (see Table 20.1). Pain is a variable feature, but may be prominent in certain toxic syndromes (e.g. thallium poisoning). Autonomic dysfunction is typically absent or mild but is prominent in some acute exposures (e.g. pyrinuron, arsenic, organophosphate, n-hexane, or acrylamide). Weakness as a general rule is a late finding, confined to distal muscles, and mild in nature, again with some exceptions (e.g. vincristine in patients with Charcot–Marie–Tooth disease, and lead and hexacarbon toxicity). Finally, in patients with preservation of distal reflexes despite significant "large-fiber" pattern sensory loss, spinal cord or brain involvement should be considered. This may coexist with peripheral neuropathy (e.g. subacute combined systems disease due to vitamin B_{12} or copper deficiency).

Ancillary testing

Electrodiagnostic testing

Nerve conduction studies and needle electromyography (EMG) examination tailored to the clinical problem provide useful diagnostic information by confirming the presence of "large-fiber" peripheral neuropathy, and determining pathophysiology (e.g. axon loss vs demyelination), severity, chronicity, and length dependency. It is important to recognize that electrodiagnostic testing will not detect a pure "small-fiber" sensory or autonomic neuropathy, for which other testing is available (see below).

Nerve and skin biopsy

Nerve biopsy is important in the diagnosis of inflammatory, infiltrative, or infectious neuropathies. The most commonly selected nerves are the sural, superficial radial, or superficial peroneal sensory nerves. The last has the advantage that the adjacent peroneus brevis muscle may also be sampled using the same incision, raising the diagnostic sensitivity of the biopsy from

Table 20.3. Considerations for laboratory investigation of neuropathy

Neuropathy type	Acute	Subacute or chronic
Demyelinating		
Symmetric	Lumbar puncture (protein, cell counts) HIV serology, Lyme disease titer, ANA	Lumbar puncture (protein, cell counts) Serum/urine protein electrophoresis, immunofixation HIV serology Antibody testing: MAG, GD1A, GD1B, sulfatide Genetic testing, e.g. *PMP22, MPZ, Cx32* Autoimmune: ANA, Ro, La Bone marrow biopsy, bone survey MRI of brain (leukodystrophy) VLCFA analysis Arylsulfatase A levels
Asymmetric/ Multifocal	Nerve biopsy Lumbar puncture Genetic testing: *PMP22* deletion	Lumbar puncture Antibody testing: GM1 (IgM) Genetic testing: *PMP22* deletion
Axonal		
Symmetric	Lumbar puncture Urine porphyrins Heavy metal screening of blood/urine/hair samples Anti-GM1 antibody (IgG) Nerve biopsy	Biochemistry: renal, liver, thyroid function, fasting glucose, GTT, glycated hemoglobin Vitamin B_{12}, thiamin assay Genetic testing for CMT II HIV, Lyme disease serology Paraneoplastic workup Tissue biopsy for amyloid deposition Genetic testing for familial amyloid polyneuropathy Autoantibody screen: ANA, RF, complements, Ro, La Salivary gland biopsy (Sjögren's syndrome) Celiac antibodies
Asymmetric/ Multifocal	Nerve biopsy Serum autoantibodies: p-ANCA, ANA Cryoglobulins ACE level Hepatitis serology Lyme disease titer Lead level Paraneoplastic workup Blood glucose testing, glycosylated hemoglobin, GTT	Nerve biopsy Lumbar puncture Lyme disease titer Tissue biopsy for amyloid deposition Genetic testing for familial amyloid polyneuropathy Body CT scan Autoantibody screen: ANA, RF, complement, Ro, La Salivary gland biopsy (Sjögren's syndrome)

ACE, angiotensin-converting enzyme; ANA, antinuclear antibodies; CMT, Charcot–Marie–Tooth disease; GTT, glucose tolerance test; MAG, myelin-associated glycoprotein; p-ANCA, perinuclear anti-neutrophil cytoplasmic antibodies; PMP22, peripheral myelin protein 22; RF, rheumatoid factor; VLCFA, very-long-chain fatty acids.

approximately 50% to 75% for peripheral nerve vasculitis. The technique of skin punch biopsy to examine epidermal nerve fiber density (ENFD) is useful in the diagnosis of suspected small-fiber sensory polyneuropathies. Reduced ENFD supports the diagnosis, and comparison of ENFD at proximal (thigh) and distal (ankle) sites clarifies whether the loss of epidermal nerve fibers follows a length-dependent pattern.

Laboratory testing

Table 20.3 outlines considerations for laboratory testing, beginning with key clinical and electrodiagnostic features. Nerve biopsy is reserved for the diagnosis of suspected vasculitic or inflammatory neuropathy and cerebrospinal fluid (CSF) examination for suspected demyelinating polyneuropathies (e.g. acute or chronic inflammatory demyelinating polyradiculoneuropathy). Some testing is of limited utility when employed as a screening tool (e.g. heavy-metal testing), but is useful in select circumstances and performed on appropriate samples (e.g. blood, urine, or hair). The same is true for standardized antibody-based and molecular-based "panels" which are not cost-effective as screening tools but may be very helpful when the pre-test probability of an antibody mediated or genetic neuropathy is reasonably high.

Autonomic and quantitative sensory testing

Basic autonomic function testing may be performed at the bedside with measurement of orthostatic blood pressure and heart rate, and R-R interval during Valsalva maneuver. More detailed testing in a dedicated laboratory provides both a qualitative as well as quantitative assessment of vasomotor and sudomotor function, sympathetic skin response, and thermoregulatory sweat test. QST allows quantitation of large-fiber function (via vibration detection threshold measurement) and small-fiber function (via heating/cooling/pain detection threshold measurement) and compares individual responses with those of age-matched controls.

References

Asbury AK, Gilliat RW, eds. The clinical approach to neuropathy. In: *Peripheral nerve disorders*. Butterworths, London, 1984: 1–20.

Dyck PJ, Litchy WJ, Lehman KA, et al. Variables influencing neuropathic endpoints: The Rochester Diabetic Neuropathy Study of Healthy Subjects. *Neurology* 1995;**45**:1115.

Griffin JW, Hseih S-T, McArthur JC, Cornblath DR. Laboratory testing in peripheral nerve disease. *Neurol Clin* 1996;**14**:119–33.

Kennedy WR, Said G. Sensory nerves in skin answers about painful feet? *Neurology* 1999; **53**:1614–15.

Lewis RA, Sumner AJ. The electrodiagnostic distinctions between chronic familial and acquired demyelinative neuropathies. *Neurology* 1982;**32**:592–6.

Light AR, Perl ER. Peripheral sensory systems. In: Dyck PJ, Thomas PK, Griffin JW, Low PA, Poduslo JF (eds), *Peripheral Neuropathy*, 3rd edn. Philadelphia, PA: WB Saunders Co., 1993: 149–65.

Logigian EL. Approach to and classification of peripheral neuropathy. In: Samuels MA, Feske S. (eds), *Office Practice of Neurology*. Edinburgh: Churchill Livingstone Inc., 1996: 492–7.

Logigian EL, Kelly JJ, Adelman LS. Nerve conduction studies and biopsy correlation in over 100 consecutive patients with suspected polyneuropathy. *Muscle Nerve* 1994;**17**:1010–20.

Low PA. Quantitation of autonomic function. In Dyck PJ, Thomas PK, Lambert EH, Bunge R (eds), *Peripheral Neuropathy*. Philadelphia, PA: WB Saunders Co., 1993: 729–45.

Lynch DR, Chance PF. Inherited peripheral neuropathies. *The neurologist* 1997;**3**:277–92.

Mendell JR, Cornblath DR. Evaluation of the peripheral neuropathy patient using quantitative sensory testing. In: Mendell JR, Kissell JT, Cornblath DR. *Diagnosis and Management of Peripheral Nerve Disorders*. New York: Oxford University Press, 2001: 38–42.

Neundorfer B, Grahmann F, Engelgardt A, Harte J. Postoperative effects and value of sural nerve biopsies: a retrospective study. *Eur Neurol* 1990;**30**:350–2.

Periquet MI, Novak V, Collins MP, et al. Painful sensory neuropathy prospective evaluation using skin biopsy. *Neurology* 1999;**53**:1641–7.

Said G, Lacroix-Ciaudo C, Fujimura H, Blas C, Faux N. The peripheral neuropathy of necrotizing arteritis: a clinicopathological study. *Ann Neurol* 1988;**23**:461–5.

Hereditary Motor Sensory Neuropathies (Charcot–Marie–Tooth Disease)

Araya Puwanant and David N. Herrmann

Department of Neurology, University of Rochester Medical Center, Rochester, NY, USA

Hereditary motor and sensory neuropathies (HMSNs) are the most common inherited neuropathy (IN) with a prevalence of about 1 in 2500 (Table 21.1.) The term "HMSN" is used interchangeably with Charcot–Marie–Tooth (CMT) disease, although increasingly HMSNs are being described in terms of genetically specific CMT disease subtypes. This chapter focuses on diagnosis and care of patients with CMT, and a related disorder, hereditary neuropathy with liability to pressure palsies (HNPP).

Charcot–Marie–Tooth disease: signs and symptoms

CMT is a genetically heterogeneous family. Most patients share features of the "classic CMT disease phenotype" (Table 21.2). Symptoms typically begin in the first two decades, but can manifest first in late adulthood. The hallmark is insidious, symmetric, limb weakness and muscle wasting which usually begins in the feet/distal legs. Initial motor milestones are normal with a "classic CMT phenotype." Affected individuals are often "clumsy" runners in childhood or describe "weak ankles." High arched feet with hammer toes or flat feet may become prominent during adolescence, and trigger medical attention. Later, hand weakness and sensory loss manifest with impairments such as difficulty doing up and undoing buttons.

Patients with classic CMT may note a "deadened" feeling in the feet/legs, but, unlike with acquired neuropathies, seldom report prominent positive sensory symptoms. Pain, particularly of the lower limbs/feet, may be significant and take the form of cramps or musculoskeletal or neuropathic pain.

Examination discloses weakness and atrophy involving intrinsic foot and ankle dorsiflexor more than flexor muscles. As CMT progresses, intrinsic hand muscle and more proximal limb weakness may appear. Tendon reflex loss varies with the type of CMT, but reflexes are usually absent at the ankles, and often diffusely. Vibration and pin sensation are variably impaired in a length-dependent pattern, with distal proprioception loss occurring in more severely affected individuals. As weakness and sensory loss progress, foot drop, sensory ataxia and falls ensue. Ankle foot orthoses (AFOs) are often needed, with variable requirement for a cane/walker and rarely a wheelchair.

CMT occasionally manifests other clinical features. These may include upper limb postural tremor, dsyphonia from vocal fold paresis, respiratory insufficiency from diaphragmatic dys-

Neuromuscular Disorders, First Edition. Edited by Rabi N. Tawil, Shannon Venance.

Table 21.1. Inherited neuropathies (INs)

Isolated INs	INs as part of a multisystem disorder
Hereditary motor sensory neuropathies (includes Charcot–Marie–Tooth disease neuropathies)	Familial amyloid polyneuropathy
Hereditary neuropathy with liability to pressure palsies (HNPP)	INs associated with lipid disorders (e.g. Fabry's disease)
Hereditary sensory or sensory and autonomic neuropathies	Mitochondrial disorders
Hereditary motor neuropathies	Porphyrias
Hereditary neuralgic amyotrophy	INs associated with hereditary ataxias
	INs as part of DNA-repair disorders
	Other

Adapted from Reilly MM, Shy ME. Diagnosis and new treatments in genetic neuropathies. *J Neurol Neurosurg Psychiatry* 2009;**80**:1304–14, with permission of BMJ Publishing Group Ltd.

Table 21.2. Clinical features distinguishing Charcot–Marie–Tooth disease from chronic acquired neuropathies (e.g. diabetic neuropathy)

Inherited neuropathies	Acquired neuropathies
Symptoms present for decades	Symptoms present for months
Distal weakness and atrophy prominent	Distal weakness and atrophy are late features
Positive sensory symptoms are seldom a presenting or prominent feature	Positive sensory symptoms (e.g. prickling) often an early feature
Foot deformities (high arches, hammer toes, flat feet)	No foot deformities
Family history of neuropathy or foot deformities	No family history

function, pupillary dysfunction, ulceromutilation of the distal extremities, and scoliosis. These additional clinical features may serve as clues to the specific genetic diagnosis.

Classification of CMT and HNPP

Hundreds of mutations in approximately 40 different genes have been associated with HMSNs. About 85% of patients with demyelinating forms of CMT disease and 30% with axonal CMT disease can now receive a precise genetic diagnosis. The explosion of knowledge about genetics of INs has seen a shift from clinical and electrophysiological classification (HMSN 1–7), to a system based on inheritance pattern (autosomal dominant [AD], autosomal recessive [AR], or X-linked), nerve conduction velocities (NCVs, demyelinating, axonal, or intermediate slowing) and the specific genetic defect (Table 21.3.) HNPP is classified separately from CMT1 disease because it only rarely manifests with a CMT disease phenotype, usually manifesting as an episodic multifocal neuropathy.

Specific CMT neuropathies and HNPP (Table 21.3)

CMT1

CMT1A is the most common CMT, accounting for 70–90% of CMT1 and 50% of all CMT. It is caused by duplication of a 1.5-Mb fragment on chromosome 17p.11 which includes the peripheral myelin protein 22 *(PMP22)* gene. *PMP22* overexpression underlies development of CMT1A. New duplication of *PMP22* (resulting in sporadic CMT), accounts for 10% of CMT1A. Patients usually present with a "classic CMT disease phenotype" beginning in the first two decades. Longevity is normal, but disease severity variable. Affected individuals commonly require bracing or other gait-assistive devices, but rarely become wheelchair bound.

Table 21.3. Evolving classification of hereditary motor sensory neuropathies

Pre-genetic diagnosis	Era of genetic diagnosis
HMSN1: median or ulnar motor conduction velocity <38 m/s HMSN1A HMSN1B HMSN1X	CMT1A–F Key genes: *PMP22* duplication, mutations of *MPZ, LITAF/SIMPLE, EGR2, NEFL* CMT1X (X-linked) Key gene: *GJB1*
HMSN2 (dominant axonal): median or ulnar motor conduction velocity >38 m/s	AD-CMT2A–N Some key genes: *MFN2, KIF1B, RAB7, TRPV4, GARS, NEFL, HSPB1* and *-8, MPZ, DNM2, YARS, BSCL2* AR-CMT2 (very rare): Some involve lamin A/C, *GDAP1*
HMSN3: Déjérine–Sottas syndrome/congenital hypomyelinating neuropathy – severe early onset, conduction velocity <10 m/s	HMSN3 or CMT3 Key genes: point mutations in *PMP22, MPZ, EGR2, PRX*
HMSN4: recessive demyelinating	CMT4A-J More common genes include: *GDAP1 (CMT4A), SH3TC2 (CMT4C), PRX (CMT4F)*
HMSN5: dominant axonal neuropathy with spastic paraparesis	*MFN2* and *BSCL2* mutations account for some patients
HMSN6: axonal neuropathy with optic atrophy	*MFN2* mutations account for some patients
HMSN7: axonal neuropathy with retinitis pigmentosa	?
Other, e.g. tomaculous neuropathy	HNPP *PMP22* deletion, point mutations

AD, autosomal dominant; AR, autosomal recessive; BSCL2, Berardinelli–Seip congenital lipodystrophy 2; CMT, Charcot–Marie–Tooth disease; DNM2, dynamin 2; EGR2, early growth response protein 2; GARS, glycyl-tRNA synthetase; GDAP1 ganglioside-induced differentiation-associated protein 1; *GJB1*; gap junction beta-1 protein; HMSN, hereditary motor sensory neuropathy; HNPP, hereditary neuropathy with liability to pressure palsies; HSP, heat shock protein; KIF1B, kinesin family member 1B; *LITAF*, lipopolysaccharide-induced tumor necrosis factor-α factor; MFN2, itofusin-2; *MPZ*, myelin p zero gene; *NEFL*, neurofilament light polypeptide; *PMP22*, peripheral myelin protein 22 gene; PRX periaxin; SH3TC2 SH3 domain and tetratricopeptide repeats 2; TRPV4, transient receptor potential cation channel, subfamily V, member 4; YARS, tyrosyl-tRNA synthetase.

Occasional patients develop scoliosis, upper extremity postural tremor, or hearing and respiratory impairment. Nerve conduction studies (NCSs) disclose a demyelinating neuropathy, with upper limb motor NCVs that are almost invariably between 10 and 38 m/s, with uniform slowing.

CMT1B is due to mutations in the myelin protein zero gene *(MPZ)*, located on chromo-some 1 and accounts for about 5% of CMT1. It is essential for the normal structure and function of myelin. Over 120 *MPZ* point mutations have been associated with CMT. Patients can present with a "classic CMT disease phenotype", but are more likely to have either a severe earlier onset form with delayed ambulation and NCV <10 m/s (HSMNIII) or adult onset with variable NCV slowing.

MPZ mutations can manifest with a varying phenotype:

- CMT1B: early onset of a "classic CMT phenotype"
- HMSN III (DSN-CHN): infantile or early childhood onset, most severe form of CMT, very slow nerve conduction velocities (<10 m/s)
- CMT2I/J: late-onset CMT2, can be severe; pupillary abnormalities, deafness, and dysphagia possible
- Dominant intermediate CMT: variable severity.

Note: CHN is congenital hypomyelinating neuropathy; DSN is Déjérine–Sottas neuropathies.

X-linked dominant CMT (CMT1X) is the second most common CMT (10% of all cases) and is associated with mutations in the gap junction protein beta-1 *(GJB1)* gene encoding connexin 32 which acts as a gap junction in compact myelin. Males present earlier and are usually more severely affected than females. Electrodiagnostic testing shows intermediate range NCV (25–45 m/s), with typically slower NCVs in affected males than females.

Hereditary neuropathy with liability to pressure palsies

HNPP is an AD disorder that is allelic with CMT1A, with 85–90% of cases due to a *PMP22* gene deletion and in 10% to a *PMP22* point mutation. It usually presents with recurrent painless neuropathies at compression sites (e.g. median neuropathy at the wrist, peroneal neuropathy at the knee). The focal neuropathies recover spontaneously, although fixed neuropathic deficits accrue over time. Incidental compression (e.g. leaning on an elbow, knee crossing, squatting, or positioning during surgery) can trigger the neuropathies. The focal neuropathies are typically superimposed on a mild, often asymptomatic underlying polyneuropathy. HNPP also

predisposes to painless brachial plexopathies. Occasionally a fulminant presentation of HNPP has been described that resembles mononeuritis multiplex.

The electrophysiological pattern is one of a multifocal demyelinating neuropathy with particularly slowed motor and sensory distal latencies. Conduction block is seen at typical compression sites. Sural nerve biopsy (although rarely required for diagnosis) shows frequent focal myelin thickenings known as tomaculae. A lack of awareness of HNPP can lead to unnecessary nerve decompressions, treatment with immunosuppressive agents for misdiagnosed acquired inflammatory demyelinating polyneuropathy, or failure to take precautions to avoid external peripheral nerve compression.

CMT2 (dominant axonal CMT)

CMT2 represents 25–30% of all CMT, although it may be underdiagnosed because causative mutations are identified in only 30% of families. Mutations in the mitochondrial fusion protein, mitofusin 2 (MFN2), cause CMT2A and account for about 20% of CMT2 disease cases. *MFN2* mutations typically are associated with childhood-onset CMT with distally dominant atrophy, weakness, and sensory loss in lower more than upper extremities. However. mild later onset or asymptomatic cases do occur. Some *MFN2* mutations produce optic atrophy and CMT neuropathy (HMSN6), while others display a combination of axonal neuropathy and lower limb hyper-reflexia (HMSN V) (see Table 21.3). It is unclear how *MFN2* mutations produce CMT, but they result in abnormal mitochondrial fusion and disordered mitochondrial kinetics.

Autosomal recessive CMT disease

Recessive CMT accounts for less than 10% of all CMT, but may be most CMT cases in areas with high rates of consanguinity. Recessive demyelinating CMT is more common than axonal subtypes.

CMT4 (recessive demyelinating CMT)

At least nine genes have been associated with CMT4. Most forms present in infancy or early childhood and are severe. Among these, CMT4C is emerging as the most common, and is due to

> ★ **TIPS AND TRICKS**
>
> Distinct phenotypes occur in CMT2 that are diagnostically helpful and direct genetic testing.
>
> | CMT2 disease | Associated gene | Clinical features |
> |---|---|---|
> | CMT2A | *MFN2* | Classic CMT phenotype; optic atrophy or pyramidal tract signs frequently present |
> | CMT2B | *RAB7* | Prominent sensory loss, ulceromutilation |
> | CMT2C | *TRPV4* | Early onset vocal fold and diaphragm involvement, proximal weakness |
> | CMT2D | *GARS/BSCL2* | Upper limb and motor predominance |
> | CMT2I/J | *MPZ* | Late onset; pupillary abnormalities; hearing loss, pain and possible dysphagia |
> | CMT2H/K | *GDAP1* | Early onset (<2 years); severe course; frequent vocal fold paralysis |
>
> BSCL2, Berardinelli–Seip congenital lipodystrophy 2; GARS, glycyl-tRNA synthetase; GDAP1, ganglioside-induced differentiation-associated protein; MFN2, mitofusin-2; MPZ, myelin protein zero; RAB7, small GTPase late endosomal protein; TRPV4, transient receptor potential cation channel, subfamily V, member 4.

mutations in the gene for SH3 domain and tetratricopeptide repeats containing protein 2 (*SH3TC2*). CMT4C is characterized by childhood onset of prominent scoliosis. *SH3TC2* mutations produce a neuropathy of variable severity that is often milder and more slowly progressive than other CMT4 subtypes.

AR-CMT2 (autosomal recessive axonal CMT2)

Recessive axonal CMT, variously classified under CMT4 or as AR-CMT2, is extremely rare and has been associated with mutations in the nuclear envelope protein lamin A/C and the ganglioside-induced differentiation-associated protein 1 (GDAP1).

Intermediate CMT disease (DI-CMT)

Certain CMT present with intermediate NCV slowing (25–45 m/s) and are classified as dominant intermediate (DI) CMT diseases. Several causative genes have been identified. Dynamin 2 mutations underlie DI-CMTB and manifest in the first two decades of life, with a slowly progressive CMT disease phenotype. Some mutations are associated with congenital cataracts or neutropenia. Dynamin 2 mutations also underlie some centronuclear myopathies, which can have an associated mild distal axonal neuropathy.

Mutations in the tyrosyl-tRNA synthetase gene (*YARS*) cause DI-CMTC. Neuropathy onset is from childhood to adulthood, with a slowly progressive classic CMT disease phenotype.

Strategy for definitive diagnosis of CMT

Clinical evaluation

The history should document motor and cognitive developmental milestones, onset of symptoms, time course of neuropathy progression and functional limitations. A detailed family history including first- to third-degree relatives is essential. Patients are often unaware of familial neuropathy or foot deformities which may not have been diagnosed as such. Defining the inheritance pattern is critical for efficient CMT diagnosis; male-to-male transmission, for example, excludes X-linked disease. A family history may, however, be lacking, because new mutations are frequent with some CMT. Patients should undergo a medical and neurological examination for characteristic features of CMT.

Electrophysiology

NCSs are important for CMT diagnosis. NCVs of upper extremity motor nerves have been used to differentiate CMTs. An upper limb NCV <38 m/s (suggestive of demyelination) has historically been used to distinguish HMSN1 from HMSNII (>38 m/s). As the genetics of different CMTs has been clarified, distinct electrophysiological signatures for some CMTs have been recognized. CMT show NCVs that are extremely slow: <10 m/s (HMSNIII), >10 m/s but in a demyelinating range (CMT1, some CMT4), intermediate slowing (25–45 m/s), or essentially normal (CMT2). NCSs help direct rational genetic testing but do not definitively distinguish between an inherited and an acquired neuropathy. Definitive diagnosis of CMT needs an integration of clinical, familial, electrophysiological, and genetic information.

Genetic testing

Genetic testing facilitates CMT diagnosis and guides prognosis and family counseling. Utilizing commercially available testing, a causative mutation can be identified for at least 85% of CMT1 and about 30% of CMT2 families. Genetic testing is also useful when there is a CMT disease phenotype, but a negative family history, but not in cryptogenic polyneuropathies without an IN phenotype. A targeted genetic testing approach, focusing on mutations that are likely based on inheritance pattern, phenotype, and electrophysiological findings is preferable.

Differential diagnosis of CMT

Chronic acquired neuropathies can confound the diagnosis of CMT. Patients with early onset, slowly progressive, chronic inflammatory demyelinating polyneuropathy (CIDP) may develop foot deformities, and be misdiagnosed as having CMT. Individuals with CMT disease are susceptible to acquiring superimposed neuropathies. An inflammatory demyelinating neuropathy that may respond to immunotherapy can occur with CMT1A, CMT1B, or CMT1X. Systemic disorders such as diabetes or focal processes (e.g. entrapment neuropathy) exacerbate CMT. A precipitous decline in a patient with CMT requires consideration of the above and other acquired factors. Other INs can mimic CMT. Hereditary sensory and autonomic neuropathy type 1 (SEE Table 21.1) presents with severe sensory loss and ulceromutilation that resembles CMT2B. Finally some CMTs can present acutely as if they were an acquired neuropathy, e.g. some *MPZ* mutations manifest with a late-onset, fairly abrupt, painful, predominantly sensory neuropathy. HNPP can be mistaken for an acquired entrapment neuropathy syndrome or, if it manifests with brachial plexopathy, for focal CIDP.

✋ CAUTION!

Consider factors that influence CMT severity:

- Diabetes mellitus worsens CMT1A
- Inflammatory neuropathies (e.g. CIDP) can superimpose on CMT1A, -1B, -1X, causing precipitous decline
- Neurotoxic chemotherapies, particularly vincristine, cisplatin, oxaliplatin, and paclitaxel derivatives, should be avoided in CMT. Vincristine can cause acute quadriparesis when given to CMT patients.

Management of CMT disease and HNPP

There is currently no disease-modifying therapy for CMT or HNPP. CMT care focuses on patient and family counseling regarding the diagnosis and prognosis, and on rehabilitative and symptomatic therapies to optimize function and quality of life.

Education and genetic counseling

The natural history of CMT is not well studied for subtypes beyond CMT1A and CMT2; however, patients/families can be counseled that the neuropathy is generally slowly progressive, with normal longevity for most, and rare wheelchair requirement.

Genetic counseling is essential. Carrier and prenatal testing is possible for some forms of CMT. Preimplantation genetic diagnosis (PGD) is available for CMT1A. For families harboring severe mutations or where there is a strong family preference, prenatal testing or PGD will likely be increasingly available.

Physical rehabilitation and orthotics

Several rehabilitative approaches are used in CMT. Tailored 12- and 24-week strength training programs are safe and variously improve measures of strength, gait, and activities of daily living (ADLs), and can be individualized according to patient characteristics. We advise patients about nutrition and address obesity which can compound functional limitations. Passive stretching to prevent Achilles tendon shortening is usually recommended, although evidence of its utility is lacking. Gait and dynamic balance training may be helpful in some patients with sensory ataxia.

In patients with limited weakness, and no significant ankle joint instability, shoe modification, plantar inserts, and assistive devices (e.g. foot-up or ankle-stabilizing orthoses [ASOs]) can improve foot position. AFOs are prescribed to address foot drop and ankle instability. Carbon fiber or custom-fitted AFOs are preferable because they weigh less and are better tolerated. An occupational therapy evaluation is recommended for manual impairments that interfere with ADLs. Upper-limb bracing orthoses are occasionally helpful for severe upper extremity involvement.

Symptomatic treatment

Pain in CMT can be musculoskeletal in type (osteoarthropathy or skeletal deformities), neuropathic, or due to neurogenic cramps. Custom-made orthotics are effective in reducing musculoskeletal foot pain related to pes cavus. Strategies for other pain types include physiotherapy, stretching and conditioning exercises, orthoses and judicious use of non-opiate analgesics/neuropathic pain agents, and when necessary surgical interventions.

Fatigue and excessive day-time sleepiness are commonly reported and may be related to increased work required to accomplish ADLs, respiratory muscle insufficiency, or sleep apnea. Management is best directed at precipitating causes. Bilevel positive airway pressure ventilation should be considered for CMT patients who have significant restrictive pulmonary impairment.

Restless legs syndrome (RLS) occurs in approximately 20% of cases of CMT1 and CMT2. Sleep apnea and other factors that exacerbate RLS (e.g.

iron deficiency anemia) should be addressed. For some patients a trial of nocturnal gabapentin is warranted before considering dopamine agonists. Patients who develop vocal fold paralysis, which can occur in CMT2C and CMT4A, as well as in other forms of CMT require evaluation by an ear, nose and throat specialist, and may need surgical intervention if airway obstruction is significant.

Surgical treatment

Surgical intervention should be avoided, unless patients develop progressive foot, ankle, or other joint deformities that are symptomatic and functionally limiting and fail to respond to conservative strategies. Several surgeries including plantar fasciotomy and tendon transfer and releases have been attempted to reduce mild-to-moderate cavovarus deformities. If deformities are fixed or advanced, osteotomies are considered. Triple arthodesis is a surgical fusion of the talocalcaneal, talonavicular, and calcanocuboid joints, which should be reserved for the most severe foot deformities, given the high long-term incidence of osteoarthrosis in adjacent joints. Scoliosis of varying severity occurs in about a third of patients with CMT and about a third will require surgery.

Bibliography

Aboussouan LS, Lewis RA, Shy ME. Disorders of pulmonary function, sleep and the upper airway in Charcot–Marie–Tooth disease. *Lung* 2007;**185**:1–7.

Beals TC, Nickisch F. Charcot–Marie–Tooth and the cavovarus foot. *Foot Ankle Clin* 2008;**13**: 259–74.

Bernard R, Boyer A, Nègre P et al. Prenatal detection of the 17p11.2 duplication in Charcot–Marie–Tooth disease type 1A: necessity of a multidisciplinary approach for heterogeneous disorders. *Eur J Hum Genet* 2002;**10**:297–302.

Boentert M, Dziewas R, Heidbreder A, et al. Fatigue, reduced sleep quality and restless legs syndrome in Charcot–Marie–Tooth disease: a web–based survey. *J Neurol.* 2010;**257**:646–52.

Burns J, Landorf KB, Ryan MM, Crosbie J, Ouvrier RA. Interventions for the prevention and treatment of pes cavus. *Cochrane Database System Rev* 2007;**4**:CD006154

England JD, Gronseth GS, Franklin G, et al. Practice parameter: Evaluation of distal symmetric polyneuropathy: role of laboratory and genetic testing (an evidence-based review). *Neurology* 2009;**72**:185–92.

Herrmann DN. Experimental therapeutics in hereditary neuropathies: the past, the present, and the future. *Neurotherapeutics* 2008;**5**: 507–15.

Karol LA, Elerson E. Scoliosis in patients with Charcot–Marie–Tooth disease. *J Bone Joint Surg Am* 2007;**89**:1504–10.

Nicholson GA. The dominantly inherited motor and sensory neuropathies: clinical and molecular advances. *Muscle Nerve* 2006;**33**:589–97.

Pareyson D, Marchesi C. Diagnosis, natural history, and management of Charcot–Marie–Tooth disease. *Lancet Neurology* 2009;**8**: 654–67.

Reilly MM, Shy ME. Diagnosis and new treatments in genetic neuropathies. *J Neurol Neurosurg Psychiatry* 2009;**80**:1304–14.

Shy ME, Chen L, Swan ER, et al. Neuropathy progression in Charcot–Marie–Tooth disease type 1A. *Neurology* 2008;**70**:378–83.

Shy ME, Lupski JR, Chance PF et al. Hereditary motor and sensory neuropathies: an overview of clinical, genetic, electrophysiologic and pathologic features. In: Dyck PJ, Thomas PK (eds), *Peripheral Neuropathies*, 4th edn. Philadelphia, PA: Elsevier Saunders, 2005: 1623–58.

Ward CM, Dolan LA, Bennett DL, et al. Long-term results of reconstruction for treatment of a flexible cavovarus foot in Charcot–Marie–Tooth disease. *J Bone Joint Surg Am* 2008;**90**: 2631–42.

Young P, De Jonghe P, Stögbauer F, et al. Treatment of Charcot–Marie–Tooth disease. *Cochrane Database System Rev* 2008;**23**:CD006052.

Diabetic Neuropathies

Douglas W. Zochodne

Department of Clinical Neurosciences, University of Calgary, Alberta, Canada

Diabetic mellitus (DM) targets the peripheral nervous system in several ways. Diabetic polyneuropathy (DPN) is a diffuse disorder of peripheral nerves that targets distal axon terminals, especially those of sensory neurons. Diabetes also predisposes patients to entrapment neuropathies which include carpal tunnel syndrome, ulnar neuropathy at the elbow, and meralgia paresthetica, an entrapment of the lateral cutaneous nerve of the thigh. Finally, people with diabetes may develop other isolated or focal neuropathies that involve the lumbosacral plexus, third cranial nerve, or other sites. Moreover, although each type of neuropathic complication adds substantial disability to a person with DM, some of these may exist in combination. This brief review summarizes clinical and laboratory features of diabetic neuropathies as well as the research directions designed to understand them. Although not discussed here, DM is also recognized to target the central nervous system.

Clinical features

Diabetic polyneuropathy

DPN usually presents with sensory symptoms in people with both type 1 and type 2 diabetes. These may initially be positive, such as tingling, prickling, "pins and needles," and pain, followed by negative symptoms including numbness and gait unsteadiness. Sensory symptoms have been identified in 13–20% of patients with DM.

Neuropathic pain is the presenting symptom in 7–20% of patients with diabetes. Important descriptors of neuropathic pain in diabetes include burning (especially at night), lancinating, or electrical, shock like, walking on hot sand, tightness, painful tingling, and others. Allodynia, the sensation that normally innocuous stimuli are painful, may be prominent. The touch of the bedcovers at night may be unbearable. Although DPN may be present in over 50% of patients with diabetes, a large group is classified as asymptomatic. In these patients, neuropathy may be detected using nerve conduction studies, quantitative sensory testing (QST), autonomic studies, and other types of investigation (see below). Although no clear intervention is known to arrest incipient asymptomatic polyneuropathy, its identification may assume singular importance should therapeutic interventions arise.

> ### ⬡ SCIENCE REVISITED
>
> **MECHANISMS LINKED TO THE DEVELOPMENT OF DIABETIC POLYNEUROPATHY**
>
> - Excessive flux of polyols (sugar alcohols) such as sorbitol, which alter Schwann cell and neuronal function
> - Disease of small blood vessels (microangiopathy) involving peripheral

Neuromuscular Disorders, First Edition. Edited by Rabi N. Tawil, Shannon Venance.
© 2011 John Wiley & Sons, Ltd. Published 2011 by John Wiley & Sons, Ltd.

nerves and ganglia with ischemia and hypoxia
- Damage from free radicals generated by oxidative and nitrative stress
- Insufficient support of neurons because of abnormal levels of neurotropic growth factors or their receptors
- Damage to key neuronal proteins by excessive glycosylation
- Damage from circulating advanced end-products of glycosylation (AGEs) that act on AGE receptors (RAGE) of neurons
- Failure by insulin to offer direct support to neurons through neuronal insulin receptors (with insulin resistance of neurons)
- Combinations of the above mechanisms

DPN is termed "length dependent" because the distal ends of the longest peripheral axons are involved first. As a result, sensory symptoms and signs first appear in the ends of the toes. As DPN progresses, a pattern of "glove -and-stocking" sensory loss evolves (Figure 22.1). It occasionally involves the center of the chest, the terminal innervation zones of the intercostal nerves. Sensory abnormalities may start in the tips of the fingers somewhat later than in the lower limb. If only some fingers are involved, a superimposed entrapment neuropathy should be suspected such as carpal tunnel syndrome (e.g. involvement of thumb, index, middle, and lateral ring fingers) or ulnar neuropathy at the elbow (e.g. small finger, medial ring finger).

Subclassifications of DPN have been proposed based on the involvement of small sensory axons (small fiber), large sensory axons (large fiber), or the presence of accompanying motor involvement. In small-fiber neuropathy, there may be prominent pain, loss of sensation to pinprick and thermal stimulation with preserved sensation to vibration, position, and preserved ankle reflexes. In selective large-fiber neuropathy, a less common phenotype, there is gait unsteadiness, a Romberg sign, loss of sensation to vibration and light touch with relative preservation of pinprick and thermal sensation. Selective motor involvement is rare to nonexistent in DPN and should

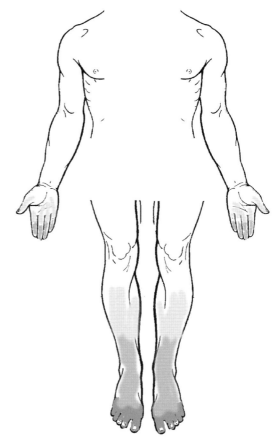

Figure 22.1. Stocking-and-glove abnormalities are the hallmark of diabetic polyneuropathy. The changes indicated may include loss of sensation, paraesthesiae, or pain. (Modified from Zochodne et al. *Diabetic Neurology* New York: Informa, 2010.)

raise suspicion of another cause of polyneuropathy. In practice, most patients with DPN have a mixture of small- and large-fiber sensory involvement including cases of painful polyneuropathy. Motor involvement tends to occur later during the course of the neuropathy with wasting of intrinsic foot muscles, and later weakness of toe and foot dorsiflexion. Prominent or asymmetric upper limb motor involvement should raise suspicion of a superimposed entrapment neuropathy such as carpal tunnel syndrome or ulnar neuropathy at the elbow.

A comprehensive clinical neurological examination is essential for the bedside evaluation of DPN. This should include assessment of distal motor muscle function, recognition of early wasting, examination of deep tendon reflexes and evaluation of sensory modalities including light touch, pinprick, thermal sensation, vibration perception. and position sensibility. The extent of sensory loss should be documented by establishing whether the patient (with eyes closed) can identify any light touch on the toe (anesthesia) or can distinguish the sharp from the dull end of a clean (not reused) safety pin (analgesia). The proximal extent of this loss should then be mapped. The gait should be assessed for antalgia (difficulty walking secondary to pain) or ataxia (loss of balance). It is important to evaluate lower limb pulses, and to check for foot ulceration. The general physical examination should include evaluation for thyroid enlargement, retinopathy, and carotid bruits. The addition of the Semmes–Weinstein monofilament testing is recommended as a predictor of later foot ulceration. This simple test involves applying a filament of bending force 10 g over the toe. Various scoring methods are described but a standard approach is to ask the patient (with eyes closed) how many times he or she can feel the monofilament pressed over the dorsum of the large toe; five trials should be attempted.

Grading scales for the severity of DPN have been generated, largely for use in research trials.

Focal neuropathies

Focal neuropathies involving either single peripheral nerves or several adjacent nerves are common in patients with diabetes. Many develop in patients with only mild or recent-onset diabetes mellitus.

Carpal tunnel syndrome

CTS is the most common entrapment in patients with diabetes and can be a source of considerable pain and disability. Female sex, repetitive hand use, previous wrist fractures, and other conditions such as hypothyroidism and connective tissue disorders are risk factors. Its symptoms are acral (finger tip) paraesthesiae as well as pain and sensory loss, with loss of hand dexterity and weakness. Early CTS may present with sensory symptoms only. Patients may awaken with pain or tingling at night or in the morning. More advanced CTS may present with thenar muscle weakness and wasting. Surgical decompression of the median nerve at the wrist benefits CTS patients with or without diabetes.

Ulnar neuropathy at the elbow

Ulnar neuropathy at the elbow (UNE) develops in approximately 2% of patients with diabetes. Its symptoms are tingling and numbness in the small finger and medial half of the ring finger, with weakness of intrinsic hand muscles. There may be pain in the elbow and hand. In some patients, considerable disability may result. The role of decompression of the ulnar nerve at the elbow, although widely used, remains controversial. Its specific benefits in diabetes mellitus are uncertain. A "Heelbo" pad, a padded arm sock fitted over the elbow, protects the nerve and may improve ulnar neuropathy during its early stages before significant axonal degeneration ensues.

Lateral femoral cutaneous entrapment neuropathy (meralgia paresthetica)

This develops from compression at the level of the inguinal ligament. Obesity, pregnancy, recent weight gain, inguinal nodes or scarring, and tight-fitting garments or belts may predispose to its development. The symptoms are tingling, numbness, and pain along the lateral thigh in the distribution of the lateral femoral cutaneous nerve. Preserved reflexes and quadriceps power distinguish this condition from femoral neuropathy, lumbosacral plexopathy, or radiculopathy. The role of decompression is not established in mild neuropathy but appears helpful to patients with intractable neuropathy.

It is unclear whether other forms of compression or entrapment neuropathy are more common in patients with diabetes mellitus. There are, however, other forms of focal neuropathy that are found in patients with diabetes including lumbosacral plexopathy, oculomotor palsy, thoracic intercostal and abdominal radicular neuropathies, and Bell's palsy (not discussed here).

Lumbosacral plexopathy

Lumbosacral plexopathy (DLSP; also known as lumbosacral radiculoplexus neuropathy, Bruns–Garland syndrome, proximal diabetic neuropathy, and diabetic amyotrophy) is a subacute motor disorder that develops in older patients, usually those with DM type 2. It presents with deep aching thigh pain, followed by weakness and wasting in the anterior thigh muscles, and occasionally involves adjacent groups of anterior compartment muscles below the knee. The quadriceps reflex disappears but sensory involvement is typically spared. Profound weight loss may accompany the disorder. Some varieties with bilateral symmetric involvement are described but usually the onset is unilateral with some patients developing contralateral involvement over time.

The course is usually protracted with a gradual decline over weeks to months followed by spontaneous recovery. The pain from DLSP can be intense, sometimes requiring opioids and hospitalization, and is described as deep, boring, and aching. No therapy has been identified to shorten the course of this condition; immunotherapy is of questionable benefit. A preliminary study has shown improvement in pain symptoms from a course of glucocorticoid therapy. DLSP may develop in patients with relatively mild DM and sometimes has followed the initiation of insulin therapy. Other causes of lumbosacral plexus damage should be routinely sought using imaging (magnetic resonance imaging or computed tomography) of the pelvis and lumbosacral spine. The etiology of DLSP is unknown, although inflammation from microvasculitis and ischemia has been considered.

Thoracic intercostal and abdominal radicular (truncal) neuropathies

These present with subacute abdominal wall or thoracic pain resembling that of herpes zoster. They may span more than one adjacent segmental territory and occasionally are bilateral. Loss of sensation to light touch and pinprick can be documented and there may be localized weakness from denervation of muscle segments, e.g. asking a patient to sit from a supine position may demonstrate bulging of a weak segment of abdominal muscle. The pain may be intense, and variously described as tingling, pricking, lancinating, aching at night, with radiation around the chest or abdomen, causing a constricting feeling. The cause of diabetic truncal radiculopathies is unknown. Slow spontaneous recovery usually occurs.

Isolated cranial nerve palsies including pupillary-sparing oculomotor palsy, and trochlear and abducens nerve palsies also occur in patients with diabetes. Imaging, including noninvasive vascular imaging, may be required to rule out a compressive lesion in all three conditions.

Diagnostic approaches

Electrophysiological studies

Electrophysiological studies are not required in all patients with diabetes and neuropathic symptoms. They are helpful however, in the presence of atypical features such as subacute progression or prominent motor involvement, especially in the setting of mild DM. Nerve conduction studies first identify declines in the amplitude of the sural sensory nerve action potential (SNAP), then sural sensory conduction velocity, and finally peroneal motor conduction slowing. Widespread loss of SNAPs with diffuse mild-to-moderate conduction velocity slowing, loss of compound muscle action potentials (CMAPs), and distal denervation by needle electromyography (EMG) develop in severe or progressive polyneuropathy. Thus, although some features of primary demyelination may occur in DPN, widespread conduction block, dispersion, or severe slowing of conduction velocity (e.g. <35 m/s in the median forearm motor nerve) are unusual and may suggest superimposed chronic inflammatory demyelinating polyneuropathy (CIDP).

Quantitative sensory testing

There are several approaches currently available for computerized testing of sensory function in the distal extremities of patients with diabetes. Examples typically include calibrated electronic interfaces for thermal thresholds (warm, cold), heat as pain, touch pressure, and vibration. The thresholds in the feet are raised in DPN.

Autonomic testing

A large number of specific autonomic tests are now available for testing cardiovascular status, erectile function, sudomotor function (sweating), gastrointestinal motility, bladder function, and pupillary responses. Several of these tests, such as sudomotor testing, are particularly useful in addressing small-fiber function in diabetes. The assessment of small axons in DM is not adequately addressed by nerve conduction studies. The reader is directed elsewhere for more detailed reviews of autonomic testing.

Pathological studies

Sural nerve biopsy is not recommended for routine clinical use. It is helpful, however, for the diagnosis of unusual or progressive neuropathies in the setting of DM to identify alternate causes such as vasculitis or amyloidosis. In diabetic lumbosacral plexopathy, biopsies of femoral cutaneous branches or the sural nerve have identified inflammation suggestive of vasculitis. The usefulness of this finding to prompt specific vasculitis therapy is uncertain. Skin biopsy, taken either by punch or blister, is a more recent form of evaluation. In diabetes, loss of epidermal axons, retraction endbulbs, and abnormal epidermal fiber length are all described. Determination of skin epidermal fiber density is useful for confirming the presence of small-fiber sensory neuropathies when routine nerve conductions are normal. A noninvasive approach toward the study of small axons in diabetes may be the use of corneal confocal microscopy, a rapid technique that identifies sensory nerve axons in Bowman's layer of the cornea.

Other

Cerebrospinal fluid (CSF) protein is often elevated in DPN but pleocytosis (the presence of white blood cells in CSF) is not expected. Biomarkers of oxidative stress in human diabetes are not specifically recognized as robust diagnostic tools for DPN.

> ### ☆ TIPS AND TRICKS
>
> * Early DPN may have minimal clinical signs despite the presence of neuropathic pain.
> * Many patients with DM may have signs of neuropathy despite being asymptomatic.
> * A full neurological examination is warranted including a Semmes–Weinstein monofilament test of mechanical sensation.
> * Loss of an ipsilateral knee reflex is an important sign of diabetic lumbosacral plexopathy.
> * Diabetic oculomotor palsy usually spares the pupil.
> * Painful sensory neuropathy can develop in patients with glucose intolerance without frank diabetes mellitus.

Mechanisms

Although extensive, the literature addressing the basic mechanisms that underlie the development of DPN offers conflicting ideas on pathogenesis. The concept that DPN is a "microvascular" or late complication of DM is debatable because DPN is well documented in early and mild DM and in children. In experimental work, the evidence for a direct role of microvascular disease in DPN is also controversial. More prominent targeting of sensory (and autonomic) axons indicates a pattern of selectivity that cannot be accounted for by blanket nerve ischemia. Models of DPN indicate that it is a gradual and progressive disorder, with prominent targeting of sensory neurons and initial loss or retraction of distal axon terminals. This feature, referred to as "length dependent" or "dying back," develops in tandem with molecular changes at the level of the cell body in dorsal root ganglia (DRG). DPN also involves aberrant signaling between axons and supporting Schwann cells of the nerve. Several major pathogenic pathways have emerged.

Excessive polyol flux through the aldose reductase pathway may contribute to DPN. These changes are linked to declines in Na^+/K^+ ATPase, rises in intra-axonal sodium, and slowing of conduction velocity in motor and sensory axons. Aldose reductase inhibitors (ARIs) that interrupt the flux improve conduction velocity in models and humans. Polyol flux has not, however, satisfactorily addressed the development of neurodegeneration.

Oxidative and nitrative stress may be generated in diabetic nerve trunks and DRG from a number of mechanisms including polyol flux, hyperglycemia, mitochondrial dysfunction, and other mechanisms. Evidence from several sources demonstrates that low-grade rises in nitric oxide synthase activity and deposition of nitrotyrosine occur in DPN models. Nitric oxide may combine with superoxide to form peroxynitrite, a particularly toxic free radical. In addition, abnormal growth factor support may impair the ability of neurons to resist neurotoxic stress from radical damage or polyols. Several studies demonstrate alterations in the levels of neurotropins but clinical trials of specific growth factors have been negative.

Abnormal AGE-RAGE neuronal signaling may trigger neurodegenerative abnormalities. AGEs are advanced glycosylation endproducts formed from proteins exposed to hyperglycemia. AGEs accumulate in diabetic tissues. They ligate several types of receptors, including RAGE, in turn activating a series of intracellular signals that include rises in the factor NFκB. RAGE expression rises in sensory neurons during experimental diabetes whereas RAGE null mice are protected from diabetic abnormalities.

In addition to these well-established mechanisms, abnormal insulin signaling may also contribute to neurodegeneration. Insulin receptors (IRs) are found on most sensory neurons and support regenerative outgrowth of neurons in vitro or after injury. Moreover, neuronal IRs are upregulated in experimental diabetes, and delivery of low doses of insulin, insufficient to alter ambient glucose levels, can correct a number of features of DPN in models. This includes local delivery of low-dose insulin near nerve, intrathecally or intranasally (intranasal injection accesses neurons through the intrathecal space). Specific insulin resistance of neurons is a new concept that is under investigation by the author.

⚠ CAUTION!

- Other types of neuropathy may occur in patients with diabetes.

- Electrophysiological studies are indicated if the features of neuropathy are atypical but are not required for routine screening.
- DPN is NOT necessarily a "microvascular" complication of diabetes and may occur in mild diabetes and in children.
- It is essential to check all patients with diabetes for foot ulcers.

Therapy

No current therapy is available to arrest or reverse DPN. Tight control of hyperglycemia through the intensive use of insulin therapy helps to reduce the prevalence of neuropathy in patients with diabetes. Aldose reductase inhibition therapy, to inhibit sorbitol accumulation, has had some success in clinical trials but its impact has been limited by attenuated potency, inadequate access to the peripheral nerve, and adverse effects.

Therapy for neuropathic pain is indicated in DPN. Evidence-based therapies include antiepileptic agents such as gabapentin and pregabalin, selective serotonin and norepinephrine reuptake inhibitors (venlafaxine, duloxetine), tricyclic antidepressants (amitriptyline), and opioids in refractory patients. Details are provided elsewhere and new guidelines from the American Academy of Neurology for the evidence-based therapy of pain in diabetic neuropathy are in press at the time of writing.

Bibliography

Barohn RJ, Sahenk Z, Warmolts JR, Mendell JR. The Bruns–Garland syndrome (diabetic amyotrophy). Revisited 100 years later. *Arch Neurol* 1991;**48**:1130–5.

Chalk C, Benstead TJ, Moore F. Aldose reductase inhibitors for the treatment of diabetic polyneuropathy. *Cochrane Database System Rev* 2007;(**4**):CD004572.

Diabetes Control and Complications Trial Research Group The effect of intensive treatment of diabetes on the development and progression of long-term complications in insulin-dependent diabetes mellitus. *N Engl J Med* 1993;**329**:977–86.

Dyck PJ, Thomas PK, eds. *Diabetic Neuropathy*. Toronto: WB Saunders, 1999.

Gries FA, Cameron NE, Low PA, Ziegler D. *Textbook of Diabetic Neuropathy*. New York: Thième, 2003.

Lauria G, Cornblath DR, Johansson O, et al. EFNS guidelines on the use of skin biopsy in the diagnosis of peripheral neuropathy. *Eur J Neurol* 2005;**12**:747–58.

Low PA. *Clinical Autonomic Disorders*. Philadelphia: PA Lippincott-Raven, 1997.

Malik RA, Kallinikos P, Abbott CA, et al. Corneal confocal microscopy: a non-invasive surrogate of nerve fibre damage and repair in diabetic patients. *Diabetologia* 2003;**46**:683–8.

Raff MC, Sangalang V, Asbury AK. Ischemic mononeuropathy multiplex in association with diabetes mellitus. *Neurology* 1968;**18**:284.

Said G, Elgrably F, Lacroix C, et al. Painful proximal diabetic neuropathy: inflammatory nerve lesions and spontaneous favorable outcome. *Ann Neurol* 1997;**41**:762–70.

Stewart J. Diabetic truncal neuropathy: topography of the sensory deficit. *Ann Neurol* 1989;**25**:233–8.

Toth C, Schmidt AM, Tuor UI, et al. Diabetes, leukoencephalopathy and RAGE. *Neurobiol Dis* 2006;**23**:445–61.

Veves A, Malik RA, eds. *Diabetic neuropathy. Clinical management*. Totowa: Humana, 2007.

Zochodne DW. Nerve and ganglion blood flow in diabetes: an appraisal. In: Tomlinson D (ed.), *Neurobiology of Diabetic Neuropathy*. San Diego, CA: Academic Press, 2002 161–202.

Zochodne DW, Kline GA, Smith E, Hill MD. *Diabetic Neurology*. New York: Informa, 2010.

Toxic and Metabolic Neuropathies

Kurt Kimpinski

Department of Clinical Neurological Sciences, University Hospital and London Health Sciences Centre, University of Western Ontario, London, ON, Canada

Toxic neuropathies

General principles

The list of chemical agents that cause neuropathy is extensive. Toxic neuropathies resulting from environmental, industrial, and occupational exposure are rare in the developed world. As a result merely trying to memorize lists of chemicals and drugs and the resulting neurological impairment is a fruitless endeavor. However, there are several principles that can help guide the clinician as to when to suspect an underlying toxic cause.

Most of the toxic neuropathies occur together with exposure to the offending agent. There are rare exceptions. Both the platinum agents (*cis*-platinum) and methyl-mercury can induce neuropathic symptoms 2 months after exposure.

The duration and degree of exposure to an offending agent corresponds to the severity of the neuropathy. The modifying factors may include gender, body mass, age and hepatorenal function. However these factors in most cases will only affect the severity but not the pattern of the neuropathy (i.e. length dependent neuropathy, sensory neuronopathy etc.).

In cases where a clear toxic etiology has been defined, withdrawal of the offending agent may not herald immediate improvement of the neuropathic symptoms. This is a result of several factors including metabolism of the offending agent and continued disruption of the peripheral nerve, primarily due to axonal degeneration. As a result the lack of immediate improvement can not always be taken as evidence that the neuropathy was not of a toxic etiology.

> ★ **TIPS AND TRICKS**
>
> **TOXIC NEUROPATHIES.**
>
> - Most toxic neuropathies occur together with exposure to the toxin.
> - The duration and level of toxin exposure usually correspond to neuropathy severity.
> - The most common pattern is a length-dependent axonal neuropathy.
> - Withdrawal of the offending agent is the primary treatment goal.

Patterns of neuropathy associated with toxic exposure

The most common pattern of neuropathy is a length-dependent axonal neuropathy. Other less common patterns associated with toxic exposure include a sensory neuronopathy pattern and toxic channelopathy. Toxic exposure can cause a distinct pattern of a sensory neuronopathy and distal (length-dependent) axonal neuropathy based on the increased permeability of the

Neuromuscular Disorders, First Edition. Edited by Rabi N. Tawil, Shannon Venance.

blood–nerve barrier at the dorsal root ganglion and distal portions of the axon. As a result chemical and pharmaceutical agents have more direct effects on the neuronal cell body and their corresponding axons at these regions. Common agents include *cis*-platinum, pyridoxine, linezolid, metronidazole, podophyllotoxin, taxanes, and thalidomide. The gold salts, oxiplatinum, and several marine toxins can affect voltage-gated sodium and potassium channels (i.e. toxic channelopathies) and are characterized by paraesthesiae, cramps, stiffness, and fasciculations.

Other patterns of neuropathy are uncommon for toxic exposures. Isolated mononeuropathies should raise the suspicion of accidental injection of agents such as analgesics or antibiotics directly into the nerve. Usually such cases are easy to distinguish based on the clinical history. Multifocal neuropathies rarely result from toxins and underlying inflammatory or vasculitic causes should be sought. The toxic demyelinating neuropathies are also uncommon. Exceptions include arsenic or diphtheria with predominantly motor neuropathies associated with areflexia and cranial nerve abnormalities.

Evaluation of toxic neuropathies

The general approach to toxic neuropathies is similar to that for all neuropathies (see Chapter 20). The main area of emphasis is on potential exposure to toxic agents. In addition, a full medication history is necessary including past pharmaceutical agents, chemotherapeutic agents, antibiotics, and other illicit drugs. The timing and duration of use of these agents in relationship to the clinical presentation must be defined as specifically as possible.

Nerve conduction studies (NCSs) and electromyography (EMG) can be useful in further determining the pattern of neuropathy. In addition, NCSs can provide clues such as patterns consistent with hereditary neuropathies such as Charcot–Marie–Tooth disease (CMT) type 1A (highly susceptible to injury with chemotherapeutic agents) or acquired inflammatory neuropathies such as Guillain–Barré syndrome (due to the acuity may prompt a search for an underlying toxic exposure).

Standard blood work to investigate the potential for vasculitic/collagen vascular disease, inflammatory processes, diabetes, vitamin deficiencies, thyroid dysfunction, and monoclonal gammopathies are of use to rule out potential causes of neuropathy.

Nerve biopsy can be of use to rule out other important causes of neuropathy, most importantly vasculitic neuropathies, infective neuropathies such as leprosy, or amyloid neuropathy. Sural nerve biopsy may provide a pattern of nerve involvement (i.e. axonal rather than demyelinating) consistent with most toxic neuropathies, but would have an extremely low likelihood of providing a specific tissue diagnosis.

Basic management principles of the toxic neuropathies

The main principle in the treatment of the toxic neuropathies is obviously the immediate withdrawal of the offending agent. Specific treatments options are discussed further under the specific individual toxic agents. Prognosis depends on both the specific agent and the severity of the neuropathy and is discussed below.

Neuropathies associated with environmental, occupational, and industrial toxins.

Ethylene oxide, methyl bromide, hexacarbons, and thallium can all cause neuropathy. These neuropathies are usually length dependent and predominantly axonal. The presentation is predominantly sensory to sensory motor dysfunction, depending on the severity of chemical exposure.

Lead neuropathy
Industrial exposure accounts for the majority of lead neuropathy, which typically causes wrist and finger extensor weakness with later involvement of other muscle groups. Sensory involvement is uncommon but length-dependent sensory and motor dysfunction has been described with more long-term exposure. Acute exposure to high concentrations of lead is associated with motor predominant neuropathy in adults. In the acute form, elevated blood lead and erythrocyte protoporphyrin levels can be measured. The rapid withdrawal of the offending agent is associated with a more favorable prognosis. Chelation therapy is controversial.

Neuropathies associated with drug and pharmaceutical agents.

Numerous pharmaceutical agents can produce a peripheral neuropathy including amiodarone, bortezomib, colchicine, disulfiram, ethambutamol, metronidazole, phenytoin, and nucleoside analogues. The neuropathy in these cases is usually sensory or sensorimotor and length dependent. Dapsone is unique because it can cause an almost isolated motor axonal neuropathy. Chemotherapeutic agents, including platinum-based compounds, taxanes, and vincristine, can all produce a sensorimotor neuropathy that is primarily axonal and length dependent.

✋ CAUTION

Pre-existing neuropathies can be worsened by toxic exposures. An important example to remember is that vincristine can cause severe neuropathic complications in patients with CMT1a (hereditary sensory motor neuropathy type 1).

Ethanol as a direct cause of neuropathy is debatable. Given the association of poor nutrition with increased alcohol intake in people with neuropathy, some authorities argue that the neuropathy is potentially related to thiamine deficiency. However, there is some evidence for a direct toxic effect of ethanol on the peripheral nerve. Irrespective, in a patient with a suspected alcohol-related neuropathy, a nutritional deficit must be ruled out.

Pyridoxine (vitamin B_6) can induce a sensory predominant neuropathy with prolonged oral intake (200–10 g/day). More significant intake, including intravenous administration, can produce a more rapid sensory neuronopathy. Symptoms can include diffuse sensory, limb ataxia, lost reflexes, and autonomic dysfunction. There is usually satisfactory neurological recovery with stopping pyridoxine in less severe cases.

Metabolic neuropathies

General principles

Metabolic neuropathies related to mineral or vitamin deficiencies are relatively limited in scope. The vast majority of these neuropathies are modest, with a length-dependent axonal pattern and are predominantly sensory. They are usually associated with malabsorption, intestinal dysfunction, or surgery/resection or malnutrition. Important clues to these types of neuropathy include the presence of ataxia in addition to the neuropathy and central nervous system involvement, which is usually more severe than the peripheral dysfunction. Features of a myelopathy in addition to the neuropathy should raise suspicion for these types of neuropathies.

Management and treatment principles are relatively straightforward. Diagnosis can be made on the basis of tests for specific mineral or vitamin deficiencies which are readily available and relatively inexpensive. Treatment is based on reversing any causative factors and replacement of the underlying nutritional deficiency.

★ TIPS AND TRICKS

METABOLIC NEUROPATHIES (NUTRITIONAL DEFICIENCIES)

- Most of these neuropathies are axonal, predominantly sensory and length dependent.
- These neuropathies are usually associated with malabsorption, intestinal dysfunction, gut surgery, or malnutrition.
- These neuropathies can include ataxia and central nervous system involvement, more severe than the peripheral dysfunction.
- Additional myelopathic features should increase the suspicion of a nutritional deficiency.
- Treatment is aimed toward replacing the nutritional deficiency.

The metabolic neuropathies related to organ or system failure are usually obvious in nature given that the organ dysfunction usually dominates the clinical picture. Treatment principles are directed at the underlying organ derangement. Treatment of the neuropathy is most often symptomatic

As for the toxic neuropathies, NCS and EMG studies can be useful in determining the pattern and severity of the neuropathy as well as ruling out other potential causes. Similarly vasculitic/collagen vascular screens, inflammatory markers, diabetes studies, and serum/urine protein electrophoresis with immunofixation should be performed to rule out other causes for neuropathy.

Neuropathies associated with vitamin deficiencies.

Thiamine (vitamin B₁) deficiency

Also known as dry beriberi, this neuropathy is usually associated with more prolonged thiamin deficiency. Initial manifestations include mild sensory loss and burning dysesthesias in the distal extremities. Progression of the neuropathy results in further distal sensory loss and weakness. Tongue and facial muscle weakness are related to cranial nerve involvement compared with ophthalmoplegia which is usually ascribed to Wernicke's disease. Hoarseness of the voice can result from recurrent laryngeal nerve involvement. NCSs reveal an axonal sensory and motor neuropathy. The mainstay of treatment is thiamin replacement (100 mg intramuscularly or intravenously) until nutritional status is improved. However, the neuropathy may respond slowly to supplementation and improvement can take up to 6–12 months and be incomplete in severe cases.

Vitamin B₁₂ deficiency

Vitamin B₁₂ deficiency as a cause of isolated neuropathy is contentious. However, it deserves mention that it is the most common cause of neurological dysfunction related to vitamin deficiency in the developed world. The classic presentation is posterior column and lateral cortical spinal tract involvement (i.e. subacute combined degeneration) with an associated sensorimotor neuropathy. The clinical features include decreased vibratory/position sense with varying paresis, hyperreflexia, and upgoing plantar responses. Distal sensory loss involving both the upper and lower limbs is common to this disorder. Causes include but are not limited to ileal disease, gastrectomy, or gastric bypass, pancreatic insufficiency, bacterial overgrowth, nitrous oxide abuse, and H₂-receptor blockers and proton pump inhibitors. Serum vitamin B₁₂ levels

can be readily measured to make the diagnosis. The addition of serum methylmalonic acid and homocysteine levels can increase the detection of vitamin B₁₂ deficiency. Treatment is accomplished by vitamin replacement either intramuscularly or orally. The neurological deficits usually respond rapidly to treatment.

Vitamin E deficiency

This vitamin deficiency is usually a result of lipid malabsorption. Rarely the disorder can be caused by hereditary disorders such as abetalipoproteinemia. Clinical features usually occur after prolonged deficiency and include ataxia, vibration, and position sensory loss. The associated polyneuropathy that rarely occurs in isolation results in hyporeflexia. The myelopathic features can, however, result in upgoing plantar responses. Other neurological manifestations include tremor, dystonia, dysarthria, ophthalmoplegia, pigmented retinopathy, and night blindness. Diagnosis is made by serum measurements of vitamin E (α-tocopherol) levels. Treatment is high-dose vitamin E replacement and dosages vary depending on etiology. Vitamin A supplementation should also be used. The progression of neurological function is usually halted with treatment and in some cases can regress.

Copper deficiency

A myeloneuropathy has been described in copper deficiency. The presentation can be similar to vitamin B₁₂ deficiency, although the sensorimotor axonal neuropathy may be more severe. Causes can include malabsorption but gastric bypass surgery has the potential to be one of the more common causes. Further clinical suspicion should be raised in those patients who do not respond to vitamin B₁₂ replacement or have a microcytic anemia with associated neutropenia or pancytopenia. Copper and zinc levels can be measured in serum. Zinc levels associated with copper deficiency are elevated and impair absorption. Copper replacement may result in rapid improvement of the neurological dysfunction but variable responses have been reported.

Bariatric surgery and neuropathy

An emerging cause of neuropathy is bariatric surgery. Autoimmune and inflammatory causes have been proposed but vitamin (thiamin, vitamin B_6 and B_{12}) and micronutrient deficiencies (copper, selenium, calcium, magnesium, etc.) likely play a significant role. The neuropathy is predominantly chronic in nature and is characterized by a generalized sensory predominant presentation, although rarely Guillain–Barré syndrome-type presentations have been described. Risk factors include prolonged gastrointestinal symptoms, no postsurgical nutritional follow-up, reduced serum albumin, prolonged hospital stay, and jejunoileal bypass. Monitoring for nutritional deficiencies (as noted above) and replacement as necessary (thiamin, vitamin B_6 and B_{12}, and multivitamins) are the primary treatment modalities.

Neuropathy associated with organ/systemic involvement

Neuropathy associated with hypothyroidism

Entrapment neuropathy, specifically carpal tunnel syndrome (CTS), is the most commonly associated neuropathy seen in hypothyroidism. Polyneuropathy can be subacute and more often sensory in nature in more than 65% of patients. More common clinical symptoms include dysesthesias distally in the limbs. Neuropathy is length dependent and predominantly sensory in nature. If weakness is a significant component of the clinical presentation a myopathy may be present. Hyporeflexia is common. The classic clinical finding is delayed relaxation of the muscle stretch reflex. Rare occurrences of polyneuropathy in hyperthyroidism have been reported. Treatment is directed at restoring normal thyroid function.

Neuropathy associated with renal failure

Neuropathy in endstage kidney disease (ESKD) is characterized by a distal symmetric motor sensory neuropathy with greater lower limb than upper limb involvement. More often the neuropathy involves large-fiber involvement with paraesthesias, reduced muscle stretch reflexes, and muscle wasting. It has a gradual onset and is associated with glomerular filtration rates >12 mL/min. The prevalence of neuropathy in ESKD has been estimated to be as high as 50–100% depending on clinical criteria.

Other less common neuropathies have been described in uremia/ESKD including an isolated small-fiber neuropathy in more than 30% of patients. In addition, a more rapid neuropathy characterized by severe muscle weakness can occur. Based on NCSs this neuropathy can have both axonal and demyelinating characteristics. Cerebrospinal fluid studies are usually unhelpful because isolated protein elevation can result as part of this neuropathy and is not necessarily indicative of an alternate inflammatory neuropathy such as chronic immune demyelinating polyneuropathy or Guillain–Barré syndrome. More recent evidence indicates that maintaining serum potassium levels within the normal range, including between dialysis therapies where applicable may reduce the occurrence and severity of uremic neuropathy. Strict glycemic control can also be of benefit in those patients whose ESKD is secondary to diabetic neuropathy.

Neuropathy associated with hepatic failure

Chronic hepatic failure as a singular cause of neuropathy has been difficult to discern given that common etiologies (i.e. hepatitis B and C, etc.) have effects on both the liver and the peripheral nerve. In general hepatic failure has usually been associated with a modest sensory and motor neuropathy which is predominantly axonal in nature. Upward of 45–50% of individuals may be affected. In late-stage hepatic disease autonomic dysfunction can become more predominant. Overall the neuropathy is mild and usually asymptomatic. More significant neuropathies associated with hepatic dysfunction should be investigated in the context of the underlying cause, including hepatitis B and C, cryoglobulinemia, amyloidosis, vitamin E deficiency, cytomegalovirus, and Epstein–Barr virus, as clinical circumstances dictate.

Other important metabolic neuropathies

Amyloid neuropathy

Neuropathy involving small-diameter fibers (pain and temperature sensation) characterized by neuropathic pain is the more common neuropathy in amyloidosis. However, patients can develop a large-fiber neuropathy and/or associated mononeuropathies including CTS or a painful peripheral neuropathy. Initially the symptoms are sensory, usually affecting the lower extremity. Amyloid neuropathy can result in significant autonomic dysfunction including neurogenic orthostatic hypotension, sudomotor abnormalities, and erectile and sexual dysfunction. Multisystem involvement can be seen with involvement of kidney, liver, heart, and gastrointestinal dysmotility. The diagnosis can be made from rectal mucosa, abdominal fat, or minor salivary gland. Additional tissue biopsy can be sought from heart, nerve, or kidney when clinically involved. Familial forms of amyloid neuropathy also exist and are usually associated with genetic mutations in the transthyretin gene and less commonly with the apolipoprotein AI and gelsolin genes. Treatment is predominantly symptomatic with the exception of liver transplantation aimed at halting disease progression.

Porphyric neuropathy

Disorders of porphyrin metabolism rarely cause peripheral neuropathy and only in hepatic porphyrias. Acute intermittent porphyria may present with a Guillain–Barré-type syndrome characterized by acute motor neuropathy with minimal sensory dysfunction. Phenytoin and phenobarbital can induce attacks, and abdominal pain, confusion, and seizures may also be present.

Conclusions

The diagnosis and management of the toxic neuropathies are relatively straightforward and determined by the basic principles of neurotoxicology, including correlation of the neuropathy with the toxic agent and its subsequent removal. The metabolic neuropathies are more diverse in their underlying cause. Obtaining a clear picture of the onset, progression, and distribution (i.e. sensory and/or motor; length dependent versus multifocal; axonal versus demyelinating, etc.) can help the clinician narrow the focus of inquiry and increase the likelihood of obtaining a specific diagnosis. The reader is referred to more comprehensive works on the metabolic and toxic neuropathies for more in-depth discussion.

Bibliography

Benson MD, Kincaid JC. The molecular biology and clinical features of amyloid neuropathy. *Muscle Nerve* 2007;**36**:411–23.

Dyck PJ, Thomas PK. *Peripheral Neuropathy*, 4th edn. Philadelphia: Elsevier Saunders, 2005.

Herskovitz S, Scelsa SN, Schaumburg HH. The toxic neuropathies: Principles of general and peripheral neurotoxicology: Pharmaceutical agents. *Peripheral Neuropathies in Clinical Practice.* New York: Oxford University Press, 2010: 287–300.

Herskovitz S, Scelsa SN, Schaumburg HH. The toxic neuropathies: Industrial, occupational and environmental agents. In: *Peripheral Neuropathies in Clinical Practice.* New York: Oxford University Press, 2010: 301–10.

Koffman BM, Greenfield LJ, Ali II, Pirzada NA. Neurologic complications after surgery for obesity. *Muscle Nerve* 2006;**33**:166–76.

Krishnan AV, Kiernan MC. Uremic neuropathy: clinical features and new pathophysiological insights. *Muscle Nerve* 2007;**35**:273–90.

Monforte R, Estruch R, Valls-Solé J, Nicolás J, Villalta J, Urbano-Marquez A. Autonomic and peripheral neuropathies in patients with chronic alcoholism. A dose-related toxic effect of alcohol. *Arch Neurol* 1995;**52**:45–51.

Schaumburg H, Kaplan J, Windebank A, et al. Sensory neuropathy from pyridoxine abuse. A new megavitamin syndrome. *N Engl J Med* 1983;**309**:445–8.

Thaisetthawatkul P, Collazo-Clavell ML, Sarr MG, Norell JE, Dyck PJ. A controlled study of peripheral neuropathy after bariatric surgery. *Neurology* 2004;**63**:1462–70.

Thomson RM, Parry GJ. Neuropathies associated with excessive exposure to lead. *Muscle Nerve* 2006;**33**:732–41.

Acute Inflammatory Demyelinating Neuropathies and Variants

Mazen M. Dimachkie and Richard J. Barohn

University of Kansas Medical Center, Kansas City, KS, USA

Clinical features

Guillain–Barré syndrome (GBS) is an acute monophasic immune-mediated polyradiculoneuropathy with an incidence of 0.6–2.4 per 100 000 people. The mean age of onset is 40 years, but all ages are affected, and slightly more males than females are involved.

The most common initial symptom of GBS is paraesthesia consisting of numbness and tingling of the distal extremities. Objective sensory loss is demonstrated in most cases only later in the course of the disease. Severe radicular back pain or neuropathic pain occurs at some point in most cases. Within days of the paraesthesiae, weakness begins following a symmetric "ascending pattern." This first involves the proximal and distal leg muscles before spreading to the arms. Most patients present initially with leg weakness with or without arm weakness, while some have onset of weakness in the arms. A descending presentation, with onset in the face or arms, is less common. In addition to marked weakness, patients are hypo- or areflexic, although reflex abnormality may be delayed by up to a week. Facial nerve involvement occurs in 50–70% of cases, and 5% may develop ophthalmoplegia, ptosis, or both. GBS may selectively affect motor axons, in up to a third of cases. Axonal GBS is more likely to be associated with antecedent *Campylobacter jejuni* infection.

Over 50% of cases evolve to their nadir of weakness by 2 weeks, 80% by 3 weeks, and 90% by 4 weeks. Symptom progression beyond the 1-month mark suggests an alternate diagnosis. Some patients have mild weakness whereas others progress to flaccid quadriplegia and respiratory failure within a few days. Overall, 30% will progress to respiratory failure. Dysautonomia affects 65% of patients. The most common manifestation of autonomic dysfunction is sinus tachycardia, but patients may experience bradycardia, labile blood pressure, with hyper- and hypotension, orthostatic hypotension, cardiac arrhythmias, neurogenic pulmonary edema, changes in sweat, and in less than 5% of cases bladder and gastrointestinal dysfunction.

GBS variants

In addition to the classic presentation of GBS, clinical variants are described based on the predominant mode of fiber injury (demyelinating versus axonal), on types of nerve fibers involved (motor, sensory, sensory and motor, cranial or autonomic), and alteration in consciousness. The first GBS variant was described by C. Miller Fisher (Miller Fisher syndrome or MFS) and consists of ophthalmoplegia, ataxia, and areflexia without any weakness. Most of the patients with MFS present with two of three features and have an elevated cerebrospinal fluid (CSF) protein.

Neuromuscular Disorders, First Edition. Edited by Rabi N. Tawil, Shannon Venance.

Many cases have features overlapping with typical GBS and some MFS cases progress to otherwise classic GBS. Five percent of typical GBS cases may have ophthalmoplegia. A paraparetic variant that affects the legs predominantly with areflexia and sparing of the arms mimics an acute spinal cord lesion. Another GBS variant is pharyngeal–cervical–brachial weakness with ptosis that mimics botulism. Pure sensory and panautonomic variants are also reported. Bickerstaff's brain-stem encephalitis is a variant characterized by alteration in consciousness, hyperreflexia, ataxia, and ophthalmoplegia.

The first report of an axonal variant of GBS was in 1986, followed in 1993 by a description of the Chinese paralytic illness, an axonal motor variant of GBS termed "acute motor axonal neuropathy" (AMAN). Soon after that, reports of an acute motor–sensory axonal neuropathy (AMSAN) were published. AMAN and AMSAN are associated with *C. jejuni* infection which is a poor prognostic factor. Patients with AMAN have a more rapid progression of weakness to an earlier nadir than in acute inflammatory demyelinating polyradiculopathy (AIDP), resulting in prolonged paralysis and respiratory failure over a few days. Although the largest number of reports is from northern China, AMAN has been also described in other countries.

Immunopathology

GBS is a complex autoimmune disease of the peripheral nerves and nerve roots. There is an intense lymphocytic mononuclear cell infiltration and segmental demyelination at the nerve roots and proximal nerve segments. Unlike AIDP, AMAN is characterized by the paucity of lymphocytic infiltration and sparing of the dorsal nerve roots, dorsal root ganglia, and peripheral sensory nerves.

⬡ SCIENCE REVISITED

PATHOGENESIS

Evidence for disease pathogenesis is derived from the animal model of GBS, named experimental allergic neuritis, which is caused by a combination of T-cell-mediated immunity to myelin proteins and antibodies

---

to myelin glycolipids. Antibodies to peripheral nerve myelin were identified in the serum of AIDP patients, with a decline in titers corresponding to clinical improvement. Antibodies to myelin glycolipids are indicative of humoral autoimmunity in GBS variants. An autopsy study supporting humoral autoimmunity demonstrated an antibody-mediated complement deposition on the Schwann cell abaxonal plasmalemma but not on the myelin sheath, followed by vesicular paranodal myelin degeneration and retraction. Macrophages are then recruited to strip off the myelin lamellae. Bystander axon loss may occur with severe inflammation. The two early changes in AMAN are the lengthening of the node of Ranvier followed by the recruitment of macrophages to the nodal region. Nodal lengthening is reversible and results in impaired electrical impulse transmission due to the absence of sodium channels. Subsequently, complement activation results in macrophage recruitment. Macrophages distort paranodal axons and myelin sheaths, separate myelin from the axolemma, and induce condensation of axoplasm in a reversible fashion. Only a minority of motor axons undergo wallerian-like degeneration in severe cases, explaining the rapid recovery in some AMAN cases. Another proposed explanation is that axonal degeneration may involve the most distal nerve terminals. In seven fatal AMAN cases, immunoglobulin G and complement activation products were identified bound to the nodal axolemma of motor fibers. The suspected target autoantigen is likely GD1a because IgG antibodies to GD1a were present in 60% of AMAN cases and only 4% of AIDP cases. Molecular mimicry is suggested as the pathogenic mechanism of AMAN based on the strong association with *C. jejuni* infection. The lipopolysaccharide capsule of *C. jejuni* shares epitopes with GM1 and GD1a, resulting in cross-reacting antibodies. AMSAN shares many similarities with AMAN, although the attack in AMSAN is more severe or longer lasting, resulting in more intense and ultimately diffuse wallerian-like degeneration of sensory and motor axons. In addition to AMAN and AMSAN, molecular mimicry may also be the most plausible mechanism in the MFS because the overwhelming majority of cases has antibodies to GQ1b.

Antecedent events

An antecedent infection is noted 2–4 weeks before the onset in three-quarters of GBS cases. Most are upper respiratory infections without any specific organism identified. Known viral precipitants are the Epstein–Barr virus (mononucleosis or hepatitis) and cytomegalovirus (CMV) in 6% of cases. CMV affects younger patients with severe disease and a higher likelihood of respiratory failure. In HIV, GBS occurs at the time of seroconversion or early in the disease. When suspected, it would be important to obtain an HIV viral load measure through the polymerase chain reaction, which is more sensitive than HIV antibodies. Bacterial infections are rarely associated with GBS and include *Mycoplasma pneumoniae* and Lyme disease.

> ✋ **CAUTION!**
>
> The earliest findings in AIDP are prolonged F-wave latencies or poor F-wave repeatability due to demyelination of the nerve roots. This is followed by prolonged distal latencies (due to distal demyelination) and temporal dispersion or conduction block. Slowing of nerve conduction velocities is less helpful because it tends to appear 2–3 weeks after the onset. However, the sensitivity of nerve conduction studies (NCSs) based on reported criteria may be as low as 22% in early AIDP, rising to 87% at 5 weeks into the illness.

C. jejuni enteritis is the most common identifiable antecedent infection and precedes GBS in approximately 33% of patients. As GBS develops about 9 days after the initial gastroenteritis, stool cultures for *C. jejuni* are often negative but serological evidence of recent infection remains. Although two million cases of *C. jejuni* infection

occur each year in the USA, only about 1 per 1000 of these patients has the genetic susceptibility to develops GBS in association with specific HLA haplotypes. Other antecedent events that have been associated with GBS include immunizations, surgery, epidural anesthesia, and concurrent illnesses such as Hodgkin's disease.

Electrophysiological features

When GBS is suspected, electrophysiological studies are essential to confirm the diagnosis and exclude mimics. The differential includes other diseases associated with quadriparesis/paralysis such as myasthenic crisis, acute presentation of the idiopathic inflammatory myopathies, and the unusual motor neuron disease patient presenting with acute respiratory failure. Associated clinical features are often helpful in distinguishing these from GBS, e.g. extraocular muscle weakness, a cutaneous rash or upper motor neuron signs.

> ✋ **CAUTION!**
>
> **MIMICS OF GBS PRESENTING AS QUADRIPARESIS**[a]
>
> - Anterior horn cell: poliomyelitis or West Nile virus infection (asymmetric weakness)
> - Peripheral nerve:
>   - critical illness neuropathy
>   - lymphoma/leptomeningeal carcinomatous meningitis
>   - toxic neuropathies: solvent or heavy metals
>   - porphyria
>   - Lyme disease
>   - diphtheria
>   - vasculitic neuropathy
> - Neuromuscular junction:
>   - myasthenia gravis
>   - botulism
>   - tick paralysis
> - Muscle:
>   - idiopathic inflammatory myopathies
>   - periodic paralysis
>   - critical illness myopathy

- rhabdomyolysis
- severe hypokalemia or hypophosphatemia
• Acute spinal cord lesion

[a]Psychogenic is an exclusion diagnosis.

LIMITATIONS OF NERVE CONDUCTION STUDIES IN AIDP

First, demyelination occurs at the level of the nerve roots, most distal nerve segments, and entrapment sites. The nerve root is outside the reach of routine NCSs, and entrapment sites are usually excluded when assessing for AIDP. However, slowed conduction velocities at multiple common entrapment sites are unusual in an otherwise normal young adult and may support the clinical impression of GBS. Second, the number of motor nerves studied or those with an elicited response may be inadequate and finding prolongation of blink reflex latencies may be helpful. Finally, changes in the sensory NCSs lag behind the motor abnormalities. However, a potential clue is the preservation of a normal sural nerve response when the median and/or ulnar sensory potentials are reduced or absent. A variety of motor NCS criteria has been published in an attempt to optimize sensitivity while maintaining specificity. A recent comparison of 10 published sets of criteria yielded a 72% sensitivity and 100% specificity. Clinicians should not expect each AIDP patients to meet strict research criteria for demyelination.

In AMAN, compound muscle action potential (CMAP) amplitudes are significantly reduced in the first few days and then become absent. It is difficult in AMAN to ascertain if the absence of CMAP is due to axon loss, conduction block due to sodium channel dysfunction distal to the most distal stimulation site, or an immune attack on the nodes of Ranvier. For this reason, fibrillation potentials may occur early on in the course of AMAN and needle electrode examination is helpful. The sensory responses are normal and demyelinating conduction findings are lacking. However, in AMSAN the sensory and motor potentials are reduced in amplitude and often absent. In MFS, NCSs are often normal.

Laboratory features

Routine laboratory testing is unrevealing in GBS. Values of creatine kinase and/or transaminases may be mildly and nonspecifically elevated. Hyponatremia should raise the suspicion of porphyria. Testing for heavy metal poisoning is not routinely indicated in the absence of other findings (vomiting, delayed hair loss, or Mee's lines). Cerebrospinal fluid (CSF) analysis is essential in all GBS cases. This reveals albuminocytological dissociation, i.e. an elevated protein with 10 or fewer white cells/mm in most cases. Half of GBS cases may have a normal CSF protein in the first week, but that proportion declines to 10% if the test is repeated a week later. If there are more than 50 cell/mm^3, one should consider early HIV infection, leptomeningeal carcinomatosis, CMV polyradiculitis, and sarcoidosis. In HIV, GBS occurs at the time of seroconversion or early in the disease. Stool cultures or antibody measurements of *C. jejuni* do not change management of GBS cases but may indicate a poor prognosis for recovery.

Antibodies to GM1 gangliosides have been described more frequently in AMAN and correlate with greater functional disability at 6 months. IgG antibodies to GD1a were present in 60% of AMAN cases and only 4% of AIDP cases. GT1a antibodies correlate with the presence of bulbar signs and symptoms and may be seen with Bickerstaff's brain-stem encephalitis. Although the authors do not recommend antibody testing in GBS, MFS is a notable exception. GQ1b antibodies are highly sensitive and specific to MFS but may be seen in GBS cases with marked ophthalmoparesis.

Treatment

General supportive care

As 30% of GBS cases progress to respiratory failure, supportive care is the most important element of management. Patients must frequently be monitored for impending respiratory failure. Expiratory forced vital capacities <15 mL/ kg of ideal body weight (adjusted for age) or a negative inspiratory force <60 cmH$_2$O indicates the need for urgent intubation and mechanical ventilation before hypoxemia supervenes. This is associated with marked weakness of neck muscles and inability to count out loud till 20. Patients with severe dysphagia may require nasogastric or feeding tubes. It is important when managing autonomic instability to be conservative and avoid chasing blood pressure fluctuations. Use of long-acting antihypertensives is contraindicated. Bedridden patients should have deep venous thrombosis prophylaxis with compressive hose and/or anticoagulants in the form of subcutaneous heparin or enoxaprin. Bedside passive range of motion can help prevent muscle contractures in paralyzed patients. It is important to be mindful that these patients are most often alert and cognitively intact. Vigilance towards infections is important because most severe cases develop urinary or pulmonary infections.

Treatment with plasmapheresis or intravenous immunoglobulin (IVIG) is indicated for patients with weakness impairing function or any respiratory involvement. Patients and their family should be educated about the fact that it takes on average 2–3 months for patients to walk without aids no matter what therapy is used. A valid approach in milder GBS cases is to closely observe patients for progression in the first 2 weeks while reserving treatment for those who become nonambulatory or unable to stand unaided.

Plasma exchange

Plasma exchange (PE) was the first treatment shown to be effective in GBS through the removal of antibodies, complement, immune complexes, and likely proinflammatory cytokines.

The volume of PE is 50 mL/kg administered five times daily or every other day over 5–10 days, totaling 250 mL/kg. PE beyond the standard amount will not offer additional benefits. The replacement fluid should preferably be albumin. Complications of PE include hypotension, pulmonary embolism, anemia, low platelets, delayed clotting, hypocalcemia, and citrate toxicity, as well as those related to the need for a large double-lumen intravenous catheter.

SCIENCE REVISITED

THE EVIDENCE BEHIND PE AND IVIG
Studies consistently demonstrated a statistically significant reduction in the time to weaning from the ventilator by 13–14 days and time to walk unaided by 32–41 days. In addition the French Cooperative Group showed a reduction in the proportion of patients who required assisted ventilation, a decrease in the time to onset of motor recovery, and a reduction in time to walk with assistance. The Guillain–Barré syndrome Study Group identified similar benefits with more PE recipients improved at 4 weeks, and the 1 grade improvement occurring 3 weeks earlier. The Dutch Guillain–Barré Study Group demonstrated in 1992 a favorable response to IVIG and suggested superiority of IVIG over PE. A subsequent study by the Plasma Exchange and Sandoglobulin Guillain–Barré Syndrome Trial Group confirmed the equivalence of both therapies in GBS

Intravenous immunoglobulin

The precise mechanisms of action of IVIG in neuromuscular disorders are unknown. Infused IVIG interferes with costimulatory molecules involved in antigen presentation. IVIG modulates antibody, cyotokines, and adhesion molecule production as well as macrophage Fc receptor. It also interferes with complement activation and membrane attack complex formation.

The total dose of IVIG is 2 g/kg administered over 3–5 days. The common reactions are usually infusion-related side effects such as nausea, vomiting, fever, myalgia, chest tightness, and headache. These can be minimized with pretreatment with acetaminophen and an antihistamine, and by slowing down the infusion rate. Less common reactions include rash, aseptic meningitis, and neutropenia. Renal insufficiency, stroke, or myocardial ischemia is rare. Total IgA deficiency is extremely rare but such patients may experience anaphylaxis when given IVIG. However, obtaining quantitative IgA levels is not practical in this urgent scenario.

Both PE and IVIG are equally effective, but, in the hemodynamically unstable patient, PE is contraindicated. IVIG is more often readily available in most hospitals. There is no added benefit in treating PE recipients subsequently with IVIG. A recent randomized controlled trial of corticosteroids in GBS revealed no added benefit.

Prognosis

Most patients with GBS start to recover spontaneously after 28 days. The mean time to complete recovery is 200 days in 80% of cases. However, many (65%) have minor residual signs or symptoms, making recovery less than complete. Major residual neurological deficits affect 10–15% of patients. The mortality rate is 5% and results from complications of critical illness (infections, adult respiratory distress syndrome, pulmonary embolism), and rarely dysautonomia. The relapse rate is 5% and it usually occurs within the first 8 weeks. Relapsing–remitting chronic inflammatory demyelinating polyneuropathy should be suspected in those who continue to progress after 8 weeks from onset.

Most AMAN patients have more delayed recovery than AIDP. Some AMAN cases recover quicker due to reversible changes of the sodium channels at nodes of Ranvier or by degeneration and regeneration of intramuscular motor nerve terminals. Most MFS patients recover by 6 months.

★ TIPS AND TRICKS

POOR PROGNOSTIC FACTORS IN GBS

- Rapid onset before presentation (<7 days)
- Mechanical ventilation
- Severely reduced distal CMAP amplitudes (<20% lower limit of normal values)
- Preceding infection with CMV
- Preceding diarrheal illness/*C. jejuni*
- Older age
- Ventilator dependence at 2 weeks

Bibliography

Albers JW, Donofrio PD, McGonagle TK. Sequential electrodiagnostic abnormalities in acute inflammatory demyelinating polyradiculoneuropathy. *Muscle Nerve* 1985;**8**:528–39.

Albers JW, Kelly JJ Jr. Acquired inflammatory demyelinating polyneuropathies: clinical and electrodiagnostic features. *Muscle Nerve* 1989; **12**:435–51.

Asbury AK, Cornblath DR. Assessment of current diagnostic criteria for Guillain–Barré syndrome. *Ann Neurol* 1990;**27**(suppl):S21–4.

French Cooperative Group on Plasma Exchange in Guillain–Barré syndrome. Efficiency of plasma exchange in Guillain–Barré syndrome: role of replacement fluids. *Ann Neurol* 1987;**22**:753–61.

Griffin JW, Li CY, Macko C, et al. Early nodal changes in the acute motor axonal neuropathy pattern of the Guillain–Barré syndrome. *J Neurocytol* 1996;**25**:33–51.

Guillain–Barré syndrome Study Group. Plasmapheresis and acute Guillain–Barré syndrome. *Neurology* 1985;**35**:1096–104.

Hadden RD, Cornblath DR, Hughes RA, et al. Electrophysiological classification of Guillain–Barré syndrome: clinical associations and outcome. Plasma Exchange/Sandoglobulin Guillain–Barré Syndrome Trial Group. *Ann Neurol* 1998;**44**:780–8.

Hafer-Macko C, Sheikh KA, Li CY, et al. Immune attack on the Schwann cell surface in acute inflammatory demyelinating polyneuropathy. *Ann Neurol* 1996;**39**:625–35.

Ho TW, Mishu B, Li Cy, et al. Guillain–Barré syndrome in northern China: Relationship to Campylobacter jejuni infection and antiglycolipid antibodies. *Brain* 1995;**118**:597–605.

Plasma Exchange and Sandoglobulin Guillain–Barré Syndrome Trial Group. Randomized trial of plasma exchange, intravenous immunoglobulin and combined treatments in Guillain–Barré syndrome. *Lancet* 1997;**349**:225–30.

Ropper AH. The Guillain–Barré syndrome. *N Engl J Med* 1992;**326**:1130–6.

Van den Bergh PY, Piéret F. Electrodiagnostic criteria for acute and chronic inflammatory demyelinating polyradiculoneuropathy. *Muscle Nerve* 2004;**29**:565–74.

van der Meché FG, Schmitz PI, and the Dutch Guillain–Barré Study Group. A randomized trial comparing intravenous immune globulin and plasma exchange in Guillain–Barré syndrome. *N Engl J Med* 1992;**326**:1123–9.

van Koningsveld R, Schmitz PI, Meché FG, et al. Effect of methylprednisolone when added to standard treatment with intravenous immunoglobulin for Guillain–Barré syndrome: randomised trial. *Lancet* 2004;**363**:192–6.

van Koningsveld R, Steyerberg EW, Hughes RA, et al. A clinical prognostic scoring system for Guillain–Barré syndrome. *Lancet Neurol* 2007; **6**:589–94.

Chronic Immune-mediated Demyelinating Polyneuropathies

Agnes Jani-Acsadi and Richard A. Lewis

Department of Neurology, Wayne State University, School of Medicine, Detroit, MI, USA

Chronic immune-mediated polyneuropathies (CIMPs) encompass a spectrum of peripheral nerve disorders defined by common pathophysiological features, chronicity of their clinical presentation, and their response to immune -modulating treatments. Chronic immune-mediated neuropathies may be further divided into three major groups based on their clinical and pathophysiological features:

(1) the chronic immune-mediated demyelinating polyneuropathies (CIMDPs)
(2) chronic immune-mediated axonal neuronopathies/neuropathies
(3) neuropathies associated with vasculitis, connective tissue, and granulomatus disorders.

In this chapter we review the current approach in the diagnosis and management of the demyelinating forms of chronic acquired immune polyneuropathies.

Recent years have brought forth an increased awareness of CIMDPs primarily due to wider availability of diagnostic laboratory and neurophysiological tests and advances in available treatment modalities. Broad international collaborations have repeatedly attempted to ease the diagnostic process by defining clinically meaningful diagnostic criteria and management strategies. Familiarity with these disorders is necessary for the neurologist and general practitioner alike because the neuropathies lead to progressive disability of affected patients and an increased economic and healthcare burden. The latter is related to patient disability, and the need for prolonged and often expensive treatment, the association with concomitant other illnesses, and the potential for severe adverse drug reactions. Defining diagnostic criteria is helpful for earlier diagnosis and monitoring treatment outcome. However, there remain a lack of controlled, prospective, randomized treatment trials for newer immunomodulatory drugs, as well as good biomarkers and predictors of treatment outcome and prognosis.

Chronic immune-mediated demyelinating polyneuropathies

History

Chronic progressive and recurrent polyneuropathies (polyneuritis) have been increasingly recognized since the 1950s but it was Dyck and colleagues who in 1975 first described a cohort of 53 patients with "chronic inflammatory polyradiculoneuropathy." The same group subsequently reported that these patients were steroid

Neuromuscular Disorders, First Edition. Edited by Rabi N. Tawil, Shannon Venance.

responsive, underscoring the immune pathogenesis of the disorder. The demyelinating aspect of the disorder was then added to the diagnosis, now called chronic inflammatory demyelinating polyradiculoneuropathy (CIDP). These reports emphasized the progressive or relapsing evolution, and the nonlength-dependent pattern of weakness in which symmetric proximal and distal muscles were involved. This remains the characteristic features of "classic" CIDP.

In some aspects CIDP might be considered as the chronic equivalent of acute inflammatory demyelinating polyradiculoneuropathy (AIDP), the most common form of Guillain–Barré syndrome (GBS). Similarities between AIDP and CIDP include the symmetry of clinical symptoms, hypo-/areflexia, the albuminocytological dissociation in cerebrospinal fluid (CSF), and the electrodiagnostic evidence of slowed nerve conduction velocities and conduction block that is consistent with the segmental demyelination seen in some nerve biopsies. Furthermore, acute-onset CIDP and CIDP relapses may be preceded by inflammatory, infectious, or other antecedent events, as is seen in patients with GBS. Differentiating between acute-onset/recurrent CIDP and AIDP remains a differential diagnostic and management challenge. The temporal differentiation between the subacute, monophasic GBS, which typically progresses over 3 weeks, plateaus, and then improves, and CIDP which has progression or relapses over periods of more than 8 weeks is somewhat arbitrary. However the 8-week demarcation has proven to be very useful in determining treatment plans. Some have applied the term "subacute demyelinating neuropathy" (SIDP) if the symptoms peak between 4 and 8 weeks, although in the authors' experience these tend to evolve later into a more typical CIDP presentation.

For many years CIDP was considered a specific disease. However, it is now clear that there are a number of immune-mediated demyelinating neuropathies with varying degrees of similarity to CIDP. The authors prefer to use chronic acquired demyelinating polyneuropathies (CADPs) or CIDMPs (chronic immune demyelinating polyneuropathies) to describe the large group of disorders, and apply CIDP only to the subgroup with the classic presentation described above. Consistent with this is the approach taken in the guidelines by the European Federation of Neurological Societies/Peripheral Nerve Society (EFNS/PNS), in which CIDP is described as typical or atypical (still CIDP but with unusual features) and CIMDP that is distinct from CIDP.

Clinical heterogeneity of CIMDP (Box 25.1) necessitates the use of electrodiagnostic studies in diagnosis and performance of supportive laboratory studies, including spinal fluid analysis and, although less frequently, nerve biopsy (Box 25.2.).

Epidemiology

Obtaining epidemiological data on CIDP and the different variants was limited in the past due to variability in applied diagnostic criteria and lack of comparative data on the individual subtypes.

Box 25.1. Chronic immune-mediated demyelinating polyneuropathies (CIMDPs)

1. **Classic/typical CIDP**
2. **CIDP variants/atypical CIDP**

Sensory predominant

Distal acquired symmetric form/DADS

Associated with paraprotein IgA and IgG

Associated with multiple myeloma

Associated with other systemic disease

Associated with central nervous system
  demyelination

Lewis–Sumner Syndrome; multifocal
  sensorimotor demyelinating
  polyneuropathy with persistent
  conduction block (MADSAM)

3. **CIMDP distinct from CIDP**

POEMS (polyneuropathy, organomegaly,
  endocrinopathy, M-protein, and skin)

Demyelinating neuropathies associated with
  IgM MGUS:
  – with anti-MAG
  – without anti-MAG

Chronic ataxic neuropathy ophthalmoplegia
  M-protein agglutination disisalosyl
  antibodies (CANOMAD)

Multifocal motor neuropathy (MMN) with
  persistent conduction block

See text for abbreviations.

Box 25.2. Diagnostic approach to CIDP

1. **Clinical course/examination findings**
   Inclusion criteria:
   Typical CIDP: symmetric proximal and distal weakness with sensory involvement, hyporeflexia
   Atypical CIDP: DADS, L-SS, focal CIDP, pure motor or pure sensory
   Exclusion criteria
   CIMDP distinct from CIDP (see Box 25.1)
   Evidence of Lyme disease; diphtheria, drug or other toxins or hereditary neuropathies
2. **Electrodiagnosis**
   a. Motor nerve conduction studies of at least four motor nerves with proximal motor conduction studies as needed, showing prolonged distal latencies and temporal dispersion, variable nerve conduction slowing to less than 70% of normal; secondary axonal degeneration may be present
   b. Sensory nerve conduction studies with somatosensory evoked potentials to assess proximal sensory conductions
3. **Supportive testing**
   Laboratory studies:
   a. CSF analysis for protein and cell count: elevated protein in 80% of patients (50–200 mg/dL); 10% with mild pleocytosis (<50 cells); may have elevated γ-globulin (HIV infection)
   b. Exclusion of other systemic illnesses by ESR, CBC, ANA, ENA, urine/serum immunoelectrophoresis
   c. Genetic testing to rule out hereditary demyelinating neuropathies if needed
      – Imaging studies: MRI with gadolinium enhancement of plexus and/or roots/cauda equina
      – Pathology: nerve biopsy of clinically affected nerve (most often sural, superficial peroneal, or radial sensory or gracilis motor nerve) showing segmental demyelination and remyelination, onion-bulb formation in relapsing forms, and interstitial and endoneurial/perivascular infiltration
      – Clinical treatment response with objective endpoint assessment

ANA, antinuclear antibody; CBC, complete blood count; CSF, cerebrospinal fluid; ENA, extractable nuclear antigen; ESR, erythrocyte sedimentation rate. see text for other abbreviations.
Modified from EFNS/PNS guidelines (2010).

In practice, diagnosis may have also been hindered by the lack of availability of supportive testing such as electrodiagnosis and serology, and as such the prevalence was undervalued. The estimated prevalence of CIDP in populations from the UK, Australia, Norway, and Japan is 0.8–7.7 per 100000. Using EFNS/PNS criteria of 2006 the prevalence of CIDP was 4.77 per 100000 whereas applying the American Academy of Neurology (AAN) Diagnostic Criteria of 1991 gave the prevalence as 1.97 per 100000. Both sets of criteria appeared to *equally* identify patients requiring treatment, although the EFNS/PNS criteria may be able to further delineate epidemiological data for the variant forms of CIDP. Nevertheless, the striking difference in prevalence and incidence depending on which diagnostic criteria are used underscores some of the controversy in finding the optimal approach to diagnostic sensitivity and specificity.

CIDP has no gender or racial predilection. Age of onset is variable but prevalence increases with age (fifth to seventh decades). Childhood forms of idiopathic CIDP appear to have a more precipitous onset similar to that seen in GBS. Preceding viral or bacterial infection or other events are less frequent when compared with AIDP (30% versus approximately 60–70% in GBS) but relapses may be triggered by infections, immunization (controversial), surgery, or trauma.

Typical and atypical CIDP

CIDP is an acquired disorder that may present as chronically progressive or relapsing. Classic clinical features are symmetric motor predominant symptoms and involve all extremities, both proximally and distally. Atypical CIDP includes the multifocal disorder, Lewis–Sumner syndrome, a distal symmetric form of CIDP (DADS), monoclonal mammopathy of undetermined significance (MGUS)-related CIDP with IgA and IgG paraproteins, and CIDP associated with central nervous system (CNS) demyelination and other systemic disorders. *In contrast*, other similar disorders are considered distinct from CIDP because of significant differences in clinical, laboratory, electrodiagnostic, and treatment features, including immunoglobulin M paraproteinemia-associated demyelinating neuropathies, particularly myelin-associated glycoprotein (anti-MAG) neuropathies, POEMS syndrome (**p**olyneuropathy, **o**rganomegaly, **e**ndocrinopathy, **m**onoclonal gammopathy, and **s**kin changes), and multifocal motor neuropathy (see Box 25.1).

The AAN diagnostic criteria of 1991 were designed for research purpose and have been criticized for being too restrictive for clinical use. Since then numerous approaches have been suggested, all using a combination of clinical, CSF, and elecromyographic (EMG) findings. More recently, international guidelines spearheaded by the European Federation of Neurologic Societies/Peripheral Nerve Society (EFNS/PNS) have focused on combining clinical and neurophysiological features to enhance diagnostic accuracy, along with using supportive evidence including spinal fluid protein, magnetic resonance imaging (MRI) abnormalities, and response to therapy (see Box 25.2). The EFNS/PNS clinical criteria focused on typical and acceptable atypical features and stress the importance of exclusion criteria. The EFNS/PNS electrodiagnostic criteria establish probability of diagnosis at three different levels as definite, probable, and possible.

The consensus group led by Koski took a different approach. Based on a review of over 50 cases of CIDP as well as 100 cases of other neuropathies, this group developed two relatively simple separate rules to diagnose CIDP. Validation studies showed very high sensitivity and specificity, particularly if the Lewis–Sumner syndrome cases were excluded. The most striking finding of this approach was that, if a patient had the "classic" presentation of symmetric, proximal, and distal weakness, the chances of the diagnosis being CIDP were so high that electrodiagnostic studies, although confirming the diagnosis, did not add to the diagnostic yield.

⚗ SCIENCE REVISITED

An autoimmune–inflammatory etiology for CIDP has been proposed based on: (1) clinical observations describing infections and immunizations triggering onset and exacerbations of various forms of the disorders; (2) association with systemic immune disorders; (3) similarities with rodent models of autoimmune experimental neuritis; (4) detection of both T- and B-cell-mediated responses to certain myelin antigens, perivascular endoneurial infiltration by lymphocytes, and macrophages; (5) spinal fluid cytoalbuminological dissociation in some of the forms; and (6) response to immunomodulation. No specific common autoantigens have so far been identified. Certain human leukocyte antigens (HLAs) occur more frequently in patients with CIDP (HLA-Dw3, -DRw3, -A1, and -B8).

Clinical features of CIDP

The clinical presentation of CIDP is heterogeneous and varies from purely motor to purely sensory forms to a multifocal (Lewis–Sumner syndrome) presentation, although most typically patients present with a combination of proximal and distal muscle weakness and paraesthesia. The patients complain of difficulty with gait such as tripping and unexplained falling, may have trouble taking stairs, and/or hand dexterity may be impaired. Loss of sensory function is more frequent than pain but paraesthesiae are fairly common. Rarely, extremely high CSF protein levels have been associated with pseudotumor cerebri syndrome, with headache, papilledema, visual loss, and field cuts. *Clinical examination* needs to include a thorough general physical examination to look for evidence of disorders that have been associated with CIDP (skin changes, lymph nodes, malignancy, etc.) *Neurological examination* needs to extend to all levels of the neuraxis to detect not only peripheral but also CNS pathology. Cranial nerve III–VII palsies may be suggested by diplopia (occurs in at least 10%) and lower face weakness, but bulbar muscle dysfunction as an initial presentation has also been described.

Gait abnormalities depend on the extent and combination of motor and sensory deficits, and may vary from steppage to slapping gait due to foot drop and proprioceptive deficits or inability to ambulate due to marked proximal weakness. Confrontational strength exam usually shows symmetric weakness of both proximal and distal muscles in both arms and legs. Atrophy points to secondary axonal degeneration which accounts for the persistent deficits that lead to longstanding disability. Fasciculations may be observed, including some in the tongue, which would lead one to consider the diagnosis of amyotrophic lateral sclerosis. Coordination is consistent with the extent of weakness, and patients may have superimposed sensory ataxia due to large-fiber involvement. Muscle stretch reflexes are absent or diminished. Sensory exam reveals mainly reduced large-fiber modalities such as diminished proprioception and vibration often in a glove-and-stocking distribution. Usually no pathological reflexes are obtained. Autonomic dysfunction and respiratory failure are rare (<10%).

✋ CAUTION!

Distinguishing acute and chronic immune neuropathies is important due to potential treatment implications: although patients with CIDP typically respond to corticosteroids, hence the historic name of steroid-responsive polyneuropathy, AIDP/GBS patients may worsen. Detailed clinical, electrodiagnostic, and supportive laboratory testing, including spinal fluid analysis, is necessary to establish diagnosis. Only about 16% of patients with CIDP present acutely or subacutely, 60% typically progress slowly, and 30% develop a relapsing–remitting presentation.

Atypical forms of CIDP

Despite the heterogeneity in the clinical presentation of the different CIDP variants in terms of the pattern of distribution of their symptoms and signs, they share a similar dysimmune demyelinating mechanism. Their identification is important because they are as amenable to treatment modalities as the classic form.

Pure sensory CIDP/CISP

A significant proportion of patients (about 15%) have a pure sensory form of CIDP due to isolated/primary involvement of the sensory roots or sensory nerve fibers (CISP). Some patients show marked sensory ataxia, with normal nerve conduction studies but somatosensory evoked potentials may show sensory root involvement. Some patients have marked slowing of motor nerve conduction despite normal strength. It can be very difficult to distinguish this form of CIDP from sensory neuronopathies. The benefit of treatment of this form of CIDP is unclear.

Pure motor CIDP

This is much more uncommon than pure sensory CIDP and is considered by some to be part of the spectrum of multifocal motor neuropathy, However, the disorder is symmetric, proximal, and distal, and is otherwise similar to classic CIDP. It typically responds to treatment with intravenous immunoglobulin (IVIG).

Distal acquired demyelinating symmetric polyneuropathy

These patients present similar to the idiopathic length-dependent polyneuropathies with overwhelmingly sensory complaints, but show marked demyelinating features on nerve conduction studies. Many patients with DADS have an IgM paraprotein, and about half of these patients have antibodies directed against myelin-associated glycoprotein (MAG). This latter group is considered distinct from CIDP in the EFNS/PNS guidelines but the other IgM DADS patients are considered atypical CIDP. The authors' experience differs with this approach as they find IgM DADS with and without anti-MAG to behave identically.

CIDP associated with concurrent illnesses

Concurrent illness-associated CIDP is clinically similar to classic CIDP. The exact pathophysiology is not known. The multifocal variants of illness-associated CIDP feature segmental demyelination and remyelination on teased fiber preparation and biopsy, *in contrast* to the wallerian degeneration of vasculitic mononeuropathy multiplex. Nerve conduction studies may show conduction block, an electrodiagnostic marker of segmental demyelination, and disorders of the node of Ranvier.

CIDP may occur with human immunodeficiency virus (HIV) infection, frequently at the time of conversion with typical CSF pleocytosis, chronic active hepatitis B and C without cryoglobulinemia, CNS demyelination/multiple sclerosis, systemic lupus erythematosus, inflammatory bowel disease (IBD), and the use of tumor necrosis factor α (TNF-α) blockers in patients with rheumatoid arthritis (etanercept and infliximab).

There have been reports of CIDP in patients with diabetes mellitus and Charcot–Marie–Tooth disease (CMT), but whether there is a clear increase in incidence is unclear. Pregnancy has also been associated with CIDP in the third trimester or postpartum.

Monoclonal gammopathy of undetermined significance-associated CIDP

A small but significant proportion of CIDP patients (up to 20% according to some estimates) have MGUS. The M protein is mostly IgA or IgG based on serum immunofixation. Response to therapy is similar to classic CIDP and better than IgM MGUS CIDP patients. IgM MGUS patients usually have a distally predominant clinical presentation (DADS) and may respond to immunomodulatory treatment less, although they may respond to rituximab. MGUS may also be associated with *axonal* polyneuropathies requiring a different therapeutic approach.

Multifocal CIDP

Lewis–Sumner syndrome/MADSAM (atypical CIDP) and multifocal motor neuropathy (distinct from CIDP)

In 1982, Lewis, Sumner, Brown, and Asbury described five patients who presented as a

★ **TIPS AND TRICKS**

- Lymphoproliferative disease needs to be ruled out by skeletal bone survey and bone marrow evaluation if M protein is identified.
- The M protein of malignant paraproteinemias, such as the ones associated with Waldenström's macroglobulinemia and multiple myeloma, consist typically of λ light chains.
- IgG and IgA paraproteinemia-associated CIDP is rare and similar in phenotype and treatment response to classic CIDP.

sensorimotor mononeuropathy multiplex and, rather than having electrodiagnostic and pathological findings of vasculitis, these patients had persistent conduction block and evidence of segmental demyelination. This was considered to represent a multifocal variant of CIDP. Subsequent reports have consistently shown response to treatments in a similar manner to "classic CIDP" and the terms Lewis–Sumner syndrome (L-SS) and MADSAM (multifocal acquired demyelinating sensory and motor) are used interchangeably.

In 1988, Clark and Parry and, in a separate paper, Pestronk et al described patients with a pure lower motor neuron disorder, initially diagnosed as motor neuron disease, who also had persistent conduction block. This pure motor disorder, now called multifocal motor neuropathy, has been associated with elevated serum antibody to GM1 in 35–83% of patients and has been shown to respond to IVIG but not to plasmapheresis. Corticosteroids actually tend to cause symptomatic worsening of the disease.

The interrelationship of CIDP, L-SS, and multifocal motor neuropathy (MMN) remains a topic of considerable discussion. Some authors argue that L-SS and MMN are part of a continuum because some patients with otherwise typical MMN have some sensory symptoms and signs, particularly as the disease progresses. Others argue that the sensory changes on clinical and electrodiagnostic examination, the lack of associated anti-GM1 antibodies, and the similar response to all CIDP treatments set L-SS apart from MMN. There is also one pathology report of fascicular biopsies that show differences between MMN and L-SS (J Peter Dyck, personal communication). The biopsy of L-SS patients at the site of conduction block shows inflammatory infiltrates and evidence of segmental demyelination and remyelination, including onion-bulb formations. Similar biopsies of MMN patients show no inflammation and no evidence of myelin pathology. Other evidence is developing to suggest that MMN is likely to be due to an immune attack on the nodes of Ranvier and/or possibly the paranodal region.

Diagnoses of L-SS and MMN both rely on the demonstration of conduction block but some authors have described patients with typical clinical features without block. In this circumstance, the possibility of vasculitic mononeuropathy multiplex should be investigated. The conduction block, when found, should be seen in segments that are not typical sites of compression. If found in the ulnar nerve at the elbow, peroneal nerve at the knee, or radial nerve at the humeral neck, it would be important to determine if the patient has hereditary neuropathy with liability to pressure palsies (HNPP). Typically, HNPP has other characteristic electrodiagnostic features but a finding of a *PMP-22* deletion would be diagnostic. It should also be noted that rarely a point mutation of *PMP-22* that prevents protein formation may also cause the HNPP phenotype.

CSF protein tends to be slightly higher in L-SS than MMN but, in both disorders, the protein is rarely over 100 mg%, pointing to minimal involvement of nerve roots. Besides the conduction block there may be very little other signs of segmental demyelination in MMN and in some cases of L-SS, pointing to the very restricted localization of the disease.

The prognosis for L-SS tends to be similar to CIDP, with 33% of patients going into remission after treatment with IVIG, corticosteroids, or immunosuppressants. MMN has been shown to respond to IVIG but many patients progress despite initial response and there is some evidence that axonal loss continues despite symptomatic and physiological response.

Diagnosis and treatment approaches

The diagnosis of CIDP is based on clinical and electrophysiological examinations plus the supportive evidence of spinal fluid. MRI of the roots and plexus and nerve biopsy studies may also be performed depending on the clinical picture. Although Koski's criteria state that "typical CIDP" may not require electrodiagnostic evidence of demyelination, the authors still find EMG important in the evaluation of all patients. Box 25.2 summarizes a practical approach to diagnosis.

Treatment must be individualized and relate to the severity of disease, rapidity of progression, and general state of health. It is important that the physician and patient develop realistic expectations of treatment response. Randomized clinical trials have established IVIG, plasma exchange, and corticosteroids as primary treatment modalities. The authors refer the reader to current reviews, such as the EFNS/PNS guidelines, for details of initial and maintenance treatment strategies as well as a discussion of emerging therapies.

Conclusion

Recognizing and treating CIDP and its variants are frequently a challenge for the practicing neurologist. It is important that the clinician develop an approach that will lead to accurate and timely diagnosis. Randomized controlled trials have proven that the standard practice of using IVIG, plasma exchange, and corticosteroids is efficacious in many patients. However, the ultimate goals of reducing long-term disability and attaining clinical remission remain elusive. Further treatment trials are necessary to determine the efficacy of new therapies.

Bibliography

American Academy of Neurology AIDS Task Force. Research criteria for diagnosis of chronic inflammatory demyelinating polyneuropathy (CIDP). *Neurology* 1991;**41**;617–18.

Austin JH. Recurrent polyneuropathies and their corticosteroid treatment *Brain* 1958;**81**:192.

Bril V, Banach M, Dalakas MC, et al., on behalf of the ICE Study Group. Electrophysiologic correlations with clinical outcomes in CIDP. *Muscle Nerve* 2010;**42**:492–7.

Dyck PJ, O'Brien PC, Oviatt KF, et al. Prednisone improves chronic inflammatory demyelinating polyradiculopathy more than no treatment. *Ann Neurol* 1982;**11**:136-41.

Jacob S, Rajabally YA. Current proposed mechanisms of action of intravenous immunoglobulins in inflammatory neuropathies. *Curr Neuropharmacol* 2009;**7**;337–42.

Joint task force of the European Federation of Neurological Societies and the Peripheral Nerve Society European Federation of Neurological Societies/Peripheral Nerve Society. Guideline on management of chronic inflammatory demyelinating polyradiculoneuropathy – First Revision *Eur J Peripheral Nerv Syst* 2010;**15**:1–9.

Koski CL, Baumgarten M, Magden LS, et al. Derivation and validation of diagnostic criteria for chronic inflammatory demyelinating polyneuropathy. *J Neurol Sci* 2009;**277**:1–8.

Latov N, Gorson KC, Brannagan TH, et al. Diagnosis and treatment of chronic immune-mediated neuropathies. *J Clin Neuromusc Dis* 2006;**7**:141–57.

Lewis RA, Sumner AJ, Brown MJ, Asbury AK. Multifocal demyelinating neuropathy with persistent conduction block. *Neurology* 1982;**32**:95–164.

Parry GJ, Clarke S. Pure motor neuropathy with multifocal conduction block masquerading as motor neuron disease. *Muscle Nerve* 1988;**11**:103–7.

Pestronk A, Cornblath DR, Ilyas AA, et al. A treatable multifocal motor neuropathy with antibodies to GM1 ganglioside. *Ann Neurol* 1988;**24**:73–8.

Rajabally YA, Nicolas G, Pieret F, Bouche P, Van den Berg PYK. Validity of diagnostic criteria for chronic inflammatory demyelinating polyradiculoneuropathy: a multicentre European study. *J Neurol Neurosurg Psychiatry* 2009;**80**:1364–8.

Rajabally YA, Simpson BS, Beri S, Bankart J, Gosalakkal JA. Epidemiological variability of chronic inflammatory demyelinating polyneuropathy with different diagnostic criteria: study of UK population. *Muscle Nerve* 2009;**39**:432–8.

Ruts L, Drenthen J, Jacobs BC, van Doorn PA, the Dutch GBS Study Group Distinguishing acute-onset CIDP from fluctuating Guillian–Barré Syndrome: a prospective study. *Neurology* 2010;**74**:1680–6.

Saperstein D, Katz JS, Amato AA, Barohn RJ. Clinical spectrum of chronic acquired demyelinating polyneuropathies. *Muscle Nerve* 2001;**24**:311–24.

Taylor BV, Wright RA, Harper CM, Dyck PJ. Natural history of 46 patients with multifocal motor neuropathies with conduction blocks. *Muscle Nerve* 2000;**23**:900–8.

Vasculitic Neuropathies

W. David Arnold and John T. Kissel

Department of Neurology, Division of Neuromuscular Medicine, The Ohio State University Medical Center, Columbus, OH, USA

The vasculitides are a complex and heterogeneous group of disorders with varying features related to the distribution of blood vessel involvement. Although no universally accepted classification of vasculitis exists, many schemes were proposed on the basis of etiology, size of involved vessels, histopathology, organ involvement, and other clinical features. A useful classification of vasculitis associated with neuropathy was developed by a Peripheral Nerve Society task force, which divides the vasculitides associated with neuropathy into three main groups: primary systemic, secondary systemic, and nonsystemic (Box 26.1).

Primary systemic vasculitis includes disorders affecting small, medium, and large vessels with no known underlying cause. Primary systemic vasculitides commonly associated with neuropathy include microscopic polyangiitis, Churg–Strauss syndrome, Wegener's granulomatosis, and polyarteritis nodosa. Secondary systemic vasculitis involves immune-mediated vessel injury in the setting of a pre-existing inflammatory condition such as connective tissue disease, infections, and medication-induced inflammation. In both primary and secondary systemic vasculitides, the neuropathy occurs with other features of systemic involvement, and neuropathy is a common feature when small arteries and arterioles are involved. In contrast, nonsystemic vasculitic neuropathy (NSVN) presents with vasculitic involvement predominantly confined to the blood supply of the peripheral nervous system, although muscle is also occasionally involved. NSVN includes localized variants of vasculitic neuropathy including diabetic and nondiabetic radiculoplexus neuropathy, which are usually non-life threatening and follow a limited and monophasic, although occasionally recurrent, course that differs significantly from other subsets of vasculitis.

Presentation

The clinical presentation of vasculitis depends on the distribution and severity of blood vessel involvement. In primary and secondary systemic vasculitis, systemic signs and symptoms related to renal, gastrointestinal, or other organ involvement may be prominent, but occasionally neuropathy may be a heralding feature before the development of systemic involvement. By definition, NSVN is not associated with prominent systemic features, but mild associated systemic symptoms such as fatigue, malaise, and weight loss can occur. The classic presentation of vasculitic nerve involvement includes sensory and motor deficits as multiple individual nerve mononeuropathies, overlapping mononeuropathies, and much less frequently a distal symmetric polyneuropathy (Figure 26.1). A pattern of pure multiple mononeuropathy is by far the easiest to recognize but is only rarely present.

Neuromuscular Disorders, First Edition. Edited by Rabi N. Tawil, Shannon Venance.

© 2011 John Wiley & Sons, Ltd. Published 2011 by John Wiley & Sons, Ltd.

Box 26.1. Peripheral Nerve Society classification of vasculitides associated with neuropathy

Primary systemic vasculitides

Predominantly small vessel vasculitis
    Microscopic polyangiitis[a]
    Churg–Strauss syndrome[a]
    Wegener's granulomatosis[a]
    Essential mixed cryoglobulinemia (non-HCV)
    Henoch–Schönlein purpura

Predominantly medium vessel vasculitis
    Polyarteritis nodosa (PAN)

Predominantly large vessel vasculitis
    Giant cell arteritis

Secondary systemic vasculitides associated with one of the following

Connective tissue diseases
    Rheumatoid arthritis
    Systemic lupus erythematosus
    Sjögren's syndrome
    Systemic sclerosis
    Dermatomyositis
    Mixed connective tissue disease

Sarcoidosis

Behçet's disease

Infection (such as HBV, HCV, HIV, CMV, leprosy, Lyme disease, HTLV-I)

Drugs

Malignancy

Inflammatory bowel disease

Hypocomplementemic urticarial vasculitis syndrome

Nonsystemic/localized vasculitis

Nonsystemic vasculitic neuropathy
    Includes nondiabetic radiculoplexus neuropathy
    Includes some cases of Wartenberg's migrant sensory neuritis (provisional)

Diabetic radiculoplexus neuropathy

Localized cutaneous/neuropathic vasculitis
    Cutaneous PAN
    Others

[a]Anti-neutrophil cytoplasmic antibody (ANCA)-associated vasculitides; CMV, cytomegalovirus; HBV, hepatitis B virus; HCV, hepatitis C virus; HIV, human immunodeficiency virus; HTLV, human T-lymphotropic virus.

Asymmetric weakness and sensory loss not clearly following the pattern of distinct nerves is the most common presentation of vasculitic neuropathy. Although vasculitic neuropathy does not typically follow a length-dependent pattern, distal and lower limb nerves are more commonly affected.

The diabetic and nondiabetic radiculoplexus neuropathies are now commonly included in the spectrum of nonsystemic/localized variants of vasculitis associated with neuropathy. The typical presentation of radiculoplexus neuropathy includes that of acute to subacute buttock, hip, or thigh pain followed by weakness and atrophy that typically affect the thigh muscles but can also affect other regions, including the distribution of the brachial plexus and thoracic nerve roots. Neuropathic pain is a prominent feature of all types of vasculitis and appears to be more common and severe in vasculitic neuropathy than in any other type of neuropathy, occurring in over 90% patients.

> **SCIENCE REVISITED**
>
> In the largest series of NSVN, the most common presentation was an asymmetric polyneuropathy occurring in 77% followed by multifocal neuropathies in 13%, asymmetric radiculoplexus neuropathies in 8%, and a distal symmetric polyneuropathy in 2%.

Diagnosis

The extent of testing in a patient with suspected vasculitic neuropathy depends largely on the presenting signs and symptoms. The workup for possible vasculitis includes a thorough history and physical examination, neurophysiological testing with electromyography (EMG) and nerve conduction studies (NCSs), specific laboratory testing to identify or exclude coexistent or associated disorders, and usually nerve biopsy. EMG and NCSs are indicated for essentially all patients presenting with suspected vasculitic neuropathy, because they define the distribution of involvement (focal, multifocal, or length dependent), fiber type involved (sensory and/or motor), neuropathophysiology (axonal loss

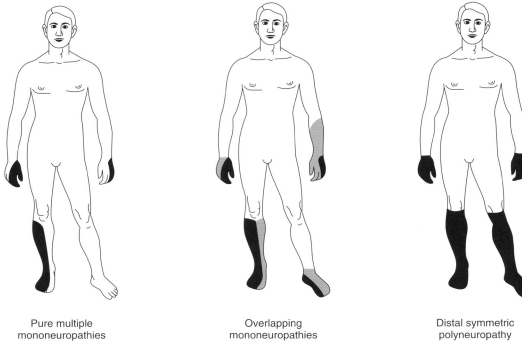

| Pure multiple mononeuropathies | Overlapping mononeuropathies | Distal symmetric polyneuropathy |

Figure 26.1. The classic patterns of vasculitic neuropathy are represented here. The most characteristic presentation is that of true multiple mononeuropathies, but due to accumulated nerve involvement the deficits may merge into an asymmetric neuropathy or, in the occasional patient, a nearly symmetric distal polyneuropathy.

versus demyelination), and the most appropriate nerve for biopsy. NCSs in vasculitic neuropathy usually demonstrate reduced sensory and motor amplitudes, signifying axonal loss, with normal or mildly reduced conduction velocities. The needle electrode examination demonstrates findings of active and/or chronic denervation depending on the chronicity of the patient's symptoms. Findings of axonal loss in the distribution of an asymmetric length-dependent pattern or in the distribution of multiple named nerves (i.e. multiple mononeuropathy) on electrodiagnostic studies are strongly suggestive of an underlying vasculitic neuropathy. Conversely, a symmetric distribution of findings by EMG/NCSs makes vasculitis much less likely. Significantly reduced conduction velocities or other findings of demyelination including temporal dispersion or persistent conduction block should also prompt the clinician to look for alternative diagnoses, although rarely a pseudocon-

duction block may be seen in the acute phase of nerve injury with ongoing nerve ischemia.

EMG and NCSs are helpful in excluding other peripheral nerve disorders which may present with asymmetric or multifocal features. Hereditary neuropathy with predisposition to pressure palsies (HNPP) is a relatively rare, autosomal dominantly inherited neuropathy related to *PMP-22* deletion on chromosome 17 which can mimic the presentation of vasculitic neuropathy. Patients with HNPP present with asymmetric complaints of multiple nerve entrapments but do not typically present with the pain characteristic of vasculitis. The presence of demyelinating changes on neurophysiological testing typically makes HNPP easily distinguished from vasculitis. Similarly, diabetic neuropathy is associated with increased susceptibility to compression or entrapment neuropathies, which may lead to a neuropathy with asymmetric clinical and examination features. Findings of mononeuropathies with features of demyelination only at common sites of nerve entrapment usually help to distinguish this from a vasculitic process.

The presentation of sensory loss and weakness in the distribution of multiple individual nerves or an asymmetric neuropathy should always prompt consideration of vasculitic neuropathy. This is particularly true if significant pain or discomfort is present.

The laboratory evaluation of vasculitic neuropathy should include testing for any systemic conditions suggested by the history and examination. The typical evaluation of vasculitic neuropathy includes complete blood count with differential, renal and hepatic panels, urinalysis, erythrocyte sedimentation rate (ESR), C-reactive protein (CRP), antinuclear antibody (ANA), antineutrophil cytoplasmic antibody (ANCA), rheumatoid factor, serum electrophoresis with immunofixation, glucose tolerance testing, cryoglobulins, and serum complement. Hepatitis B surface antigens and hepatitis C antibodies are also usually obtained because vasculitis can occur in the setting of hepatitis. Testing for other infectious agents associated with secondary systemic vasculitis, including human immunodeficiency virus (HIV), rickettsiae, *Mycobacterium tuberculosis*, Lyme disease, and syphilis, should be considered in select cases.

ESR is elevated in about 70% of patients with vasculitis. Mild-to-moderate elevation may be seen in both systemic and nonsystemic vasculitic neuropathy, but severely elevated ESR is essentially always seen with systemic involvement; in fact, ESR >100 mm/h is considered an exclusion criterion for NSVN.

Nerve biopsy remains a critical part of the evaluation of suspected vasculitic neuropathy because the toxicity associated with chronic immunomodulatory therapy used in vasculitic neuropathy demands diagnostic certainty. Commonly biopsied nerves include the sural, superficial peroneal, and superficial radial nerves, but the clinical examination and electrodiagnostic evaluation should guide the biopsy site. A normal examination and nerve conduction response in the nerve to be biopsied significantly lessens the chance of abnormal findings and thus the diagnostic yield of a nerve biopsy. A nerve that is clinically involved should be selected, keeping in mind the morbidity that is associated with a nerve biopsy which can include pain, dysesthesia, and persistent numbness. When feasible, a combined nerve and muscle biopsy may increase diagnostic sensitivity. In systemic vasculitis multiple organs may be involved in addition to the peripheral nervous system. If the patient's symptoms, examination, and diagnostic testing suggest involvement of other organs, consideration should be given to obtaining tissue in the least invasive manner.

A definite histological diagnosis requires endoneurial or epineurial vessel wall infarction in association with perivascular or transmural infiltration by inflammatory cells (Plate 26.1). In the absence of true vessel wall infarction and necrosis, a presumptive diagnosis of probable vasculitis is reasonable if transmural or perivascular inflammation is associated with at least one of the following: chronic thrombosis, hemosiderin deposition, asymmetric nerve fiber loss, or prominent wallerian degeneration.

Treatment

The initiating factors for most cases of vasculitic neuropathy remain incompletely understood, although the disorder is presumed to be an immune-mediated process, most likely related to both immune complex deposition and cellular-mediated mechanisms. In the case of the hypersensitivity vasculitides associated with cancer, medications, or infection, antigen removal through treatment of the primary underlying process is an important therapeutic strategy. Otherwise, nonspecific immunomodulation is the cornerstone of therapy for vasculitic neuropathies of any cause.

Most patients with vasculitic neuropathy require treatment. The major determinations to be considered in the management of vasculitic neuropathy include the need for monotherapy with corticosteroids alone versus combination therapy with a cytotoxic agent, the length of induction treatment using corticosteroids with or without combination therapy before transitioning to maintenance therapy with less toxic agents, and the length of treatment with maintenance therapy after a clinical remission is apparent. Corticosteroids remain the primary modality of treatment during induction therapy, most often as monotherapy in patients with mild primary systemic vasculitic neuropathy and NSVN. Typically steroids are initiated orally with prednisone at 1.5 mg/kg per day as a single, morning dose for mild cases or intravenously with methylprednisolone in particularly severe or fulminant cases. In some cases continued progression will be observed despite high-dose corticosteroid management, and combination therapy is necessary.

The presence of rapidly progressive weakness or multiorgan involvement, particularly renal or central nervous system, should also prompt consideration for combination therapy. The use of combination therapy carries additional risk and should be used only by clinicians familiar with prescribing precautions. Cyclophosphamide is the best studied agent for combination therapy. Traditionally, cyclophosphamide has been administered orally at 1.5–2.5 mg/kg per day, but pulsed intravenous dosing has demonstrated benefits of less toxicity, improved tolerability, and decreased cumulative dose with nearly equal efficacy. A typical protocol for intravenous pulse cyclophosphamide administration is $0.6 \, \mathrm{g/m^2}$ every 2 weeks for three doses, followed by $0.7 \, \mathrm{g/m^2}$ every 3 weeks for three to six additional doses. In elderly patients or patients with renal impairment the dose should be decreased ($0.5 \, \mathrm{g/m^2}$). Patients should also be administered mesna or aggressive hydration to help reduce the risk of bladder toxicity.

After a period of induction therapy, typically 6 months, using corticosteroids with or without combination therapy, patients should be transitioned to less toxic maintenance immunomodulatory treatment. Azathioprine and methotrexate are both considered first-line agents for maintenance immunomodulatory therapy. The standard dose of azathioprine is 2.0–2.5 mg/kg per day. Methotrexate is typically initiated at a starting dose of 15 mg/week and titrated to 25 mg/week over a period of 1–2 months. The ideal length of maintenance immunomodulatory treatment after clinical remission is not entirely clear, but treatment should continue until improvement maximizes. If there is no evidence of recurrence after 6 months of clinical stability, discontinuation of immunomodulation can be considered. Continued treatment with low dose prednisone (5–7.5 mg daily) and/or a steroid-sparing agent such as methotrexate or azathioprine for 18–24 months may be considered in the hope of reducing the risk of future disease recurrence.

✋ CAUTION!

Vasculitic neuropathy is associated with axonal loss that may be severe. Despite aggressive immunomodulatory treatment, reinnervation and clinical recovery of sensory and motor function are typically slow and may be incomplete in severely affected nerves. Caution should be used to avoid overtreatment if ongoing disease activity is not apparent.

A major difficulty for clinicians treating patients with vasculitic neuropathy is that there are no precise ways to monitor disease activity and remission, but close follow-up with monitoring of objective measures of the motor and sensory examination, repeat EMG and NCSs, and inflammatory markers such as ESR or CRP may be helpful to identify disease recurrence.

Neuropathic pain is a typical aspect of vasculitic neuropathy and can be severe and debilitating. Treatment usually includes some combination of the usual anticonvulsant medications (calcium channel α2δ ligands such as gabapentin and pregabalin) and antidepressants (tricyclic antidepressants and serotonin/norepinephrine reuptake inhibitors), and occasionally opiates. The pain with vasculitis is most severe during disease activity and usually responds dramatically to immunomodulation. In general, once the disease process has been treated, symptomatic pain management can be reduced and sometimes discontinued. In patients with vasculitic neuropathy with no other evidence of ongoing vasculitis, worsening pain may be a clue to re-emerging disease activity.

Prophylaxis against the toxic effects of immunomodulatory therapy is another and often neglected aspect to managing these patients. Corticosteroids should be used in conjunction with agents for bone health maintenance and a low calorie, low salt diet. Blood pressure and glucose status need to be monitored, along with periodic eye examinations for cataracts. Antibiotic *Pneumocystis jiroveci* pneumonia prophylaxis should be considered in patients with risks factors for infection or when multiple immunomodulatory agents are implemented. Typically double-strength sulfamethoxazole and trimethoprim is administered three times weekly to patients on ≥20 mg prednisone daily in combination with an additional immunomodulatory agent. Prophylaxis should be considered in patients with coexistent pulmonary disease administered >20 mg daily of prednisone alone. Dapsone is an alternate agent that can be used in patients with sulfa allergy or intolerance. Due to the reasonably low cost and risk of antibiotic prophylaxis, most clinicians err on the side of caution when considering antibiotic prophylactic measures.

There is limited research about specific therapeutic rehabilitation recommendations, but rehabilitation with the help of a physical and/or occupational therapist should be initiated as early as possible, usually after the severe pain has subsided. Orthotic interventions, such as ankle–foot orthoses, are frequently necessary. Functional recovery should be viewed as combined improvement on the basis of rehabilitation efforts, modification of activities of daily living, as well as neurological recovery on the basis of axonal sprouting and collateral reinnervation.

Bibliography

Collins M, Dyck P, Gronseth G, et al. Peripheral Nerve Society Guideline on the classification, diagnosis, and investigation of nonsystemic vasculitic neuropathy. *J Peripher Nerv Syst* 2010;**1**:20–9.

Collins MP, Mendell JR, Periquet MI, et al. Superficial peroneal nerve/peroneus brevis muscle biopsy in vasculitic neuropathy. *Neurology* 2000;**55**:636–43.

Collins MP, Periquet MI, Mendell JR, Sahenk Z, Nagaraja HN, Kissel JT. Nonsystemic vasculitic neuropathy: insights from a clinical cohort. *Neurology* 2003;**61**:623–30.

Dyck PJ, Benstead TJ, Conn DL, Stevens JC, Windebank AJ, Low PA. Nonsystemic vasculitic neuropathy. *Brain* 1987;**110**(Part 4):843–53.

Dyck PJ, Engelstad J, Norell J. Microvasculitis in non-diabetic lumbosacral radiculoplexus neuropathy (LSRPN): similarity to the diabetic variety (DLSRPN). *J Neuropathol Exp Neurol* 2000;**59**:525–38.

Dyck PJ, Norell JE. Non-diabetic lumbosacral radiculoplexus neuropathy: natural history, outcome and comparison with the diabetic variety. *Brain* 2001;**124**(Part 6):1197–207.

Jennette JC, Falk RJ, Andrassy K, et al. Nomenclature of systemic vasculitides. Proposal of an international consensus conference. *Arthritis Rheum* 1994;**37**:187–92.

Kernohan JWWH. Periarteritis nodosa: a clinicopathologic study with special reference to the nervous system. *Arch Neurol Psychiatry* 1938;**39**:655–86.

Kissel JT, Slivka AP, Warmolts JR, Mendell JR. The clinical spectrum of necrotizing angiopathy of the peripheral nervous system. *Ann Neurol* 1985;**18**:251–7.

Kissel JT, Riethman JL, Omerza J, Rammohan KW, Mendell JR. Peripheral nerve vasculitis: immune characterization of the vascular lesions. *Ann Neurol* 1989;**25**:291–7.

Lovshin LaK. Peripheral neuritis in periarteritis nodosa. *Arch Intern Med* 1948;**82**:321–38.

McCluskey L, Feinberg D, Cantor C, Bird S. "Pseudo-conduction block" in vasculitic neuropathy. *Muscle Nerve* 1999;**22**:1361–6.

Said G, Lacroix C, Lozeron P, et al. Inflammatory vasculopathy in multifocal diabetic neuropathy. *Brain* 2003;**126**(Part 2):376–85.

Satoi HM, Oka NM, Kawasaki TM, et al. Mechanisms of tissue injury in vasculitic neuropathies. *Neurology* 1998;**50**:492–6.

Vital C, Vital A, Canron MH, et al. Combined nerve and muscle biopsy in the diagnosis of vasculitic neuropathy. A 16-year retrospective study of 202 cases. *J Peripher Nerv Syst* 2006; **11**:20–9.

Paraneoplastic Neuropathies

Pariwat Thaisetthawatkul

Department of Neurological Sciences, University of Nebraska Medical Center, Omaha, NE, USA

Neuromuscular disorders associated with malignancies result from several mechanisms:

- Direct invasion of cancer into the neuromuscular tissues
- Iatrogenic effects from the treatment
- Factors closely related to but not the direct effect of the underlying cancer or its treatment
- Paraneoplastic neuromuscular disorders.

Direct invasion of cancers into the neuromuscular tissues is infrequent compared with its occurrence in the central nervous system but it is probably underdiagnosed. Primary malignancies can directly invade or compress nerve roots, plexus, individual peripheral nerves, or muscles. The clinical manifestations are focal or multifocal, usually asymmetric, and include weakness, muscle atrophy, sensory changes, and pain. The diagnosis can be achieved by appropriate electrophysiological testing, neuroimaging, and, if necessary, biopsy of the nerves or muscles involved. Certain cancers have tendencies to directly invade particular peripheral neural elements. Breast and lung cancers frequently cause brachial plexopathy. Colorectal and cervical cancers cause lumbosacral plexopathy. Lymphoma can affect peripheral nerves in a more generalized manner. Tumors or metastasis to the vertebral bodies or the paravertebral area can cause local nerve root or plexus compression.

Effects of chemotherapy and radiation therapy are a consideration in neuromuscular presentation in cancer patients. Iatrogenic effects from cancer treatment, especially from chemotherapy, is probably the most common cause of peripheral neuropathy in cancer patients. The clinical symptoms are those of generalized, acute, or subacute symmetrical sensorimotor or pure sensory neuropathy. The diagnosis can be made by clinical symptoms and signs, history of the use of chemotherapy, the dose and duration of treatment and the development of symptoms during the course of treatment.

Certain chemotherapeutic agents, such as paclitaxel, have coasting effects in which the symptoms develop and progress even after the course of chemotherapy is completed. Vinca alkaloids cause length-dependent axonal sensorimotor and autonomic neuropathy. Cisplatin directly affects sensory ganglion neurons and can cause a pure sensory ganglionopathy or neuronopathy. Paclitaxel affects neuronal cell body and its axon, causing a sensory-predominant neuropathy. Cytosine arabinoside has been reported to cause a Guillain–Barré syndrome (GBS)-like neuropathy. Local radiation therapy can cause brachial or lumbosacral plexopathy and cauda equina syndrome many years after

Neuromuscular Disorders, First Edition. Edited by Rabi N. Tawil, Shannon Venance.

treatment. The symptoms are therefore asymmetric, often unilateral, slowly progressive weakness with atrophy and sensory symptoms in the affected limb. In radiation-induced plexopathy or radiculoplexopathy, pain is usually less common than in metastatic disease. Myokymic discharges (high-frequency repetitive discharges) may be seen on electromyographic (EMG) studies. Other causes of neuromuscular problems that do not arise directly from cancer or its treatment include nutritional deficiency and metabolic disorders such as thiamin or cobalamin deficiency. Carcinoid tumor can cause niacin deficiency. Cancer patients who have malnutrition and become cachectic could develop neuromuscular complications when critically ill.

☆ TIPS AND TRICKS

NEUROPATHIES SECONDARY TO THE DIRECT EFFECTS OF MALIGNANCIES

- The most common cause of neuropathy in patients with cancers is chemotherapy-induced neuropathy
- An infiltrative brachial plexopathy is more likely due to breast and lung cancers whereas infiltrative lumbosacral plexopathies are associated with colorectal and cervical cancers
- The presence of myokymic discharges on EMG are suggestive of radiation-induced plexopathy rather than metastatic disease.

Most physicians refer to paraneoplastic syndromes as "remote effects" of cancer on the nervous system that are not caused by direct invasion or other nonmetastatic complications. Paraneoplastic neurological syndromes usually precede the identification of cancer and, even if the related cancer is finally found, the cancer is usually small, indolent, and nonmetastatic. Often, the symptoms of the paraneoplastic neurological syndrome predominate while the cancer itself remains asymptomatic. Paraneoplastic syndromes may simultaneously involve the central nervous system, resulting in a clinical picture of a multifocal neurological disease further complicating the diagnosis. Paraneoplastic neurological syndromes are rare but exact frequency remains uncertain. Nevertheless, as paraneoplastic syndromes precede the detection of a neoplasm, early recognition can lead to detection of a cancer at an earlier and potentially more curable stage. Paraneoplastic syndromes are thought to be due to an immune-mediated process arising from cross-reacting antibodies against tumor antigens and the antigens in the neural tissues. Paraneoplastic neuromuscular disorders include paraneoplastic neuropathy, myopathy, motor neuron diseases, and neuromuscular junction diseases. This chapter addresses only paraneoplastic neuropathies.

⌘ SCIENCE REVISITED

Most paraneoplastic neuropathies are thought to be an immune-mediated process resulting from antibodies directed against tumor antigen that cross-react with peripheral neural tissues

---

Paraneoplastic neuropathies

There are five major clinical presentations of the paraneoplastic neuropathies:

1. Sensory neuronopathy or ganglionopathy
2. Autonomic neuropathy
3. Sensorimotor neuropathy
4. Pure motor neuropathy
5. Acquired neuromyotonia.

Although mixed sensorimotor neuropathies are more frequent paraneoplastic manifestations of cancer, pure sensory neuropathies due to neuronopathies and ganglionopathies are more specific and therefore more highly suggestive of the presence of an underlying malignancy.

Sensory neuronopathy or ganglionopathy

The symptoms are acute or subacute, progressive numbness, tingling, paraesthesiae, and loss of sensory functions. Pain can be prominent. Unlike length-dependent neuropathies, symptoms do not typically start in the toes or lower extremities but often start in the upper limbs, and progress to the lower limbs. In addition, sensory symptoms are often asymmetric and can involve the face, chest, or trunk. As the neuronopathy progresses, sensory ataxia and pseudoathetosis in the limbs can be seen. Motor symptoms are typically absent even though profound loss of proprioceptive sense can be mistaken for motor weakness, especially when a patient is unable to walk. Deep tendon reflexes are usually absent. Sensory deficits involve all modalities. Nerve conduction studies show a pattern of severe pure sensory involvement, often with absence of all sensory responses, whereas motor studies are normal or minimally changed. Cerebrospinal fluid (CSF) analysis may show elevated protein or other inflammatory findings. Although infrequently done, a nerve biopsy might reveal severe loss of myelinated fibers without evidence of inflammation. This syndrome is most commonly associated with small cell lung cancer (SCLC) or neuroendocrine tumors. Other tumors that have been reported also include breast and ovarian cancer and lymphoma. The sensory neuronopathy syndrome can precede the identification of the cancers for many months or years.

Paraneoplastic sensory neuronopathy is a disorder of the dorsal root ganglion sensory neurons. Pathology shows marked inflammatory infiltration around dorsal root ganglion neurons, which degenerate and are replaced by satellite cells (Nageotte's nodule) suggesting an immune-mediated process as a likely pathogenesis. Serum anti-Hu antibodies are detected in about 80% of cases and are therefore an important diagnostic test. The main target of the antibody is the antigen Hu-D, which is expressed in both the sensory neurons and on the surface of the tumors.

★ TIPS AND TRICKS

PARANEOPLASTIC NEUROPATHIES

- Pure sensory neuropathies, neuronopathies, or ganglinopathies are the most specific paraneoplastic nerve manifestation
- SCLCs are the most common cause of paraneoplastic neuropathies

---

The differential diagnosis of paraneoplastic sensory neuronopathies includes:

- Toxic, cisplatin-induced sensory neuronopathy. Although paraneoplastic sensory neuropathies are often asymmetric and usually painful, affecting small-fiber as well as large-fiber nerves, cisplatin neuronopathy is symmetric, usually large fiber, rarely painful, with sparing of pain and temperature sensation. Cisplatin neuronopathy usually stops progressing several months after the medication is stopped, although "coasting "may be seen initially. Paraneoplastic neuronopathy continues to progress.
- Dysimmune neuronopathies associated with Sjögren's syndrome.
- Excessive intake of vitamin B_6 (pyridoxine toxicity).
- Friedreich's ataxia, an inherited spinocerebellar disorder.
- Idiopathic sensory neuronopathy.

The prognosis of paraneoplastic sensory neuronopathy is poor. Despite an immune-mediated pathogenesis, the neuronopathy does not respond to immunotherapy and continues to progress relentlessly. Early detection and treatment of underlying cancer arrest progression but do not reverse the neuropathy. In cases presenting with the neurological syndrome alone, especially when anti-Hu is present, vigorous and continuous search for an underlying cancer is recommended. A positron emission tomography (PET) scan could be helpful in identifying an underlying cancer when computed tomography (CT) or magnetic resonance imaging (MRI) fail.

Autonomic neuropathy

Paraneoplastic autonomic neuropathy presents with acute or subacute onset of orthostatic symptoms, ocular involvement, gastrointestinal dysmotility, bladder dysfunction, and anhidrosis. Orthostatic symptoms are found in more than 70% of cases and include lightheadedness, dizziness, and syncope on standing up. Ocular involvement includes abnormal pupillary reaction and dry eyes. Gastrointestinal dysmotility is prominent and causes early satiety, weight loss, bloating, intestinal pseudoobstruction, chronic constipation, recurrent vomiting, and ileus. Symptoms of autonomic neuropathy are more commonly associated with other paraneoplastic syndromes including sensory neuronopathy, limbic encephalitis, Lambert–Eaton myasthenic syndrome, and cerebellar degeneration. Autonomic dysfunction as the sole manifestation occurs in less than 10% of cases.

An autonomic reflex screening test assessing postganglionic sudomotor (sweat), cardiovagal, and cardioadrenergic functions usually shows varying abnormalities from limited autonomic neuropathy to widespread panautonomic failure. Gastrointestinal manometry often shows hypomotility, uncoordinated motility, and intense tonic contraction. In most cases, anti-Hu antibodies can be detected (less than 10% of anti-Hu-positive cases have autonomic symptoms) but other paraneoplastic antibodies such as CRMP-5 can also be seen. Most anti-Hu-positive cases will be associated with SCLC.

Recently, a specific antibody directed against the α_3 subunit of the acetylcholine receptor (AChR) was discovered in patients with dysautonomia. About 50% of those who have ganglionic AChR antibodies have underlying cancers, again most commonly SCLC. Other cancers associated with this antibody include thymoma, and bladder and rectal cancers. Ganglionic AChR antibody was shown to reduce the number of synaptic AChRs at the autonomic ganglia, possibly by crosslinking and internalization of the receptors, an effect that is reversible. Similar to other paraneoplastic syndromes, prognosis of paraneoplastic autonomic neuropathy is related to the underlying cancer. In cases of ganglionic AChR antibody-mediated cases, treatment of the underlying cancer has been shown to improve the autonomic symptoms as well as to lower the level of the antibody. Spontaneous remission of the symptoms without cancer treatment can also occur. It is unclear if treatment with immunotherapy helps improve the autonomic symptoms, although would seem to be warranted in light of the pathogenesis. In patients of Lambert–Eaton myasthenic syndrome, treatment with 3,4-diaminopyridine and of the underlying cancer has been shown to improve the autonomic symptoms.

Sensorimotor neuropathy

Paraneoplastic sensorimotor neuropathy presents with acute, subacute, or chronic progressive weakness and sensory symptoms and deficits.

Acute sensorimotor neuropathies

An acute demyelinating neuropathy clinically identical to GBS is associated with Hodgkin's disease. Other cancers associated with GBS include SCLC, and kidney, esophageal, and tongue cancer as well as melanoma. The typical syndrome consists of acute or subacute onset of progressive symmetric motor greater than sensory symptoms in an ascending pattern over 4–6 weeks, accompanied by loss of deep tendon reflexes, unilateral or bilateral facial weakness, elevated CSF protein, and demyelination on EMG. Treatment of GBS associated with cancers is the same as GBS without cancers.

Subacute sensorimotor neuropathies

Chronic inflammatory demyelinating polyradiculoneuropathy (CIDP) is rarely associated with pancreatic, colon, liver, and breast cancers. CIDP presents with subacute onset of weakness and sensory symptoms progressing over more than 8 weeks associated with elevated CSF protein and demyelination on EMG. Again, treatment is the same as CIDP without cancers.

Chronic sensorimotor neuropathies

Sensorimotor neuropathies associated with hematological malignancies are frequently associated with monoclonal gammopathy of uncertain significance and, less commonly, anti-MAG (myelin-associated glycoprotein) antibody. Lymphoma, multiple myeloma, osteosclerotic myeloma, and Castleman's disease are all associated with paraproteinemic neuropathies. Most cases present with subacute or chronic progressive weakness and sensory symptoms, elevated CSF protein, and demyelinating or axonal changes on EMG. In cases of anti-MAG neuropathy, sensory symptoms, especially large-fiber symptoms, are more pronounced. The patients typically present with gait disturbance with minimal weakness but frequently tremor in the upper limbs. It is important to screen for monoclonal proteins in unexplained neuropathies in patients aged >50 and complete a skeletal survey looking for underlying hematological malignancy in patients who have an acquired demyelinating polyneuropathy.

In multiple myeloma, a predominantly small-fiber "amyloid" neuropathy can be seen in which case electrodiagnostic studies may be normal or minimally abnormal. Amyloid neuropathy seen in the setting of multiple myeloma is due to AL protein and typically present with a painful, subacute, progressive axonal sensorimotor neuropathy with weight loss, prominent autonomic symptoms, and involvement of other organs, such as heart, kidneys, and liver. Diagnosis requires tissue biopsy for diagnosis, and biopsy of peripheral nerves, rectum, kidney, bone marrow, or omental fat pad may be helpful.

Osteosclerotic myeloma may be challenging to diagnose. The hematological diagnosis may become more readily apparent when the features of POEMS (**p**olyneuropathy, **o**rganomegaly, **e**ndocrinopathy, monoclonal gammopathy, **s**kin changes) are appreciated. A patient with POEMS typically presents in the fifth to seventh decades with weakness and paraesthesiae, and electrodiagnostic studies consistent with distal, sensorimotor, demyelinating polyneuropathy. Papilledema and hyperpigmented macules can be seen. Organomegaly usually involves the liver but splenomegaly and lymphadenopathy can be found. Hypogonadism, thyroid dysfunction, and diabetes mellitus are the more common features of endocrine involvement. Unlike multiple myeloma, hypercalcemia and renal failure are rarely seen in POEMS. Bone marrow biopsy showing abnormal plasma cell infiltration, lymph node biopsy showing angiofollicular hyperplasia (Castleman's disease), bone biopsy showing osteosclerotic myeloma, or a blood test showing elevated plasma vascular endothelial growth factor is helpful in diagnosis.

Treatment of sensorimotor neuropathy associated with hematological malignancy usually requires treatment of the underlying cancers. Even if the cancer is in remission, the neuropathy may or may not improve. Focal diseases such as osteosclerotic myeloma may require local radiation but more diffuse diseases warrant systemic therapy. Treatment directed at neuropathy itself, such as intravenous immunoglobulin or plasmapheresis, is usually not helpful. It is also important to avoid cancer treatment that can affect peripheral nerves in these patients. Amyloid neuropathy seen in the setting of multiple myeloma has a poor prognosis with an unsatisfactory response to treatment and short survival.

☆ TIPS AND TRICKS

- Always obtain a skeletal survey looking for lytic or sclerotic bone lesions and serum immunofixation looking for monoclonal protein when evaluating a demyelinating polyneuropathy

---

Paraneoplastic pure motor neuropathy

This is a very rare syndrome and described in a small number of patients with breast cancer, lung cancer, and lymphoma. The clinical features could be either a pure lower motor neuron syndrome or combined upper and lower motor neuron disease mimicking amyotrophic lateral sclerosis. A patient typically presents with rapidly progressive subacute weakness starting asymmetrically and progressing to generalized weakness, mostly without sensory loss. Muscle atrophy is prominent. Deep tendon reflexes are decreased or absent, but may be brisk in cases with upper motor neuron involvement. In cases with a coexisting paraneoplastic sensory or autonomic involvement, making a specific diagnosis can be difficult.

The major differential diagnosis is diffuse meningeal carcinomatosis, which can give similar clinical and electrodiagnostic pictures. Most cases will not have a paraneoplastic antibody marker but, rarely, anti-Hu and anti-Yo antibodies have been reported, especially in cases associated with lung and breast cancers, respectively. Electrophysiological studies usually reveal findings of an active and diffuse neurogenic process similar to motor neuron disease. Treatment with immunotherapy is unsatisfactory and prognosis varies. Some patients with predominantly lower motor neuron syndrome have a relatively benign course whereas other patients progress to respiratory failure and short survival.

Paraneoplastic acquired neuromyotonia

This rare syndrome is characterized by the insidious onset of continuous muscle twitching, cramps, myokymia, muscle stiffness, and pain (Isaac's syndrome). In some cases, there is additional involvement of the central nervous system with seizure, behavioral changes, and encephalopathy (Morvan's syndrome). Electrophysiological study shows repetitive afterdischarges following the compound muscle action potentials and repetitive firing of F waves. Repetitive stimulation reveals high-frequency cramp discharges. Needle EMG shows spontaneous activity such as fasciculations, myokymia, neuromyotonia, and doublet and triplet firing of motor units. About half of these patients have antibody against voltage-gated potassium channels. This syndrome has been reported with SCLC and thymoma. In mild cases, treatment with membrane stabilizers such as phenytoin or carbamazepine can be helpful. More severe cases with more disabling symptoms may require immunotherapy such as intravenous immunoglobulin or plasmapheresis.

Bibliography

Briemberg HR, Amato AA. Neuromuscular complications of cancer. *Neurol Clin North Am* 2003;**21**:141–65.

Chalk CH, Windebank AJ, Kimmel DW et al. The distinctive clinical features of paraneoplastic sensory neuronopathy. *Can J Neurol Sci* 1992;**19**:346–51.

Dispenzeri A. POEMS syndrome. *Blood Rev* 2007;**21**:285–99.

Freeman R. Autonomic peripheral neuropathy. *Lancet* 2005;**365**:1259–70.

Kelly JJ, Kyle RR, Miles JM, et al. The spectrum of peripheral neuropathy in myeloma. *Neurology* 1981;**31**:24–31.

Kuntzer T, Antoine J, Steck A. Clinical features and pathophysiological basis of sensory neuronopathies. *Muscle Nerve* 2004;**30**:255–68.

Low PA, Vernino S, Suarez G. Autonomic dysfunction in peripheral nerve disease. *Muscle Nerve* 2003;**27**:646–61.

Rudnicki SA, Dalmau J. Paraneoplastic syndromes of the peripheral nerves. *Curr Opin Neurol* 2005;**18**:598–603.

Vernino S. Autoimmune and paraneoplastic channelopathies. *Neurotherapeutics* 2007;**4**:305–14.

Vernino S. Antibody testing in peripheral neuropathies. *Neurol Clin* 2007;**25**:29–46.

Vernino S, Adamski J, Kryzer T, et al. Neuronal nicotinic ACh receptor antibody in subacute autonomic neuropathy and cancer-related syndromes. *Neurology* 1998;**50**:1806–13.

Vernino S, Low PA, Fealey RD, et al. Autoantibodies to ganglionic acetylcholine receptors in autoimmune autonomic neuropathies. *N Engl J Med* 2000;**343**:847–55.

Brachial and Lumbosacral Plexopathies

Kristine M. Chapman[1] and Amanda Sherwin[2]

[1]Division of Neurology, University of British Columbia, Vancouver, British Columbia, Canada
[2]Vancouver Hospital, Vancouver, British Columbia, Canada

Brachial plexopathy

Brachial plexus anatomy

The brachial plexus is a complex network of nerve fibers that supply the upper limb (Figure 28.1). The ventral rami (roots) merge to become the upper (C5, C6), middle (C7), and lower (C8, T1) trunks. The trunks divide into anterior and posterior divisions. The divisions regroup to form the lateral, posterior, and medial cords. The cords form the five major terminal branches of the upper limb: the musculocutaneous, median, ulnar, radial, and axillary nerves.

> ### ☆ TIPS AND TRICKS
>
> "Run to drink cold beer" is a mnemonic that can be used to remember the basic anatomic organization of the brachial plexus: **r**oots, **t**runk, **d**ivisions, **c**ords, **b**ranches.

Trauma

Traumatic injuries are the most common cause of brachial plexopathy. Motorcycle or automobile accidents, knife or gunshot wounds, iatrogenic injuries, obstetric injury, and other stretch injuries can result in brachial plexopathy.

Rarely, the whole plexus is injured due to severe trauma. The entire arm is paralyzed and muscles undergo rapid atrophy. There is usually complete anesthesia of the arm with sparing of the medial upper arm (T1 innervated). The arm is areflexic.

The **upper plexus** (C5, C6 fibers) is predominantly affected when the head is pushed forcefully away from the shoulder. The arm may be internally rotated and adducted, the forearm extended and pronated, and the palm facing out and backward in the "porter's tip" position (Erb's palsy). Sensation over the deltoid region may be impaired. The biceps and brachioradialis reflexes are affected.

Lesions to the **middle trunk** are rare but occasionally occur with trauma, resulting in primarily radial nerve involvement with weakness of the C7 extensors of the forearm, hand, and fingers. The triceps reflex may be depressed. Sensation over the dorsum of the forearm and hand may be reduced.

When the arm and shoulder are pulled upward, the **lower plexus** (C8, T1 fibers) is stretched. The patient has weakness of the intrinsic hand muscles and wrist/fingers (Déjerine-Klumpke's palsy); a claw hand deformity may develop. Sensation may be altered over the medial arm and ulnar aspect of the hand. If the first thoracic root is injured, the sympathetic nerve fibers may be involved, resulting in ipsilateral Horner's syndrome (ptosis, miosis, and anhidrosis).

Neuromuscular Disorders, First Edition. Edited by Rabi N. Tawil, Shannon Venance.
© 2011 John Wiley & Sons, Ltd. Published 2011 by John Wiley & Sons, Ltd.

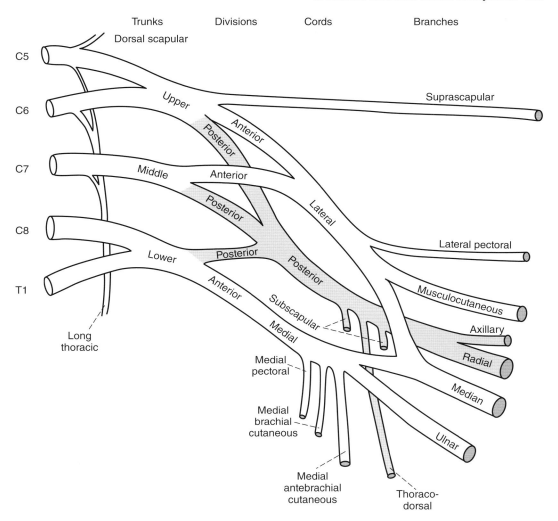

Figure 28.1. Anatomy of the brachial plexus. (Reproduced from Hollinshead WH. *Anatomy for Surgeons*, Vol 3. *The Back and Limbs*, 2nd edn, New York: Harper & Row, 1969, with permission from Harper & Row.)

⭐ **TIPS AND TRICKS**

- Timing of electrodiagnostic testing (EMG): It is best to delay neurophysiological testing for 10–14 days after an acute nerve injury, to allow time for Wallerian degeneration to occur. Axonal loss results in the loss of amplitude in motor responses and denervation potentials on electromyography (EMG).
- Primarily neuropraxic injuries (which have a better prognosis for earlier recovery) can be distinguished from injuries with axonal loss.
- A plexopathy can be distinguished electrophysiologically from a radiculopathy: sensory responses are affected in plexopathy (a postganglionic injury) but not in radiculopathy, and EMG of the paraspinal muscles may be abnormal in radiculopathy but not in plexopathy.

☆ **TIPS AND TRICKS**

TIMING OF SURGICAL REFERRAL
Preganglionic lesions and nerve root avulsion have no potential for spontaneous recovery, so early surgical intervention is warranted to maximize functional recovery. Nerve transfers (neurotization) can be performed to accelerate recovery from preganglionic injuries.

For postganglionic injuries, conservative management for the first 3–5 months will allow any element of neurapraxia to resolve and permit axonal regeneration to occur beyond the point of injury. If there is no evidence of muscle reinnervation at that time, surgical exploration is recommended. Postganglionic neuromas or ruptures may benefit from nerve grafting.

Box 28.1. Current treatment recommendations for acute brachial plexus neuropathy

- Pain management often requires a combination of neuropathic pain medication, an anti-inflammatory, ± an opioid analgesic. Options for neuropathic pain treatment include nortriptyline 10 mg, titrated to 40 mg, or pregabalin 75 mg twice daily titrated to 150 mg twice daily
- Early physical therapy to maintain range of motion
- Consider prednisone 60 mg day for 7 days, followed by tapering dose by 10 mg/day for 5 days, initiated within the first month after symptom onset to improve strength and possibly reduce duration of pain if no contraindications exist

Acute brachial plexus neuropathy

Idiopathic

Idiopathic acute brachial plexus neuropathy (ABN) is caused by an autoimmune-mediated attack on the plexus. Also called brachial neuritis, ABN has a reported annual incidence of 2–3 per 100 000 but is likely underrecognized. Over half of patients with ABN report an antecedent event, which can include infection or immunization.

Patients report acute, severe pain in the cervical, retroscapular region or shoulder, lasting from days to weeks. The acute pain is followed within weeks by rapidly progressive weakness and atrophy of the affected muscles. The distribution of affected muscles is characteristically "patchy." Phrenic and cranial neuropathies (nerves IX, X, XI, and XII) can occur. Sensory changes are often mild. ABN is typically unilateral, but may be bilateral in 10–30% of cases.

Nerve conduction studies (NCSs)/EMG demonstrate axonal involvement in most cases. Computed tomography (CT) or magnetic resonance imaging (MRI) of the cervical spine rules out a surgically remediable cause of radiculopathy, but imaging of the plexus is typically normal. If there is a positive family history, or a history of compressive neuropathies, genetic testing for hereditary neuropathy with predisposition to pressure palsies (HNPP) can be considered. The

initial acute pain is often severe and should be aggressively treated; often a combination of anti-inflammatory, neuropathic medication and opiate analgesics is needed. Early implementation of physical therapy to prevent frozen shoulder is important. Current treatment recommendations are given in Box 28.1.

EVIDENCE AT A GLACE

A systematic Cochrane Review found only anecdotal evidence on intravenous immunoglobulin (IVIG), intravenous steroids, and plasmapheresis in the treatment of neuralgic amyotrophy. There is currently no evidence from randomized trials on any form of treatment for neuralgic amyotrophy. A prospective, randomized trial is under way.

Most patients show significant improvement. However, in a large series of 246 patients with ABN, almost a third had chronic pain, and most patients had some persisting functional deficits at 6-year follow-up. The recurrence rate is reported to be between 5 and 26%, with a median time to recurrence of 2 years.

The distribution of weakness in acute brachial plexus neuropathy is often patchy. Commonly affected nerves include:

- Suprascapular nerve → supra- and infraspinatous muscles → weak shoulder abduction/external rotation
- Anterior interosseous nerve → inability to do the "OK sign" with the fingers
- Long thoracic nerve → serratous anterior muscle → scapular winging
- Axillary nerve→ deltoid muscle → weak arm abduction
- Phrenic nerve → diaphragm muscle → dyspnea, elevated hemidiaphragm on imaging

Hereditary brachial plexus neuropathy

Hereditary brachial plexus neuropathy (HBPN) is a rare, autosomal dominant condition characterized by recurrent, painful brachial neuropathy. Mutations in the *SEPT9* gene on chromosome 17q25 have been identified. Minor dysmorphic features can be seen in some patients, and there is a higher rate of recurrence.

Hereditary neuropathy with predisposition to pressure palsies

HNPP is autosomal dominantly inherited due to a deletion involving the peripheral myelin protein-22 gene locus (*PMP22*) on chromosome 17p11.2. Ten percent have brachial plexus involvement; this can be the first or only clinical expression of HNPP. The plexopathy may be recurrent and is often painless. Patients often have a history of compressive mononeuropathies, and may have a mild generalized polyneuropathy.

Thoracic outlet syndrome

The neurovascular structures (brachial plexus, subclavian artery, and vein) pass from the base of the neck into the axilla through the thoracic outlet, which is bordered by the anterior and middle scalene muscles, first rib, and clavicle. Thoracic outlet syndrome (TOS) is best thought of as three distinct clinical syndromes:

1. True neurological TOS is uncommon. The lower trunk is usually affected. Wasting and weakness of the hand involves the C8–T1 innervated hand muscles (thenar > hypothenar eminence). Sensory changes involve the medial forearm and hand. Anatomical abnormalities such as a cervical rib or fibrous band may predispose a patient to TOS.
2. Vascular TOS (arterial or venous). In arterial TOS, compression or injury to the subclavian artery can result in a cool and pale arm and hand.
3. Nonspecific TOS, also known as functional or disputed TOS. This condition is controversial, lacking specific diagnostic criteria. Nonspecific TOS may be preceded by trauma or a whiplash-type injury. The main feature is pain in the

Scapular winging is commonly seen in brachial plexus lesions due to involvement of the long thoracic nerve. However, it also may be seen in trapezius and rhomboid muscle paralysis, and some muscular dystrophies.

	Medial winging	Lateral winging	
Injured nerve	Long thoracic	Spinal accessory	Dorsal scapular
Muscle weakness	Serratus anterior	Trapezius	Rhomboids
Exam	Arm flexion; push-up motion against a wall	Arm abduction	Arm extension from full flexion
Scapula	Entire scapula displaced more medial and superior	Superior angle more laterally displaced	Inferior angle more laterally displaced

Martin RM and Fish DE. Scapular winging: anatomical review, diagnosis, and treatment *Curr Rev Musculoskel Med* 2008;**1**:1–11 with permission from Humana Press.

shoulder and arm that may be provoked by certain arm positions or activity. Patients often have subjective paraesthesiae not confined to a specific anatomical localization. The neurological examination is typically normal. High false-positive rates for provocative tests (Adson's and EAST maneuvers) make the clinical utility of these tests questionable.

> ⚠ CAUTION!
>
> Although surgery may be indicated in true neurogenic TOS, caution should be used in nonspecific TOS because the outcome of surgical intervention has been poorly studied and there is risk of damage to the brachial plexus. In addition, there are no studies comparing natural progression with active intervention in TOS. A Cochrane review on **treatment for TOS** found only very-low-quality evidence that a specific treatment is better than no treatment.

Cancer

Tumors of the brachial plexus

Tumors of the brachial plexus are rare and most are benign. Schwannomas and neurofibromas are the most common tumors arising in the bra-chial plexus. Approximately a third occur in patients with neurofibromatosis type 1. Tumors may arise as a sequela to prior irradiation. More often, tumors spread to the plexus via direct extension from adjacent structures or metastasize. Pancoast's tumor is a tumor of the superior pulmonary sulcus of the lung which can directly invade the lower plexus. Most patients present with a local mass, local pain, or paraesthesiae (Table 28.1).

A chest radiograph or CT scan may show a primary lesion. In over 80% of patients with brachial plexus metastases, contrast-enhanced CT scan or MRI of the plexus shows a circumscribed soft tissue mass or diffuse soft tissue infiltration. Bone scans and radiographs can provide evidence of malignant bony metastasis. In cases of malignant tumors, a metastatic workup is indicated.

> ⚠ CAUTION!
>
> Some patients have no obvious tumor mass on MR scans and have changes consistent with "fibrosis" or radiation injury, but they later turn out to have plexus metastases.
>
> There is overlap in the clinical presentation between radiation plexopathy and neoplastic involvement.

Table 28.1. Features that help distinguish between radiation-induced plexopathy (RIP) and metastatic infiltration of the plexus

	Radiation	Metastasis
Distribution	More often involves the upper trunk C5–6 distribution	More often involves the lower trunk, C8–T1 distribution
Pain	Less frequent, later in delayed RIP	More likely early and severe
Latent period	Longer	Shorter
Horner's sign (ptosis, myosis, anhidrosis)	Infrequent	Frequent. (C8–T1 or lower trunk)
Skin changes, lymphedema	More common; ±radiation damage to overlying skin	Less common
Imaging: CT or MRI	May have low or high signal intensities in the plexus on T_2-weighted images, ±gadolinium enhancement	Circumscribed soft tissue mass or diffuse soft tissue infiltration in up to 90% of patients, epidural lesions
Myokymia on EMG	+	−

Radiation plexopathy

With improved survival, more attention is being paid to complications of cancer treatment, including radiation-induced plexopathy. Three forms of radiation plexopathy are recognized:

1. Acute radiation-induced brachial plexopathy, seen during or shortly after radiotherapy for Hodgkin's disease.
2. Early delayed radiation plexopathy, which typically occurs within 6 months of treatment. It is characterized by pain in the shoulder and axilla, paraesthesiae in the forearm and hand, and, in some patients, mild weakness. It is often reversible, improving over several months.
3. Delayed radiation plexopathy, which presents over 12 months after treatment. The average onset is 1.5–4 years after treatment but may present 10 years or more after treatment. Delayed radiation injury is reported to be related to vascular injury, although direct damage to peripheral axons and myelin sheaths occurs as well. Clinically, numbness or paraesthesiae are most prominent, with weakness typically developing later. Most patients do not have pain at the outset, although they may develop some pain over time. Deficits gradually worsen over several years, but symptoms plateau in about a third of patients.

There is a rough correlation between the risk of radiation-induced brachial plexopathy and the total dose of radiation administered to the plexus. Although clinical, electrophysiological, and imaging features can help distinguish between radiation-induced plexopathy and metastatic infiltration, there is considerable overlap (see Table 28.1). There is no effective treatment for radiation injury and management is symptomatic. Physical therapy to prevent frozen shoulder may be helpful.

Lumbosacral plexopathy

Lumbar and lumbosacral plexus anatomy

The **lumbar plexus** is derived from the ventral rami of L1–4 whereas the **lower lumbosacral plexus** is primarily derived from the ventral rami of L5 and S1–3 with a contribution from L4.

The lumbar plexus is located in the retroperitoneum posterior to the psoas muscle.

The femoral nerve arises from the posterior divisions of L2, L3, and L4, and the obturator nerve arises from their anterior divisions. The iliohypogastric (L1), ilioinguinal (L1), genitofemoral nerve (L1, L2) and lateral femoral cutaneous nerve (L2, L3) also arise from the lumbar plexus. The L5, S1–3 nerve roots make up the lower lumbosacral plexus with a component of the L4 nerve root that continues with L5 as the lumbosacral trunk. The lower lumbosacral plexus gives rise to the remaining peripheral nerves of the lower limb including the sciatic nerve (L4, L5, and S1–3), superior (L4, L5, and S1) and inferior (L5, S1, and S2) gluteal nerves, and the posterior cutaneous nerve of the thigh (S1, S2) (Figure 28.2).

Lumbosacral plexopathy (LSP) is in the differential diagnosis for patients presenting with low back, hip or pelvic pain, and sciatica. In a **lower lumbosacral plexopathy** (L4–S1) patients report pain, numbness, and tingling on the posterolateral leg and foot. Over time they may develop weakness in the knee flexors, hip extensors, hip abductors, and ankle dorsiflexors/plantar flexors. They may catch their toe walking or develop a "foot drop." The ankle jerk may be absent.

In an **upper lumbar plexus lesion** (L1–4) patients experience pain and paraesthesiae in the low back, hip, and thigh. They may develop weakness in the hip flexors, knee extensors, and hip adductors, and complain of difficulty walking up stairs or rising from a low chair. The knee jerk may be affected but ankle jerk reflexes should be present.

Trauma

The lumbosacral plexus is anatomically protected, so lumbosacral plexopathies are typically seen in high-energy traumas associated with fractures of the pelvic ring, acetabulum, or dislocations of the sacroiliac joint. Mild nerve injury usually recovers with conservative treatment. In severe nerve injuries, surgical repair of the lumbar plexus can be considered. Reconstructive surgery has the most favorable outcome when there is a short delay between the injury and surgical intervention.

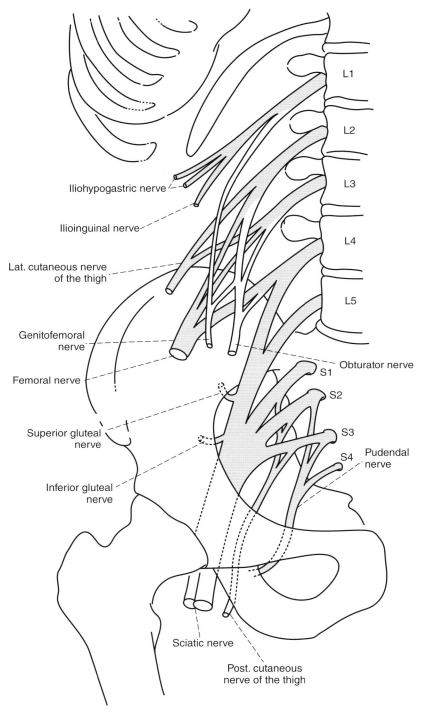

Figure 28.2. Anatomy of the lumbosacral plexus. (Adapted from Hollinshead WH. *Anatomy for Surgeons*, Vol 3. *The Back and Limbs*, 2nd edn, New York: Harper & Row, 1969, with permission from Harper & Row.)

Intra- or postpartum lumbosacral plexopathy

Intrapartum lumbosacral plexopathies are uncommon and typically caused by compression of the lumbosacral trunk between the maternal pelvic rim and the fetal head. Clinical symptoms generally begin during active labor as the fetus descends into the pelvis. The most common presentation is unilateral foot drop with weakness in dorsiflexion and eversion of the ankle, and toe extension. Numbness and tingling are present on the anterolateral aspect of the leg and top of the foot (L5 distribution).

Short stature and large birth weight are risk factors. Imaging is negative, but can be used to rule out other pathology such as a disc herniation. Prognosis is favorable with resolution of symptoms in 3–5 months, in keeping with a primarily demyelinating compressive neuropathy. However, lengthy and incomplete recovery associated with axonal loss can occur if there is prolonged compression of the nerve.

Iatrogenic

The incidence of intraoperative injury is very low; mononeuropathies such as femoral or sciatic neuropathies are more common. A plexopathy can be caused by direct instrumentation or postoperative development of scar tissue. Abdominal aortic aneurysm repair may be associated with ischemic injury to the plexus.

Retroperitoneal hematoma

Retroperitoneal hematomas are typically associated with anticoagulant therapy, but they also occur with bleeding disorders, aortic aneurysm, and occasionally idiopathically.

A large hematoma can compress the entire lumbar plexus. More commonly, a smaller hematoma will affect the intrapelvic portion of the femoral nerve, localizing the weakness to hip flexion and knee extension with numbness and tingling on the anterolateral thigh. CT scans of the pelvis reveals the presence of blood whereas EMG localizes the lesion to the femoral nerve or lumbar plexus. Treatment is usually conservative.

Cancer

Cancer is a common cause of lumbosacral plexopathy. Primary neoplasms of the plexus, such as neurofibromas, are rare. The lumbosacral plexus is affected more frequently by metastasis (primarily breast) or direct extension from the terminal gastrointestinal tract or genitourinary system. Lymphoma or sarcoma can infiltrate the lumbosacral plexus.

The primary complaint is often pain. Over time, paraesthesiae and weakness develop. Lower extremity edema may occur, but this is more common in bilateral plexopathies. Urinary and fecal incontinence is uncommon, although rectal masses are found in more than a third of patients with neoplastic lower lumbosacral plexopathies.

CT or MRI may provide evidence of a mass pressing on or surrounding the plexus. Electrodiagnostic studies may demonstrate denervation in muscles innervated by different nerves and help with prognostication. The treatment of neoplastic lumbosacral plexopathies includes radiation, surgical removal of the tumor, or chemotherapy.

Radiation-induced lumbosacral plexopathies (RILSPs) can occur months to several decades after radiation, arising after abdominal or pelvic radiation for colon cancer, lymphoma, or testicular or gynecological cancers. Vascular changes can cause axonal loss, and development of fibrosis may lead to entrapment and compression neuropathies. It can be difficult to differentiate clinically between a cancer recurrence and a radiation plexopathy.

Diabetic versus nondiabetic lumbosacral radiculoplexus neuropathy

Diabetic lumbosacral radiculoplexus neuropathy (DLRPN), also known as diabetic amyotrophy, most commonly occurs in patients with well-controlled, recent-onset, type 2 diabetes mellitus (DM). A similar syndrome seen in nondiabetic patients is known as nondiabetic radiculoplexus neuropathy (NDLRPN), and has a similar clinical presentation. Both NDLRPN and DLRPN often affect middle-aged individuals, and typically follow an unintentional weight loss of >4 kg. The patient initially experiences rapid onset of severe burning or deep aching pain in the pelvis or proximal thigh. As the pain subsides the patient will often develop significant proximal weakness and atrophy affecting muscles innervated by the femoral and obturator nerves (typically unilaterally, but occasionally bilaterally). Although the patient may report numbness and tingling over the thigh, pain and motor deficit often predominate. The patellar tendon reflex is commonly absent. Electrodiagnostic studies show axonal loss in femoral and obturator innervated muscles. Diagnostic imaging is not useful for identifying lesions in DLRPN and NDLRPN.

Recovery without medical intervention takes place in most patients, but it can take up to several years and may leave residual deficits.

EVIDENCE AT A GLANCE

A controlled trial using intravenous methylprednisolone in DLRPN showed that there was no significant improvement in neurological deficits; however, there was marked improvement in pain-related symptoms. A 2009 Cochrane Intervention Review determined that there was insufficient clinical evidence from randomized trials to endorse the use of immunosuppressive therapies for the treatment of DLRPN. Current treatment guidelines include pain management and physical therapy.

Meralgia paresthetica

Patients experience numbness, and sometimes paraesthesias or neuropathic pain over a discrete region of the anterolateral thigh in the distribution of the lateral femoral cutaneous nerve. Patients can be reassured that weakness will not develop. Patellar and ankle jerk reflexes should be present. The nerve is most commonly affected as it exits the pelvis under the inguinal ligament.

Meralgia paresthetica is a clinical diagnosis. Electrodiagnostic are mainly used to rule out a femoral nerve injury or lumbar radiculopathy. Treatment is usually conservative.

EVIDENCE AT A GLANCE

The 2008 Cochrane Review of treatment for meralgia paresthetica found four treatment options based on observational studies that were at least 69% effective: spontaneous recovery (69%), injection of a corticosteroid and local anesthetic (83%), surgical decompression (88%), and neurectomy (94%).

Bibliography

Dubuisson A, Kline DG. Brachial plexus injury: a survey of 100 consecutive cases from a single service. *Neurosurgery* 2002;**51**:673–82.

Harper CM, Thomas JE, Cascino TL, Litchy WJ. Distinction between neoplastic and radiation-induced brachial plexopathy, with emphasis on the role of EMG. *Neurology* 1989;**39**:502–6.

Johannson S, Svensson H, Denekamp J. Timescale of evolution of late radiation injury after postoperative radiotherapy of breast cancer patient. *Int J Rad Oncol Biol Phys* 2000;**48**:745–50.

Katirji B, Wilbourn AJ, Scarberry SL, Preston DC. Intrapartum maternal lumbosacral plexopathy. *Muscle Nerve* 2002;**26**:340–7.

Khalil N, Nicotra A, Rakowicz W. Treatment of meralgia paresthetica. *Cochrane Database System Rev* 2008;(3):CD004159.

Lang EA, Borges J, Carlstedt T. Surgical treatment of lumbosacral plexus injuries. *J Neurosurg Spine* 2004;**1**:64–71.

Martin RM, Fish DE. Scapular winging: anatomical review, diagnosis, and treatments. *Curr Rev Musculoskelet Med* 2008;**1**:1–11.

Planner AC, Donaghy M, Moore NR. Causes of lumbosacral plexopathy. *Clin Radiol* 2006;**61**: 987–95.

Povlsen B, Belzberg A, Hansson T, Dorsi M. Treatment for thoracic outlet syndrome. *Cochrane Database System Rev* 2010; (1): CD007218.

Preston DC, Shapiro BE. *Electromyography and Neuromuscular Disorders: Clinical-electrophysiologic correlations*, 2nd edn. Philadelphia, PA: Elsevier, 2005.

Stewart JD. *Focal Peripheral Neuropathies*, 4th edn. West Vancouver, British Columbia: JBJ Publishing, 2009.

Thaisetthawatkul P, Dyck PB. Treatment of diabetic and nondiabetic lumbosacral radiculoplexus neuropathy. *Curr Treatment Opt Neurol* 2010;**12**:95–9.

van Alfen N, van Engelen BG. The clinical spectrum of neuralgic amyotrophy in 246 cases. *Brain* 2006;**129**:438–50.

van Alfen N, van Engelen BM, Hughes RC. Treatment for idiopathic and hereditary neuralgic amyotrophy (brachial neuritis). *Cochrane Database System Rev* 2009;(**3**):CD006976.

Wilbourn AJ. Plexopathies. *Neurol Clinics* 2007; **25**:139–71.

Part IV

Disorders of Motor Neurons

Approach to Diseases of the Motor Neurons

Christen Shoesmith

London Health Sciences Centre Motor Neuron Diseases Clinic, and University of Western Ontario, London, Ontario, Canada

Motor neuron diseases are a group of acquired and hereditary diseases that primarily affect the motor neurons of the spinal cord and brain. Degeneration of motor neurons in the spinal cord causes lower motor (LMN) neuron findings and degeneration of cerebral motor neurons produces upper motor neuron (UMN) signs and symptoms. When approaching a patient with suspected motor neuron disease (MND), it is most important to first evaluate whether the deficits are isolated to the motor system, or whether they involve other neurological systems. The next step is to determine if this is solely a UMN syndrome, solely a LMN syndrome, or mixed UMN and LMN syndrome. The most common motor neuron disease, amyotrophic lateral sclerosis (ALS), affects both the spinal cord and the cerebral motor neurons producing mixed UMN and LMN findings. The final step is to rule out conditions that are MND mimics and are potentially treatable, before assigning a diagnosis of MND (Box 29.1).

When diagnosing a patient with an MND, it is best to be able to give as specific a diagnosis as possible to help with treatment options, prognosis, and hereditary factors. There is no single test that is highly sensitive and specific for MND, with the exception of the genetic confirmation of the inherited MNDs. The diagnosis of most MNDs is based on a combination of the clinical history, physical examination, electrophysiology,

imaging, and serology. This chapter focuses on a general approach to adult-onset MND. Chapters 30 and 31 give more specific details about spinal muscular dystrophy and amyotrophic lateral sclerosis, respectively.

Clinical history

Clues that can help narrow the diagnosis include age of onset, site of onset, rate and pattern of progression, and nonmotor symptoms. Although there are exceptions, the symptoms should be predominately motor symptoms, with, at most, only minor cognitive, sensory, autonomic, or sphincter symptoms. Toxic exposures and infections such as Lyme disease, human immunodeficiency virus (HIV), human T-lymphotropic virus type I (HTLV-I), West Nile virus, and previous polio, can cause motor neuron disease.

Physical examination

Examination of MND patients reveals UMN and/or LMN signs. UMN findings include weakness, hyperreflexia, spasticity, spastic dysarthria, re-emergence of primitive reflexes (snout, root, palmomental reflex), and pseudobulbar affect. LMN findings include weakness, focal muscle atrophy, fasciculations, and hyporeflexia. UMN and LMN signs should be searched for in the craniobulbar region, upper extremities, thoracoabdominal region, and the lower extremities (Table 29.1).

Neuromuscular Disorders, First Edition. Edited by Rabi N. Tawil, Shannon Venance.
© 2011 John Wiley & Sons, Ltd. Published 2011 by John Wiley & Sons, Ltd.

Box 29.1. Differential diagnosis of motor neuron disease (MND)

Hereditary *MND*
Familial amyotrophic lateral sclerosis (ALS)
Spinobulbar muscular atrophy (Kennedy's disease)
Spinal muscular atrophy (SMA)
Hereditary spastic paraplegia (HSP)
Hereditary distal motor neuropathies
Frontotemporal dementia with ALS
Hexosaminidase A deficiency
Adrenomyeloneuropathy (AMN)

Acquired *MND*
Amyotrophic lateral sclerosis (ALS)
Primary lateral sclerosis (PLS)
Progressive muscular atrophy (PMA)
Progressive bulbar palsy
Hirayama variant
Spinal cord pathology (multilevel radiculopathies, cervical spondylosis, syrinx, dural arteriovenous fistula)
Paraneoplastic
Toxic (electrical injury, lead, cycad, lathyrism, konzo)
Metabolic (hyperparathyroidism, hyperthyroidism, copper deficiency)
Infectious (polio, West Nile virus, HIV, HTLV-1)
Inflammatory (multifocal motor neuropathy, sarcoidosis)
Other degenerative central nervous system disorders (cortical basal ganglionic degeneration, multiple system atrophy, polyglucosan body disease)

Although some MNDs demonstrate pure motor system dysfunction, others demonstrate dysfunction of other central and peripheral nervous system components. For example, with amyotrophic lateral sclerosis (ALS), frontotemporal cognitive and behavioral findings are common and patients with Kennedy's disease can have a sensory polyneuropathy.

SCIENCE REVISITED

Spinal bulbar muscular atrophy (Kennedy's disease) is an X-linked inherited disease

caused by a trinucleotide expansion in the androgen receptor gene. The abnormal protein forms aggregates that are toxic to motor neurons. The affected male patients have diffuse fasciculations, cramping, proximal muscle weakness, dysarthria, and dysphagia. They also have gynecomastia, testicular atrophy, and reduced fertility. Nerve conduction studies will often demonstrate a coexistent sensory neuropathy. With this disease, the lifespan is only mildly shortened and treatment, at present, is only symptomatic. Recent clinical trials assessed the use of testosterone inhibitors to prevent translocation of the mutant androgen receptor into the nucleus. However, no significant beneficial effect was observed.

Investigations

All patients with a suspected MND should have nerve conduction studies and electromyography (EMG), to confirm or exclude LMN involvement. EMG should show evidence of acute and chronic denervation. Fibrillation potentials and positive sharp waves are evidence of acute denervation. Fasciculations have also been proposed as evidence of acute denervation, particularly when a diagnosis of ALS is being considered (Awaji criteria). Signs of chronic denervation on EMG include the presence of large-amplitude motor units, reflecting the presence of reinnervation. Convincing EMG evidence of motor neuron degeneration requires pathological findings in at least two muscles innervated by different nerves and roots. Excluding multifocal motor neuropathy (MMN) is very important in the evaluation of individuals with predominately LMN findings; MMN is diagnosed by identifying conduction block in motor nerves across noncompressible sites with preserved sensory responses.

An MND workup should include imaging of the neuroaxis in most patients to exclude structural lesions that can mimic MND. Findings suggestive but not pathognomonic for ALS include corticospinal tract hyperintensities and a T_2-weighted hypointense rim in the precentral cortex on magnetic resonance imaging (MRI).

Table 29.1. Upper (UMN) and lower (LMN) motor neuron signs

Region	LMN signs	UMN signs
Bulbar	Flaccid dysarthria	Spastic dysarthria
	Tongue fasciculations	Hyperactive gag reflex
	Tongue atrophy	Palmomental reflex
		Snout reflex
		Routing reflex
		Hyperactive jaw jerk
		Pseudobulbar affect
		Forced yawning
Cervical	Fasciculations in arm muscles	Upper extremity spasticity
	Atrophy of arm muscles	Upper extremity hyperreflexia
		Hoffman's or Tromner's reflex
		Preserved reflexes in a weak and wasted limb
Thoracic	Fasciculations in paraspinals	Loss of abdominal reflexes
	Fasciculations in abdominal muscles	
Lumbar	Fasciculations in leg muscles	Leg spasticity
	Atrophy of leg muscles	Leg hyperreflexia
		Babinski's sign
		Crossed hip adductor reflex
		Retained reflexes in a weak and wasted limb

Box 29.2. Tumors associated with paraneoplastic motor neuron disease

Non-Hodgkin's lymphoma
Hodgkin's lymphoma
Small cell lung cancer (anti-Hu)
Testicular germ cell tumors
Renal cell carcinoma
Breast cancer
Ovarian cancer (anti-Yo)

The need for other body imaging depends on the clinical history. As there have been several case reports of paraneoplastic MND improvement after removal of a renal cell carcinoma, abdominal ultrasonography would be reasonable in most patients to exclude that diagnosis. Other investigations for paraneoplastic disorders include a chest radiograph, testicular ultrasonography, mammography, and pelvic ultrasonography (Box 29.2).

Blood work should be drawn to rule out potentially treatable causes of MND mimics. All patients should have a creatine kinase (CK), vitamin B_{12}, thyroid-stimulating hormone (TSH), and calcium done. If there is any hint of an inflammatory condition present (i.e. prior history of rheumatological condition, rash, substantial night sweats, or rapid weight loss), then inflammatory serum markers should also be drawn (erythrocyte sedimentation rate [ESR], C-reactive protein [CRP], p- and c-anti-neutrophilic cytoplasmic antibody [ANCA], antinuclear antibody [ANA], rheumatoid factor [RF] complement levels, and an anti-ENA [extractable nuclear antigen] screen). If a patient has a predominately LMN presentation with hyporeflexia, anti-GM1 antibodies should also be tested to rule out MMN. Although anti-GM1 antibodies can be positive in degenerative MND, strongly positive anti-GM1 antibodies raise the suspicion of MMN and argue for a therapeutic trial of intravenous immunoglobulin (IVIG). If the history is suggestive of a paraneoplastic syndrome, one could consider testing for anti-Hu and anti-Yo (if female) antibodies.

Cerebrospinal fluid (CSF) evaluation in the workup of an individual with MND serves to exclude MND mimics. Degenerative MNDs demonstrate normal CSF cell counts, and so an elevated cell count raises the suspicion of an alternative diagnosis such as HIV, lepotomeningeal carcinomatosis, or an inflammatory process such as vasculitis or sarcoidosis. Patients with rapidly progressive motor neuron degeneration can have elevated protein in their CSF, but rarely would this protein be >80 mg/dL. Muscle and nerve biopsies are rarely indicated. Genetic testing for specific MNDs is indicated only if there is a family history of a similar MND.

Once an MND is confirmed and mimics excluded, the patient can be classified with regard to their specific MND diagnosis (Figure 29.1).

UMN-predominant disorders

Patients with isolated UMN findings need to have nerve conduction studies (NCSs) and EMG to rule out associated LMN involvement and imaging to exclude structural causes of the presentation. Isolated bulbar involvement is seen in spastic progressive bulbar palsy, which is usually a harbinger of ALS. Isolated extremity spasticity is seen in hereditary spastic paraplegia (HSP), infectious myelopathies (HTLV-I and -II, and HIV), inflammatory myelopathies (transverse myelitis, vasculitis) and metabolic causes (vitamin B_{12} deficiency, adrenomyeloneuropathy and its female carriers, and copper deficiency). HSP can be autosomal dominant or recessive with variable penetrance, and a positive family history is not necessary for the diagnosis. HSP results in greater lower than upper extremity spasticity and no bulbar symptoms. Pure HSP presentations have only spasticity and pyramidal weakness, and complicated HSP presentations have additional symptoms such as focal amyotrophy, dysarthria, and cognitive involvement.

Generalized spasticity with or without a spastic dysarthria can be due to primary lateral sclerosis (PLS), UMN-predominant ALS, multi-infarct states, paraneoplastic syndrome, leukodystrophy, or other demyelinating condition. Once secondary causes of spasticity are excluded, PLS should be considered. A definitive diagnosis of PLS requires progressive symptoms over at least 3 years, and ideally 5 years, without the appearance of LMN signs. In PLS, bladder and bowel symptoms are minimal, and there are no sensory symptoms or signs.

LMN-predominant disorders

Pure LMN disorders should be thoroughly investigated to rule out treatable causes of MNDs such as MMN, multilevel radiculopathies, or paraneoplastic causes. Infectious causes of LMN dysfunction should also be considered including poliomyelitis or West Nile virus-associated anterior horn cell dysfunction. Once secondary causes have been excluded, primary motor neuron diseases such as spinobulbar muscular atrophy (SBMA, also known as Kennedy's disease), progressive muscular atrophy (PMA), spinal muscular atrophy (SMA), and hereditary motor neuropathy (HMN; also called distal SMA) should be considered. SBMA is considered in male patients who have prominent facial and upper extremity fasciculations and a flaccid dysarthria. SMA is most often considered in children, but adult-onset SMA does occur, typically presenting with slowly progressive proximal muscle weakness. HMNs can be associated with distal weakness.

When no other cause for generalized and progressive LMN weakness can be identified, patients are labeled as having PMA. With time, some PMA patients will convert to ALS when UMN signs develop but most remain as a generalized LMN disease. PMA usually confers a similar prognosis to ALS, regardless of whether the patient converts to ALS. When LMN findings

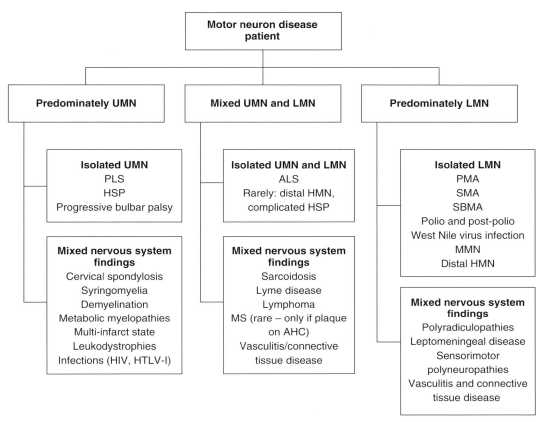

Figure 29.1. Diagnostic approach to a patient with motor neuron disease. AHC, anterior horn cell; ALS, amyotrophic lateral sclerosis; HMN, hereditary motor neuropathy; HSP, hereditary spastic paraplegia; LMN, lower motor neuron; MMN, multifocal motor neuropathy; MS, multiple sclerosis; PLS, primary lateral sclerosis; PMA, progressive muscular atrophy; SBMA, spinobulbar muscular atrophy; SMA, spinal muscular atrophy; UMN, upper motor neuron.

remain isolated to a single spinal segment over time, the patient is considered to have the flail arm or flail leg variant of MND, which confers a better prognosis than typical ALS.

SCIENCE REVISITED

The Hirayama variant is a variant of focal MND that deserves special mention. This condition generally affects young males (ages 15–25), often of Asian descent, with progressive distal arm amyotrophy. The weakness progresses over 1–4 years, then plateaus. Weakness is usually confined to a single limb, but may be bilateral. On autopsy,

some cases have evidence of ischemia in the region of the anterior horn cells, and it is hypothesized that neck flexion in these cases triggers partial spinal cord compression, possibly due to altered dura elasticity, causing impaired blood flow to the spinal cord.

Mixed UMN and LMN disorders

ALS is the most common diagnosis within this category. However, secondary causes should be considered, including spinal cord compression with multilevel radiculopathies and a syrinx causing both spasticity and anterior horn cell loss. Primary causes of mixed UMN and LMN findings include both sporadic and familial ALS, HSP associated with amyotrophy (Silver's and Troyer's syndromes), and uncommon presentations of distal HMNs.

> ★ **TIPS AND TRICKS**
>
> Diffuse fasciculations is a common presentation at neuromuscular clinics. Patients have frequently "Googled" their symptoms and are worried that they have ALS. If their neurological examination and EMG are normal, then these patients most likely have benign cramp fasciculation syndrome. Fasciculations may be seen on EMG, but these are usually rare and are not large amplitude or complex fasciculations. These patients should be seen in follow-up in 6–12 months to ensure that their examination remains normal.

Final comments

Unfortunately, we still do not have a full understanding of the cause(s) of primary sporadic MND including PLS, PMA, progressive bulbar palsy, and ALS. It is likely that a combination of environmental factors in the presence of specific susceptibility gene polymorphisms triggers MND. It is uncertain at this stage whether the primary sporadic MNDs are separate diseases with distinct pathophysiology or just different presentations of the same disease. Until we have a better understanding as to the cause of these primary MNDs, they will continue to be classified separately, particularly as there are differences with regard to prognosis in these diseases.

Bibliography

Andersen PM, Borasio GD, Dengler R, et al. EFNS task force on management of amyotrophic lateral sclerosis: guidelines for diagnosing and clinical care of patients and relatives. *Eur J Neurol* 2005;**12**:921–38.

Brooks BR, Miller RG, Swash M, Munsat TL. El Escorial revisited: revised criteria for the diagnosis of amyotrophic lateral sclerosis. *Amyotroph Lateral Scler Other Motor Neuron Disord* 2000;**1**:293–9.

de Carvalho M, Dengler R, Eisen A, et al. Electrodiagnostic criteria for diagnosis of ALS. *Clin Neurophysiol* 2008;**119**:497–503.

Filippi M, Agosta F, Abrahams S, et al. EFNS guidelines on the use of neuroimaging in the management of motor neuron diseases. *Eur J Neurol* 2010;**17**:526–e20.

Finsterer J. Bulbar and spinal muscular atrophy (Kennedy's disease): a review. *Eur J Neurol* 2009;**16**:556–61.

Gordon PH, Cheng B, Katz IB, Mitsumoto H, Rowland LP. Clinical features that distinguish PLS, upper motor neuron-dominant ALS, and typical ALS. *Neurology* 2009;**72**:1948–52.

Irobi J, Dierick I, Jordanova A, Claeys KG, De Jonghe P, Timmerman V. Unraveling the genetics of distal hereditary motor neuronopathies. *Neuromol Med* 2006;**8**:131–46.

Katsuno M, Banno H, Suzuki K, Adachi H, Tanaka F, Sobue G. Clinical features and molecular mechanisms of spinal and bulbar muscular atrophy (SBMA). *Adv Exp Med Biol* 2010;**685**:64–74.

McKee AC, Gavett BE, Stern RA, et al. TDP-43 proteinopathy and motor neuron disease in chronic traumatic encephalopathy. *J Neuropathol Exp Neurol* 2010;**9**:918–29.

Shook SJ, Pioro EP. Racing against the clock: recognizing, differentiating, diagnosing, and referring the amyotrophic lateral sclerosis patient. *Ann Neurol* 2009;**65**(suppl 1):S10–16.

Talman P, Forbes A, Mathers S. Clinical phenotypes and natural progression for motor neuron disease: analysis from an Australian database. *Amyotroph Lateral Scler* 2009;**10**:79–84.

Turner MR, Scaber J, Goodfellow JA, Lord ME, Marsden R, Talbot K. The diagnostic pathway and prognosis in bulbar-onset amyotrophic lateral sclerosis. *J Neurol Sci* 2010;**294**:81–5.

Valdmanis PN, Daoud H, Dion PA, Rouleau GA. Recent advances in the genetics of amyotrophic lateral sclerosis. *Curr Neurol Neurosci Rep* 2009;**9**:198–205.

Van den Berg-Vos RM, Visser J, et al. A long-term prospective study of the natural course of sporadic adult-onset lower motor neuron syndromes. *Arch Neurol* 2009;**66**:751–7.

Verma A, Bradley WG. Atypical motor neuron disease and related motor syndromes. *Semin Neurol* 2001;**21**:177–87.

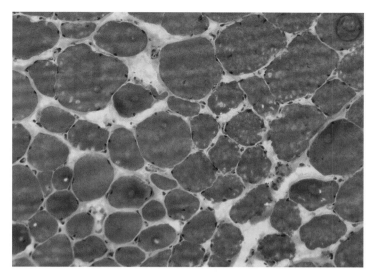

Plate 2.1. Axial views of a muscle biopsy from a boy with limb girdle muscular dystrophy type 2I stained with hematoxylin and eosin demonstrating substantial variability in fiber size, increased endomysial fat, and fibrous deposition, along with occasional fibers with internal nuclei.

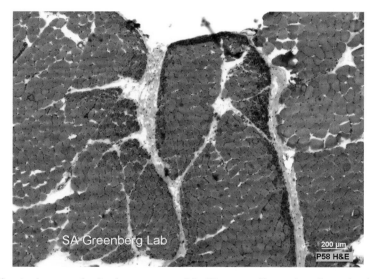

Plate 3.1. Perifascicular atrophy in dermatomyositis. Hematoxylin and eosin stain shows small, bluish myofibers at borders between muscle fascicles and perimysial connective tissue.

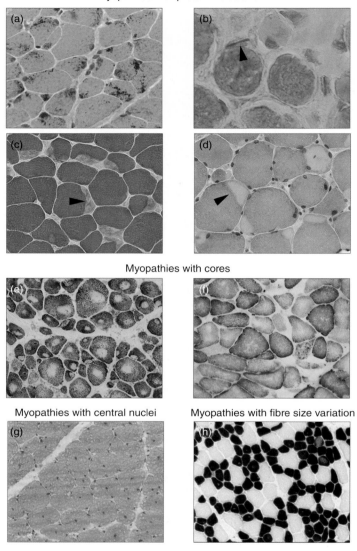

Myopathies with protein inclusions

Myopathies with cores

Myopathies with central nuclei

Myopathies with fibre size variation

Plate 14.1. Light microscopy examples of the subtypes of congenital myopathy. (a–d) Myopathies with protein accumulations: (a) nemaline myopathy: Gomori trichrome stain demonstrating cytoplasmic rods; (b) intranuclear rod myopathy: Gomori trichrome stain demonstrating intranuclear rods (arrow) – patient with *ACTA1* mutation; (c) cap disease: ATPase stain demonstrating light staining "caps" (arrow); (d) myosin storage myopathy: hematoxlin and eosin (H&E) stain. (e, f) Myopathies with cores: (e) central core disease: cytochrome oxidase stain, also demonstrating fiber-type uniformity – patient with *RYR1* mutation; (f) multi-minicore disease: cytochrome oxidase stain – patient with *SEPN1* mutation. (g) Myopathies with central nuclei: centronuclear myopathy: H&E stain – patient with *DNM2* mutation. (h) Myopathies with fiber size variation: congenital fiber type disproportion – patient with *TPM3* mutation. (Reproduced from North KN. What's new in the congenital myopathies. *Neuromusc Disord* 2008;**18**:433–22, with permission from Elsevier.)

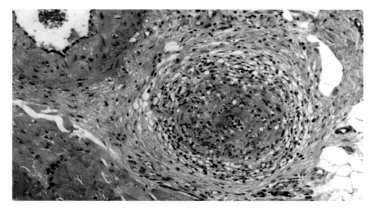

Plate 26.1. Epineurial blood vessel showing intense transmural inflammation and fibrinoid necrosis in a patient with nonsystemic vasculitis (hematoxylin and eosin stain).

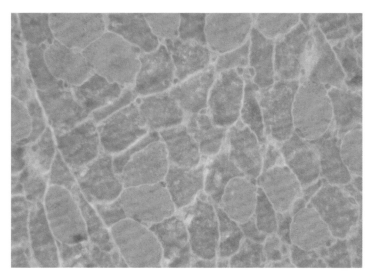

Plate 32.1. Acute myosin-loss myopathy (acute quadriplegic myopathy). Light microscopy shows areas of myofibrillar loss: Gomori's trichrome.

Spinal Muscular Atrophy

Jacqueline Montes[1] and Petra Kaufmann[2]

[1]SMA Clinical Research Center, Department of Neurology, Columbia University, New York, NY, USA
[2]National Institute of Neurological Disorders and Stroke (NINDS), National Institutes of Health, Bethesda, MD, USA

Spinal muscular atrophy (SMA) is a genetically determined motor neuron disease that typically presents in infancy or childhood and, in its most severe form, is the leading genetic cause of infant death. The disease affects an estimated 10–16 of 100 000 infants and children who have progressive muscle weakness caused by degeneration of lower motor neurons in the spinal cord and brain stem. It is an autosomal recessive disorder genetically characterized by the absence of the survival motor neuron (SMN1) gene located on chromosome 5q13. Despite identification of a single mutation, SMA is phenotypically heterogeneous, ranging from a life-threatening to life-altering disease. As a result, a classification system based on motor function is used for clinical purposes.

There are no curative treatments available for patients with SMA to date. Clinical management is focused on prevention and treatment of complications due to muscle weakness. Since multiple body systems can be affected, a multidisciplinary approach to management is necessary. Recently published consensus derived practice guidelines were established to address five care areas; diagnostic/new interventions, pulmonary, gastrointestinal/nutrition, orthopedics/rehabilitation, and palliative care. Furthermore, practice parameters were categorized into three clinical groups; non-sitters, sitters and walkers, to address the specific needs and complications based on disease severity and function.

SMA pathogenesis and clinical features

Lack of the SMN1 gene is embryonically lethal in the absence of the duplicate modifying gene named SMN2. This duplicated gene has a single nucleotide substitution that alters RNA splicing and, as a result, only about 10% of the SMN2 gene product represents full-length SMN protein. The remaining 90% represents a truncated protein with little residual function. Consequently, SMN2 copy number determines SMA clinical severity, with the greatest number of copies associated with the mildest symptoms.

Although SMN is expressed in all tissues, deficiency selectively affects lower motor neurons. Degeneration affects proximal and distal segments of the motor neuron. Defects of the pre- and postsynaptic terminals of the neuromuscular junction, and impaired axonal outgrowth, may precede motor neuron cell death and are associated with symptoms of weakness.

Symptoms of SMA can rarely be present at birth or manifest only in adulthood. Commonly, the symptoms appear between 3 months and 3 years of age. Hypotonia, weakness, typically more prominent in proximal musculature,

Neuromuscular Disorders, First Edition. Edited by Rabi N. Tawil, Shannon Venance.
© 2011 John Wiley & Sons, Ltd. Published 2011 by John Wiley & Sons, Ltd.

Table 30.1. Clinical types of spinal muscular atrophy (SMA) defined by maximum function achieved

SMA type	Age at onset (months)	Relative incidence (%)	Life expectancy	Highest function achieved	Major complications
Type 1 Werdnig–Hoffman (severe)	0–6	60	Reduced	Never sits	Respiratory complications
Type 2 (Intermediate)	7–18	27	Near normal	Never stands	Scoliosis and contractures
Type 3 Kugelberg–Welander (mild)	>18	12	Normal	Stands and walks	Prominent proximal weakness
Type 4 (adult)	Second or third decade	1	Normal	Walks during adult years	Mild motor impairment

preserved sensation, and diminished or absent reflexes are hallmarks for the disease and should prompt evaluation for SMA. Tongue fasciculations and a fine hand tremor are often additional clues to the SMA diagnosis. To further define the disease, SMA is divided into three clinical groups defined by maximum function achieved (Table 30.1). In most SMA phenotypes, a decline in motor function occurs early on in the course, and is followed by periods of relative stability, or a slower rate of decline over time modified by influences such as growth and complications of weakness.

Disease severity is associated with age at onset, with the most severe forms of the disease presenting during infancy as first described in the late nineteenth century by Werdnig and Hoffmann. These patients, termed "type 1 SMA" patients, have minimal functional use of their limbs, and by definition never achieve the ability to sit unsupported. Although SMA type 1 has the highest incidence among SMA phenotypes, it represents a smaller portion of a typical clinic population due to the limited life expectancy. Recent advances in proactive medical care has resulted in more SMA type 1 patients surviving past 2 years of age.

The intermediate form of the disease, termed "SMA type 2," includes patients presenting between 6 and 18 months of age with hypotonia and motor delay, who are clinically classified by their ability to sit unsupported. Patients with SMA type 2 never become functional walkers but typically live into adulthood. Physical and occupational therapy are an integral part of the care of patients with SMA type 2 to maximize functional independence, integrate technology, and prevent orthopedic complications common in this cohort. Similarly, pulmonary complications are common, making proactive respiratory management essential.

The mildest SMA phenotype, type 3, also termed "Kugelberg–Welander disease," presents after 18 months of age with symptoms of proximal weakness, mostly of the legs. Patients with SMA type 3 attain the ability to walk unaided. They complain of difficulty rising from the floor or low surfaces, running, and negotiating stairs. Fatigue is most common in this phenotype. Pulmonary complications are not common in SMA type 3, and patients typically have a normal life expectancy.

Children presenting with symmetric, proximal more than distal weakness that is greater in the legs than the arms, diminished or absent deep tendon reflexes, and preserved sensation should raise high suspicion for SMA. Tongue fasciculations and hand tremors are a common finding. The first diagnostic procedure for SMA is DNA analysis for the *SMN* gene deletion which has up to 95% sensitivity and 100% specificity, to detect homozygous deletions of *SMN1* exon 7. If negative, electromyography (EMG) and nerve conduction studies, laboratory studies for muscle enzyme creatine kinase, and possibly muscle or nerve biopsy may be indicated to test for other motor neuron disorders, myopathies, neuropathies, or muscular dystrophies.

Once an SMA diagnosis has been confirmed, genetic inheritance of this autosomal recessive disorder should be reviewed with the family with referral for genetic counseling. Parental carrier testing and prenatal or preimplantation diagnosis are options for family planning. Testing of asymptomatic siblings is not recommended in the absence of a viable intervention. However, genetic counseling and carrier testing when unaffected siblings reach reproductive age are indicated.

Management of SMA

Family education is essential upon diagnosis. Multidisciplinary care should be implemented, ideally in a specialized neuromuscular clinic and, depending on disease severity, may include a neurologist, pulmonologist, gastroenterologist, physiatrist, physical and occupational therapists, and a communication specialist. For patients with infancy-onset SMA type 1, the prognosis should be discussed with the family so that they can make an informed choice between palliative multidisciplinary care and a more active approach which would include respiratory support and feeding through a gastrostomy tube. When palliative care is chosen for an SMA type 1 baby, the multidisciplinary care should ideally include a palliative care specialist, hospice care, and psychological support to the family, so that the patient's and family's suffering is minimized and a meaningful relationship and memories are encouraged. If proactive care is chosen for severe SMA type 1 patients or for all milder phenotypes, a multidisciplinary approach should be tailored to the patient and family's individual needs. The following care areas should be considered.

Pulmonary management

Impaired pulmonary function is the major cause of morbidity and mortality in SMA type 1 and more severe SMA type 2. The axial muscle weakness associated with SMA impairs chest wall mobility and development, resulting in poor lung growth. Impaired lung function is compounded by scoliosis, exacerbating respiratory compromise. Poor airway clearance, atelectasis, and potential swallowing dysfunction put SMA patients at high risk for recurrent infections. Proactive pulmonary care is an integral part of managing SMA patients. Routine immunizations including influenza, pneumococcal, and respiratory syncytial virus vaccines in those aged <2 years are highly recommended prophylaxis in this population. Maintaining adequate nutrition and hydration is also recommended to maximize pulmonary health.

Respiratory insufficiency is first manifest as nocturnal hypoventilation, with complaints of orthopnea, morning headaches, and daytime sleepiness. Typical assessments include pulse oximetry, polysomnography, end-tidal carbon dioxide, and transcutaneous CO_2 monitoring in infants and young children. Serum bicarbonate levels are typically normal despite respiratory insufficiency during sleep. Assessments of forced vital capacity in the seated and supine positions to monitor pulmonary function in patients aged >5 years with SMA types 2 and 3 should be performed routinely. Formal swallowing evaluations are indicated after acute unexplained respiratory failure or recurrent pneumonia.

If respiratory insufficiency is identified, chronic in-home treatment should be implemented. For poor airway clearance, the use of cough assist devices is recommended. High-frequency chest wall oscillation therapy is also used as an adjunct to help loosen and mobilize secretions. Hypoventilation is treated with noninvasive positive pressure ventilation. Tracheostomy and long-term mechanical ventilation is a treatment option in patients with respiratory failure who are not adequately maintained with noninvasive measures.

Overall, pulmonary issues are important to consider when managing SMA patients. For all SMA patients, perioperative care should include preoperative evaluation for respiratory status, infections, cough effectiveness, sleep-disordered breathing, asthma, aspiration, and reflux, because they are at high risk for post-anesthesia complications. These complications can include hypoventilation, atelectasis, impaired airway clearance, and poor cough, which can lead to prolonged intubation, infection, tracheostomy, and death. Postoperatively patients should be weaned to noninvasive ventilation as a transition to extubation with careful postoperative pain management.

★ **TIPS AND TRICKS**

For prevention of infection, children with SMA should receive all standard immunizations. Influenza and pneumococcal vaccines should be administered to infants aged >6 months and respiratory syncytial virus vaccines in those aged <2 years during the winter months.

During illness or perioperative period, it is important to implement aggressive airway clearance using mechanical exsufflation, chest physical therapy, and suctioning as needed. For patients with known hypoventilation, use of noninvasive positive pressure ventilation while sleeping, with daytime use as needed during the time of illness or immediately postoperatively, is recommended. Consider having a low threshold for antibiotic use in SMA patients with respiratory illness.

Gastrointestinal and nutrition management

Involvement of the bulbar cranial nerves is common in the more severe SMA types 1 and 2 phenotypes, and rare in SMA type 3. The resultant muscle weakness causes feeding and swallowing impairment which may lead to malnutrition and aspiration. Common problems related to gastrointestinal dysfunction include constipation, delayed gastric emptying, and gastroesophageal reflux. Constipation may result from weakened abdominal muscles, decreased mobility, and poor hydration.

Children with feeding difficulties and/or recurrent pneumonias should be referred for a swallowing evaluation. Treatment should be directed toward reducing the risk of aspiration and maxi-

✋ **CAUTION!**

Any child with an absent or abnormal gag reflex is at high risk for aspiration. For that reason, a Nissen funduplication together with a gastrostomy procedure is highly recommended even if reflux is not apparent.

To avoid reflux, children with feeding tubes should be fed upright a minimum of 30° and, if in bed, turned onto their right side.

mizing nutrition. Gastrostomy tube placement is indicated if swallowing function is deemed inadequate and sufficient nutrition cannot be maintained.

Conversely, patients with less severe type 2 and nonambulant type 3 SMA are at greater risk of over-nutrition and obesity in the setting of typically normal bulbar function but decreased functional mobility. Excessive adiposity places greater demands on already weakened muscles and further compromises function. Nutritional counseling and assessments of dietary intake should be incorporated in routine clinical management. As SMA patients have decreased lean body mass, children should maintain lower percentiles for weight and body mass index on growth curves. A well-balanced diet is recommended with close monitoring of nutritional status.

Orthopedic management

Weakness and limited mobility can result in poor posture, decreased extensibility of muscle, and joint contractures. Axial muscle weakness and prolonged sitting further predispose SMA patients to scoliosis. Maintaining flexibility and normal joint range of motion is essential to maximize function and positioning and to minimize pain and discomfort. Walkers are at lowest risk for joint contractures, but often show increased compensatory lordosis of the lumbar spine as a result of hip flexor weakness and altered gait mechanics. Hip flexor and knee extensor tightness and joint contractures are common in sitters. Weakness of the ankle dorsiflexors in nonambulatory SMA patients increases the risk of Achilles tendon tightness and equinovarus deformities. Shoulder girdle weakness can result in limitations at end-range shoulder motion and wrist and hand weakness in the more severe phenotypes, resulting in contractures of the elbow, wrist, and fingers.

For all SMA patients, stretching and range of motion exercises are a necessary and chronic preventive intervention. Bracing can be both preventive and corrective but is limited to distal limb segments. Scoliosis occurs in more than 50% of patients with SMA and is most prevalent in non-ambulant patients. Impaired pulmonary function, reduced mobility, and pain can be the consequences of untreated scoliosis. Spinal deformities can also make positioning and seating more difficult, further limiting overall function. Conservative approaches include physical therapy for flexibility and strengthening of axial muscles and supportive bracing. Surgical management with spinal fusion and fixation to the pelvis is typically performed in children aged >8 years to avoid limitations in cardiopulmonary and skeletal growth. Recent advances in surgical procedures such as growing rods or vertical expandable prosthetic titanium rib (VEPTR) placements provide support and maintain alignment in younger children while the skeleton matures.

Rehabilitation management

Rehabilitation therapies, together with assistive devices and technology, are the mainstay of treatment for individuals with SMA. Early intervention for range of motion, positioning, bracing, and therapeutic exercise is essential to maximize functional performance and prevent contractures. To promote or maintain independence, mobility aids such as walkers and wheelchairs, as well as communication devices, are necessary, depending on the disease type and disability. The overall goals of physical and occupational therapy is to maximize function, strength, and endurance. Early intervention is critical to prevent the sequelae of weakness and to promote achievement of developmental milestones. Aquatic therapy is highly recommended throughout the life span of all SMA phenotypes because the buoyancy of water counteracts the effects of gravity on weak muscles and often makes movement possible. Swimming and nontraditional therapies such as yoga and hippotherapy are encouraged to augment standard therapeutic interventions because they promote flexibility and strength while being enjoyable to the patient.

All patients with SMA types 1 and 2, and many patients with SMA type 3 will require wheelchairs. As the arms are weak as well, power mobility is typically required. For patients with mild weakness, small, battery-powered motors in the hubs of the rear wheels may be adequate. For most patients, power wheelchairs are required. There are many different options in terms of size, seating, controls, etc. Therefore, expert evaluation and fitting are very important to make sure that the seating system is adapted to the patient's need, that essential equipment such as ventilators can be appropriately transported, and that the controls are fully accessible and comfortable. Referrals for power mobility should be considered as early as 2–3 years of age. Early development relies in part on the interaction with and manipulation of one's environment. Unlike typically developing healthy children, infants and toddlers with SMA are not able to explore their environment and develop independent motor skills. Powered mobility promotes functional independence and has beneficial effects on cognitive and psychosocial development. Independent exploration and play as well as mobility helps offset the occurrence of learned helplessness in children with SMA. Powered mobility in SMA is feasible in children as young as 2 years old and results in developmental gains, increased independence, and decreased caregiver burden.

Exercise

Exercise is commonly prescribed to SMA patients to increase muscle strength and function. It has been shown to have neuroprotective effects in the spinal cord and prolong survival in the SMA mouse model. However, to date, there is no evidence to support exercise as an intervention or to define practice guidelines in SMA. Anecdotal experience suggests that patients who pursue daily exercise report improved quality of life and maintain function over time which is akin to reports in similar neuromuscular disorders although mostly performed in adult populations.

Energy conservation

Fatigue is a common symptom in SMA and is often described as either experienced or physiological fatigue. Experienced fatigue is the sense or subjective report of overwhelming tiredness or exhaustion that interferes with the ability to initiate or carry out routine activities. Physiological fatigue is the decrement or inability to generate maximal force in a muscle. Regardless of the type, education and management of these symptoms rely mostly on energy conservation strategies such as minimizing the effort needed to carry out activities of daily living. The symptoms of fatigue should not be confused with those of depression. However, if depression is suspected, the patient should be further evaluated and treated as needed. Although pharmacological management of fatigue in SMA is not common, potential agents used in similar disorders are being considered for study in milder, higher functioning SMA phenotypes.

Conclusion

SMA is a motor neuron disease that typically presents in infancy and childhood with a known genetic mutation in most cases. The SMA phenotype ranges from a life-threatening disease in the severely disabled infant to a mildly affected individual with a normal life expectancy. Although there are a few promising therapies on the horizon, there is no available disease-modifying treatment. As such, multidisciplinary care is needed to manage the multiple body systems and functions that, depending on disease severity, are affected by weakness. All SMA patients benefit from exercise and rehabilitation therapies, where the more moderate or severe phenotypes often need the expertise of pulmonologists, orthopedists, and gastroenterologists. In the most severe form, palliative care specialists are an integral part of the multidisciplinary model to provide supportive end-of-life care. Proactive multidisciplinary care can reduce mortality, prevent the adverse effects of weakness, and improve function in SMA patients.

Bibliography

Cobben JM, Lemmink HH, Snoeck I, Barth PA, van der Lee JH, de Visser M. Survival in SMA type I: a prospective analysis of 34 consecutive cases. *Neuromusc Disord* 2008;**18**:541–4.

Crawford TO. Spinal muscular atrophies. In: Jones RH, De Vivo DC, Darras BT (eds), *Neuromuscular Disorders of Infancy, Childhood, and Adolescence: A clinician's approach*, Philadelphia, PA: Butterworth-Heinemann, 2003:145–66.

de Groot IJ, de Witte LP. Physical complaints in ageing persons with spinal muscular atrophy. *J Rehabil Med* 2005;**37**:258–62.

Dubowitz V. Chaos in the classification of SMA: a possible resolution. *Neuromusc Disord* 1995; **5**:3–5.

Evans GA, Drennan JC, Russman BS. Functional classification and orthopaedic management of spinal muscular atrophy. *J Bone Joint Surg* 1981;**63**[B]:516–22.

Fujak A, Kopschina C, Forst R, Gras F, Mueller LA, Forst J. Fractures in proximal spinal muscular atrophy. *Arch Orthop Trauma Surg* 2010;**130**: 775–80.

Grondard C, Biondi O, Armand AS, et al. Regular exercise prolongs survival in a type 2 spinal muscular atrophy model mouse. *J Neurosci* 2005;**25**:7615–22.

Jones MA, McEwen IR, Hansen L. Use of power mobility for a young child with spinal muscular atrophy. *Phys Ther* 2003;**83**:253–62.

Kariya S, Park GH, Maeno-Hikichi Y, et al. Reduced SMN protein impairs maturation of the neuromuscular junctions in mouse models of spinal muscular atrophy. *Hum Mol Genet* 2008; **17**:2552–69.

Oskoui M, Levy G, Garland CJ, et al. The changing natural history of spinal muscular atrophy type 1. *Neurology* 2007;**69**:1931–6.

Pearn J. Classification of spinal muscular atrophies. *Lancet* 1980;**i**:919–22.

Roper H, Quinlivan R. Implementation of "the consensus statement for the standard of care in spinal muscular atrophy" when applied to infants with severe type 1 SMA in the UK. *Arch Dis Child* 2010;**95**:845–9.

Schillings ML, Kalkman JS, Janssen HM, van Engelen BG, Bleijenberg G, Zwarts MJ. Experienced and physiological fatigue in neuromuscular disorders. *Clin Neurophysiol* 2007; **118**:292–300.

Sproule DM, Montes J, Dunaway S, et al. Adiposity is increased among high-functioning, non-ambulatory patients with spinal muscular atrophy. *Neuromusc Disord* 2010;**20**:448–52.

Wang CH, Finkel RS, Bertini ES, et al. Consensus statement for standard of care in spinal muscular atrophy. *J Child Neurol* 2007;**22**:1027–49.

Amyotrophic Lateral Sclerosis

Amy Chen[1] and Hiroshi Mitsumoto[2]

[1]Department of Neurology, University of Rochester, Rochester, NY, USA
[2]Eleanor and Lou Gehrig's MDA/ALS Research Center, Columbia University, New York, NY, USA

Amyotrophic lateral sclerosis (ALS) is the most common adult-onset motor neuron disease (MND). By definition, both the lower motor neurons (LMNs) in the spinal cord and/or brain stem and the upper motor neurons (UMNs) in the motor cortex degenerate in ALS. The disease is characterized by an unrelenting loss of skeletal, bulbar, and respiratory muscle mass and function. Most patients succumb to respiratory failure in 3–5 years from the time of symptom onset. It is important for healthcare providers to recognize the signs and symptoms of ALS, for timely referral of patients to neurologists and to coordinate multidisciplinary care, in order to enhance the quality of life of patients with ALS.

Epidemiology

The incidence of ALS is 1–2 per 100 000 people per year, which has been remarkably uniform throughout the world, except for Guam where there was an endemic ALS associated with parkinsonism and dementia in the past. However, the prevalence of ALS is only 4–6 per 100 000 due to the short mean survival. At any time in the USA, ALS affects approximately 15 000–30 000 people.

ALS is mostly a sporadic disease. At most 5% of cases are familial with mainly an autosomal dominant pattern of inheritance. The disease has a slight predominance in males over females

(1.5 : 1). The mean age of onset is between 55 and 65 years, and the median age of onset is 64 years.

Clinical presentations

Weakness is the cardinal feature of ALS and usually starts focally and asymmetrically, distally more often than proximally. A classic presentation of ALS is an adult with subacute weakness in the arms or legs, where he or she may report difficulty in buttoning, turning a key, or walking, without significant sensory symptoms. They may also report muscle *cramps*, *stiffness*, and *clumsiness* with fine motor movements. On physical examination, *atrophy* is commonly seen, especially in the intrinsic hand muscles. There is wasting of the thenar and the first dorsal interosseous muscles at early stages, and the "claw hand" appearance at advanced stages of the disease. *Fasciculations* (muscle twitching) are apparent, although they are often unnoticed by the patients themselves. Hyperactive or preserved deep tendon reflexes are elicited in the weak and atrophied muscles. Approximately two-thirds of ALS patients present in this way, and they are classified as "limb-onset" ALS.

Another 25–30% of patients first experience *dysarthria* (speech difficulty) and *dysphagia* (swallowing difficulty), and they are classified as "bulbar-onset" ALS. For unclear reasons, this presentation is more commonly seen in women

Neuromuscular Disorders, First Edition. Edited by Rabi N. Tawil, Shannon Venance.
© 2011 John Wiley & Sons, Ltd. Published 2011 by John Wiley & Sons, Ltd.

than men. *Sialorrhea* (increased saliva) is often present in these patients due to swallowing difficulty rather than an overproduction of saliva. On examination, the speech may be hypophonic and flaccid, or strangulated and spastic, depending on the proportional involvement of LMN and UMN degeneration. The tongue may show atrophy and fasciculations. It may be weak against the inner cheeks and/or slow with lateral movement. The early stages of bulbar-onset ALS are often diagnostic challenges. Although respiratory failure is the main cause of death for ALS patients, it is rarely the sole initial presenting symptom of ALS, occurring in less than a few percent of patients.

Other symptoms that are commonly seen in ALS include *fatigue* and *weight loss*. This is due to the hypermetabolic state of the disease, and the reduced energy reserve in the atrophied muscles. Weight loss occurs in almost all ALS patients even in the absence of dysphagia and insufficient nutritional intake.

Emotional lability, also known as *pseudobulbar affect*, is common in ALS patients and is due to UMN degeneration. In some cases, there may also be changes in patient's personality, behavior, and judgment, manifesting as apathy, impulsivity, or social disinhibition. *Cognitive impairment* can be diagnosed in as high as 30–50% of ALS patients, if a detailed neuropsychological test is performed. These patients may have mild executive dysfunction, attention impairment, and verbal dysfluency, suggestive of frontotemporal dementia (FTD). It is well recognized that ALS, ALS-FTD, and FTD share overlapping genetic and pathological findings.

Variants of ALS

ALS may present clinically as a pure LMN syndrome or a pure UMN syndrome. Progressive muscular atrophy (PMA) is an LMN syndrome accounting for 5–10% of MNDs. It tends to affect older men, with a relatively longer mean survival at 48 months compared with that of classic ALS at 36 months. However, approximately 25% of these patients eventually develop UMN signs, suggesting that PMA is a form of ALS, but of a slower progression.

Primary lateral sclerosis (PLS) is a pure UMN syndrome without clinical LMN signs at 4 years after symptom onset. PLS is slower in disease progression and it allows patients to have a higher level of function. As some ALS patients initially present with a pure UMN syndrome, it is difficult to distinguish PLS from ALS at early stages. Clinical studies show that patients diagnosed with PLS who have focal weakness and bulbar symptoms at baseline are more likely to eventually develop LMN signs.

ALS with parkinsonism–dementia complex (ALS-PDC) is a variant of ALS that may be more in line with other neurodegenerative disease related to tau proteinopathy rather than with the classic ALS or ALS-FTD. It has the highest incidence in the Western Pacific, although it has been reported also in areas outside this region. Patients with ALS-PDC tend to be of a younger age with a longer duration of the disease compared with patients with classic ALS.

Pathomechanisms

The cause of motor neuron degeneration in ALS is still unknown. Similar to other neurodegenerative disorders, ALS likely results from a genetic predisposition that interacts with multiple environmental factors. Our current understanding of the potential molecular pathways involved in ALS is derived from epidemiological, pathological, and genetic studies.

SCIENCE REVISITED

The underlying pathomechanism of sporadic ALS remains elusive. A complex interplay of genetic and environmental factors is likely involved in the etiology of motor neuron degeneration.

Some risk factors implicated in the development of ALS include age, diet, physical activity, heavy metal and pesticides exposure, cigarette smoking, trauma, electrical injury, geographical residence, being a Gulf war veteran, and others. The exact relationship among these factors and ALS are unknown.

Of patients with familial ALS 20% are due to mutations in the superoxide dismutase gene (*SOD1*), implicating a dysfunction of *oxidative stress response.* Another 10% are due to mutations in the fused sarcoma gene *(FUS)* and transactive response DNA-binding protein gene *(TARDBP)* encoding TDP43 protein, implicating abnormalities in *RNA processing.* Abnormal FUS and TDP43 protein aggregates are found in the brain and spinal cord tissues of sporadic ALS and non-SOD1 familial ALS, whereas abnormal SOD1 protein aggregates are found only in SOD1 familial ALS cases. Other genes involved in ALS include *alsin, senataxin,* VAMP-associated protein gene, *VAPB, angiogenin,* and *optineurin.*

Several abnormalities of cellular mechanisms are implicated in ALS including protein and neurofilament aggregation, axonal transportation, glutamate excitotoxicty, mitochondrial dysfunction, glial cell pathology, and inflammatory dysfunction.

Diagnosis of ALS

ALS is a clinical diagnosis. A detailed history and physical examination are therefore paramount for an accurate diagnosis. Progressive weakness that starts asymmetrically is the clinical basis for suspecting ALS. On physical examination, the physician should detect signs of LMN degeneration, such as muscle atrophy and fasciculations, and signs of UMN dysfunction in the affected limbs, such as clumsiness in fine motor movements and pathological reflexes. These findings must be found along the neuraxis, including the bulbar/cranial, cervical, thoracic, and lumbosacral regions, to achieve a level of diagnostic certainty as defined by the original El Escorial criteria that were set forth by the World Federation of Neurology in 1994.

★ TIPS AND TRICKS IN
   DIAGNOSING ALS

Lower motor neuron signs (in bulbar/cranial or spinal muscles):
Atrophy
Fasciculations
Hyporeflexia
Hypotonia

Upper motor neuron signs (especially useful for ALS diagnosis if they are rostral to LMN signs):
Hyperreflexia or preserved reflexes in weak limbs
Babinski's sign or contraction of tensor fascia lata with plantar stimulation
Hoffmann's sign/pathologically brisk jaw jerk
Spasticity
Slow and clumsy fine motor movements
Frontal and temporal lobar degeneration signs:
Apathy
Inattention
Social disinhibition
Verbal dysfluency
Abnormal glabellar reflex and palmomental reflex

Nerve conduction study/electromyography (NCS/EMG) testing supplements the clinical and physical evaluation of LMN dysfunction, and excludes other neuromuscular disorders that may mimic ALS; they are used by ALS experts to facilitate early diagnosis of ALS.

NCSs of ALS patients typically show normal sensory nerve responses with borderline normal or low motor nerve responses. Increased distal motor latency or markedly slowed conduction velocity should raise concerns for other conditions. Focal slowing or proximal conduction block should prompt further investigation for multifocal motor neuropathy with conduction block, which can be treated with intravenous immunoglobulin.

EMG is performed to determine the characteristics and the extent of LMN dysfunction. For the diagnosis of ALS, at least two of four regions (bulbar/cranial, cervical, thoracic, and lumbar) have to show evidence of active and chronic denervation, as defined in the Airlie House criteria and the recently modified Awaji electrodiagnostic guidelines.

Routine laboratory tests, including complete blood count, chemistry (including calcium, magnesium, and phosphorus), liver function tests, erythrocyte sedimentation rate, serum VDRL (Venereal Disease Reference Laboratory) test,

Table 31.1. Variants of amyotrophic lateral sclerosis (ALS) and examples of ALS mimickers

	UMN predominant	LMN predominant
Bulbar-onset ALS	Pseudobulbar palsy	Progressive bulbar palsy
Mimickers	Brain-stem lesions	Myasthenia gravis
	Dementia	Spinobulbar muscular atrophy
	Parkinsonism	Oropharyngeal muscular dystrophy
	Neurosarcoidosis	Neurosarcoidosis
Limb-onset ALS	Primary Lateral Sclerosis	Progressive Muscular Atrophy
		Flail Arm/Leg Syndrome
Mimickers	Cervical spondylosis	Inclusion body myositis
	Subacute combined degeneration	Post-polio syndrome
	Hereditary spastic paraparesis	Spinal muscular atrophy
	HTLV spastic paraparesis	Benign monomelic amyotrophy
	Adrenomyeloneuropathy	Multifocal motor neuropathy
	Multiple sclerosis	Polyradiculopathy
		Hexosaminidase A deficiency

creatine kinase, thyroid function test, and parathyroid hormones should be obtained to exclude other conditions. Serum protein electrophoresis with immunofixation is obtained to exclude paraproteinemia. Chest radiograph and age-appropriate cancer prescreening should also be performed to exclude the rare paraneoplastic syndrome affecting predominantly the motor neurons. Neuroimaging with magnetic resonance imaging (MRI) studies is essential to exclude structural lesions or treatable conditions, such as cervical spinal spondylosis, myelopathy, cerebral or brain-stem tumors, chronic vasculopathy, or leukodystrophy, as the cause of UMN signs in presumed ALS cases. If a male patient has an LMN syndrome, gynecomastia, sensory neuropathy, and chin twitching, genetic testing for Kennedy's disease (spinobulbar muscular atrophy) would be appropriate.

Table 31.1 lists the various forms of ALS and their mimickers. However, diagnosis of ALS at an early stage remains challenging. A high incidence of cervical spondylosis and nerve entrapment in the elderly population can make it difficult to assign the symptoms to ALS; sometimes only time and progression can affirm the diagnosis.

✋ CAUTION!

Fasciculations are seen in ALS, but also in benign fasciculation syndrome. Isolated fasciculations without weakness or muscle atrophy are not diagnostic of ALS, and should not be overzealously emphasized by physicians to cause undue anxiety for the patient.

Sensory symptoms, sphincter dysfunction, autonomic dysfunction, pain, visual loss, and diplopia are not typically seen in ALS. Their presence in the early stage of the disease should prompt investigation for other conditions.

Examples of common misdiagnoses of limb-onset ALS include cervical spondylosis, inclusion body myositis, polymyositis, and multifocal motor neuropathy. Other differential diagnoses to consider for bulbar-onset ALS include myasthenia gravis, neurosarcoidosis, and brain-stem lesions.

Patients should be warned against unproven treatment in ALS that has not undergone rigorous controlled clinical trial.

Treatment and management

In 2009 the American Academy of Neurology (AAN) published updated practice parameters in ALS. Ideally, the news of a diagnosis of ALS should be given by an expert in the field, in a setting that is relaxed, with family members present for questions and support. The physician should educate patients about ALS, discuss the varied presentations and clinical course, the rationale of treatments, the associated side effects, and current progress in ALS research. It is important to show a commitment to continued collaborative treatment and care for the patient, so that hope and trust are maintained.

Pharmacological agents

Riluzole, an antagonist of glutamate transmission, is the only medication approved by the US Food and Drug Administration for ALS treatment. It should be offered to patients with ALS, because it modestly slows disease progression. Fatigue and nausea are common side effects, and elevation of serum transaminases may rarely occur with the medication. Extensive clinical trials to identify a second and better drug are currently being conducted.

ALS patients resort to taking high-dose vitamins, minerals, antioxidants, alternative medications, and supplements with the hope to "build muscles" or to curtail disease progression. Unfortunately, none has proven efficacy in ALS.

Multidisciplinary care

Referral to a multidisciplinary care (MDC) ALS clinic should be initiated as early as possible, because it facilitates the delivery of care, enhances the quality of life, and prolongs survival of ALS patients. In general, MDC clinics include neurologists, nurses, physical therapists, occupational therapists, dietitians, speech pathologists, social workers, and service coordinators from voluntary disease organizations. Other healthcare providers, critical in management of ALS, include pulmonologists, physiatrists, gastroenterologists, psychiatrists/psychologists, orthotists, prosthodontists, and research coordinators.

Respiratory management

Monitoring and management of respiratory function is essential because respiratory insuffi-ciency eventually ensues in all ALS patients. Early respiratory symptoms experienced by ALS patients may include dyspnea with light exertion, orthopnea due to diaphragm weakness, or excessive daytime sleepiness and fatigue due to nocturnal hypoventilation. Forced vital capacity (FVC) is the most commonly used respiratory measurement. Other measurements of respiratory function include nocturnal oximetry monitoring, sniff nasal pressure (SNP), and maximal inspiratory pressure (MIP), which may be evaluated by pulmonologists. Initiation of noninvasive ventilation (NIV) is recommended when the FVC falls <50% of predicted value, or when there is a difference between supine and erect FVC, which reflects orthopnea, or when SNP is <40 cmH$_2$O, or when MIP is <−60 cm, all predictive of nocturnal hypoxemia. NIV prolongs survival, slows the rate of FVC decline, and improves the quality of life for patients with ALS. As the disease progresses, NIV becomes insufficient to maintain respiratory function. Discussions about care at the end of life and advanced directives should have occurred between the physician and patient before the terminal stage of ALS, including whether long-term ventilatory support with tracheostomy and invasive ventilation are desired or appropriate.

ALS patients may also have an ineffective cough, predisposing them to respiratory infections. Such patient may benefit from mechanical in-/exsufflators which increase peak cough expiratory flow, helping to clear secretions.

Nutritional management

ALS patients with inadequate nutritional intake have a poorer prognosis so measurement of weight and assessment of dysphagia once every 3 months is recommended. Signs of dysphagia can be initially managed conservatively but, ultimately, enteral nutrition via percutaneous endoscopic gastrostomy or radiologically inserted gastrostomy will be required to maintain proper nutrition.

Symptom management

There are various nonmotor symptoms associated with ALS, which require a partnership with allied health professions, patients, and families to achieve the best treatment response (Table 31.2). Care of ALS patients needs to be holistic. Psychosocial counseling and support are

Table 31.2. Evidence-based consensus on symptomatic treatment in amyotrophic lateral sclerosis

Symptoms	Treatments
Fatigue	Modafinil, consider NIV
Insomnia	Zolpidem, amitriptyline, NIV
Cramps	Physical therapy and massage therapy
Spasticity	Baclofen, tizanadine, dantrolene, benzodiazepines, stretch exercise, physical therapy
Sialorrhea	Glycopyrrolate, atropine, scopolamine, amitriptyline, botulinum injection to the parotid glands, radiation to salivary glands, portable suction devices
Laryngospasm	Lorazepam liquid sublingual, antacids, proton pump inhibitors
Constipation	Hydration, fiber, docusate, senna, lactulose
Pseudobulbar affect	Dexromethorphin/quinidine, tricyclic antidepressants, selective serotonin-reputake inhibitors
Depression	Amitriptyline (also for sialorrhea), SSRI (also for pseudobulbar affect)
Anxiety	Anxiolytics
Cognitive impairment	Formal neuropsychological evaluation

NIV, noninvasive ventilation; SSRI, selective serotonin-reuptake inhibitor.

extremely important for patients and their families, due to the burden of care. Educational and support group sessions can empower patients and families. Participation in clinical trial studies can provide patients with unparalleled encouragement, strength, and hope. At the advanced stage of the disease, physicians work with palliative care and hospice services to address the psychosocial and spiritual issues, and to provide care at the end of life.

Bibliography

ALS and FTD

Lomen-Hoerth C. The overlap of amyotrophic lateral sclerosis and frontotemporal dementia. *Neurology* 2002;**59**:1077–9.

Strong MJ, Lomen-Hoerth C, Caselli RJ, et al. Prevalence and patterns of cognitive impairment in sporadic ALS. *Neurology* 2005;**65**:586–90.

Variants of ALS

Gordon PH, Cheng B, Katz IB, Mitsumoto H, Rowland LP. Clinical features that distinguish PLS, upper motor neuron-dominant ALS, and typical ALS. *Neurology* 2009;**72**:1948–52.

Katz JS, Wolfe GI, Andersson PB, et al. Brachial amyotrophic diplegia: a slowly progressive motor neuron disorder. *Neurology* 1999;**53**:1071–6.

Kim WK, Liu X, Sandner J, et al. Study of 962 patients indicates progressive muscular atrophy is a form of ALS. *Neurology* 2009;**73**:1686–92.

Diagnosis of ALS

Brooks BR. El Escorial World Federation of neurology criteria for the diagnosis of amyotrophic lateral sclerosis. Subcommittee on Motor Neuron Diseases/Amyotrophic Lateral Sclerosis of the World Federation of Neurology Research Group on Neuromuscular Disease and the El Escorial "Clinical limits of amyotrophic lateral sclerosis" workshop contributors. *J Neurol Sci*, 1994;**124**(suppl):96–107.

Brooks BR, Miller RG, Swash M, Munsat TL, World Federation of Neurology Research Group on Motor Neuron Diseases. El Escorial revisited: revised criteria for the diagnosis of amyotrophic lateral sclerosis. *Amyotroph Lateral Scler Other Motor Neuron Disord* 2000;**1**:293–9.

de Carvalho M, Dengler R, Eisen A, et al. Electrodiagnostic criteria for diagnosis of ALS. *Clin Neurophysiol* 2009;**119**:497–503.

Srinivasan J, Scala S, Jones HR, Saleh F, Russell JA. Inappropriate surgeries resulting from misdiagnosis of early amyotrophic lateral sclerosis. *Muscle Nerve* 2006;**34**:359–60.

Yoshor D, Klugh A 3rd, Appel SH, Haverkamp LJ. Incidence and characteristics of spinal decompression surgery after the onset of symptoms of amyotrophic lateral sclerosis. *Neurosurgery* 2005;**57**:984–9.

Management of ALS

Miller RG, Jackson CE, Kasarskis EJ, et al. Practice Parameter update: The care of the patient with amyotrophic lateral sclerosis: Drug, nutritional, and respiratory therapies (an evidence-based review): Report of the Quality Standards Subcommittee of the American Academy of Neurology. *Neurology* 2009;**73**:1218–26.

Miller RG, Jackson EJ, Kasarskis EJ, et al. Practice Parameter update: The care of the patient with amyotrophic lateral sclerosis: Multidisciplinary care, symptom management, and cognitive/behavioral impairment (an evidence-based review): Report of the Quality Standards Subcommittee of the American Academy of Neurology. *Neurology* 2009;**73**:1227–33.

Mitsumoto H, Rabkin JG. Palliative care for patients with amyotrophic lateral sclerosis: "prepare for the worst and hope for the best". *JAMA* 2007;**298**:207–16.

Mitsumoto H, ed. *Amyotrophic Lateral Sclerosis: A guide for patients and families*, 3rd edn. New York: Demos Medical Publishing, 2009.

Science revisited

Rothstein JD. Current hypotheses for the underlying biology of amyotrophic lateral sclerosis. *Ann Neurol* 2009;**65**:S3–9.

Neuromuscular Disorders in the Intensive Care Unit

Maxwell S. Damian[1] and David Hilton-Jones[2]

[1]Cambridge University Hospitals Department of Neurology, Addenbrooke's Hospital Neurosciences Critical Care Unit, Cambridge, UK
[2]Department of Clinical Neurology, University of Oxford and John Radcliffe Infirmary, Oxford, UK

Introduction to the role of the ICU in neuromuscular disease

Patients with neuromuscular disorders may require treatment on the intensive care unit (ICU) due to respiratory weakness, or, less often, cardiac involvement in the form of either cardiomyopathy or arrhythmia. Neuromuscular patients in the ICU fall into three broad groups:

1. Patients undergoing treatment for curable/reversible neuromuscular disease (e.g. Guillain–Barré syndrome/myasthenia crisis/botulism)
2. Patients with complications of chronic neuromuscular diseases (e.g. respiratory failure in muscular dystrophy/cardiac failure or dysrhythmia in cardiomyopathy)
3. Conditions specific to the ICU or initially causing critical illness (critical illness myoneuropathy/rhabdomyolysis/secondary toxic myopathies).

Effective critical care treatment demands the coordinated care of the neurologist and the intensivist. This chapter aims to give an overview of the leading intensive care issues in the different forms of neuromuscular disease that may be seen in the ICU.

ICU management of specific acute neuromuscular diseases

1. Guillain–Barré syndrome (GBS)
2. Myasthenic crisis
3. Other myasthenic syndromes
4. Principles of respiratory monitoring in acute neuromuscular disease.

Guillain–Barré syndrome

Guillain–Barré syndrome, or acute immune demyelinating polyradiculoneuropathy (AIDP), typically presents with distal paraesthesia, back pain, and ascending weakness and reflex loss. The leading reason for ICU management is respiratory failure, often compounded by infection due to inadequate airway protection in patients with bulbar weakness. Autonomic dysregulation is a second potential cause of life-threatening complications and a reason for considering ICU admission even in the absence of ventilatory insufficiency.

Most AIDP cases reach the maximum weakness around day 10 after onset, which means that patients will have been hospitalized on account of weakness for some days before they require critical care revue. Some 30% of all cases become bedbound, and a third of these will be tetraplegic and need intubation. Bedbound patients are most at risk of respiratory failure and cardiac dysrhythmia. Autonomic dysfunction may occur in up to 60% and causes orthostatic hypotension, diabetes insipidus, ileus, or cardiac arrhythmia which may require drug treatment and occasionally emergency pacing. The overall mortality rate is 5–10%, mainly due to infection (often through aspiration resulting from inadequate airway protection) or cardiac arrhythmia.

Early recognition of high-risk patients based on their rate of progression is crucial for timely admission to the ICU. Otherwise, critical care treatment may become necessary as an emergency for a patient in extremis, which is always a sign of inadequate monitoring or, in other words, lack of adequate forethought.

Regular surveillance includes measures of vital capacity and ideally inspiratory and expiratory mouth pressures, which are more specific for respiratory muscle weakness. This monitoring is possible on the ward with simple hand-held devices. In patients with facial weakness, nasal "sniff" pressures may be obtained. Objective tests should be used regularly to assess the need for intubation: critical values are a vital capacity <20 mL/kg, a peak inspiratory pressure <30 cmH₂O, and a peak expiratory pressure <40 cmH₂O. The unit should have a defined monitoring protocol to establish the patient's monitoring and airway requirements, and ICU admission criteria should be agreed. Patients unable to walk 5 m (Hughes scale score ≥3) require intensive monitoring; patients with significant autonomic dysregulation or who do not pass the "20/30/40" test should be monitored in ICU. The latter may require intubation, as do patients with bulbar dysfunction, because of the risk of aspiration.

☆ TIPS AND TRICKS

- Patients unable to walk 5 m (Hughes scale score ≥3) require intensive monitoring.
- Patients with autonomic dysregulation or who fail the "20/30/40" test should be monitored in ICU.
- Further respiratory deterioration, or with bulbar dysfunction at risk of aspiration, necessitates intubation, not noninvasive positive pressure ventilation (NIV).

Bedbound patients are more at risk of significant autonomic dysfunction, including orthostatic hypotension, dysrhythmia, and asystole. These patients should have continuous EKG monitoring, and emergency external pacing via chest pads should be readily available in patients with signs of cardioautonomic dysfunction. Bradycardia/tachycardia syndrome seen on the EKG monitor may be predictive of dysrhythmic events. The risk of autonomic complications remains even during the rehabilitation phase.

Intubation should take place earlier rather than later, and noninvasive bilevel positive airway pressure (BiPAP) ventilation, sometimes advocated as a temporizing measure, may not be safe in progressing GBS. Preferred ventilatory modes are assist control (AC) or synchronized intermittent mandatory ventilation (SIMV) with pressure support and positive end-expiratory pressure (PEEP). Of intubated patients 50% will require ventilation for more than 3 weeks. Treatment must take autonomic dysfunction into consideration, which apart from dysrhythmia can cause labile blood pressure, adynamic ileus, or bladder dysfunction. The response to commonly used medications may be excessive in these patients and vasodilators, and β blockers in particular, must be used with caution – likewise neostigmine or metoclopramide in bradycardic patients. Evidence-based specific treatments are either intravenous immunoglobulins (400 mg/kg on 5 consecutive days) or four to six plasma exchanges of 1.5–2 L each on consecutive or alternate days. Particularly younger survivors have a chance of full recovery even after very prolonged ventilation, but up to 20% of all survivors retain a long-term disability. Mortality rates are commonly cited as 5–10%, but this applies to all cases of GBS and the mortality rate may reach 20% in ventilated patients. The authors' experience suggests that mortality may vary considerably between units and outcome data should be systematically audited.

☟ CAUTION!

- Under-monitoring leads to preventable emergency ICU admissions.
- Autonomic effects of drugs and treatments may be exaggerated in GBS.
- Bad outcomes may go unrecognized in units that treat few patients.

Myasthenic crisis

Myasthenia gravis (MG) is an autoimmune condition of the neuromuscular junction in which one of several antibodies targeting postsynaptic proteins leads to loss of function of acetylcholine receptors (AChRs). In most patients the first muscles to be involved are the extraocular muscles, causing diplopia and ptosis. In some the disease remains confined to the extraocular muscles, but in most it becomes generalized and can lead to severe weakness, including ventilatory failure. There is initially no fixed weakness in myasthenia, which can mislead the inexperienced examiner into underestimating severity.

Treatment initially consists of the cholinesterase inhibitor pyridostigmine, which provides symptomatic relief. MuSK-antibody-positive MG differs from AChR-antibody-positive MG by an inferior response to cholinesterase inhibitors and often a more unpredictable course. In most cases, immunosuppressive treatment (incremental corticosteroids, with or without a steroid-sparing agent such as azathioprine) is required for sustained benefit.

Critical care teams become involved when bulbar or respiratory weakness affects airways and breathing – the "myasthenic crisis." This most often occurs during the first year or two after presentation, or may be precipitated by infections or inappropriate medications at a later stage of the disease. Rarely, a second type of crisis ("cholinergic crisis") occurs due to excessive anticholinesterase medication, in which weakness is accompanied by cholinergic features such as miosis, bradycardia, increased bronchial secretions, cramps, fasciculations, and diarrhea. Cholinergic crisis is never seen if the dose of pyridostigmine is kept below 360 mg daily.

The initial challenge is to recognize the impending myasthenic crisis early and put adequate protection in place. The team needs to monitor fatigability and not just initial strength, which means tests of sustained muscle contraction (e.g. the Quantitative Myasthenia Gravis Score – Barohn et al 1998). Respiratory function, cough, swallowing, oxygen saturation, and alveolar–arterial gradient need to be checked frequently. Myasthenic crises have a more erratic course than GBS, which critical care outreach needs to take into account when considering ICU admission.

Treatment principles on ICU include infection control, rehydration, and careful review of medication for drugs that may impair neuromuscular transmission. If the patient is intubated, pyridostigmine is often discontinued initially, then reintroduced gradually. Intravenous pyridostigmine is given at approximately a thirtieth of the oral dose; 60 mg pyridostigmine orally is also approximately equivalent to 0.5 mg neostigmine i.v. and 1–1.5 mg neostigmine i.m. or s.c. Immunomodulatory treatment with intravenous immunoglobulin (IVIG) or plasma exchange (PE) is used in standard doses, and high-dose steroids can be given in ventilated patients, because the potential transient exacerbation of weakness that may occur in response to initiating steroids is not a concern. Intensive respiratory therapy and initial noninvasive BiPAP may reduce ventilator days. In myasthenic crises often only a short period of ventilation is needed, meaning that there is no reason for early tracheostomy (i.e. before day 7). There is, however, a relatively high risk of reintubation especially in patients with atelectasis, and the standard predictors of extubation success used on ICU may not apply.

> ### ☆ TIPS AND TRICKS
>
> - Limit pyridostigmine to a maximum of 360 mg daily.
> - Hypoxemia is a late feature – measurement of the forced vital capacity is essential.
> - Myasthenia causes fatigability which may be profound – spot assessment of strength does not tell you how the patient might be even only a few minutes later.

Other myasthenic syndromes

Congenital myasthenia is due to an inherited defect affecting the neuromuscular junction. The defect can be pre- or postsynaptic or can affect cholinesterase anchored in the synaptic cleft. Most patients present in childhood with extraocular muscle involvement and proximal limb weakness. Some forms are associated with episodic respiratory arrest which can be fatal. Anticholinesterase drugs such as pyridostigmine help some forms, but exacerbate others. Other drugs that can be helpful in specific syndromes include 3,4-diaminopyridine, ephedrine, and selective serotonin reuptake inhibitors. It is extremely rare for such patients to require ICU admission in adult life.

Botulism is most often food borne and an infrequent cause of a myasthenic syndrome, with some 930 cases per year worldwide, and some 5% mortality rate. However, patients are disproportionately prone to require critical care due to frequent bulbar weakness, and less often to respiratory failure. ICU monitoring is advised for all progressing cases, because respiratory weakness can develop rapidly. Attempts may be made to remove unabsorbed botulinum toxin from the gut, although most of the toxin will be absorbed in the upper intestine. Antitoxin may prevent progression. Further intensive care is supportive, and recovery may be very protracted. Although autonomic features are typical for botulism, there have been no reports of life-threatening autonomic complications.

ICU management of complications in chronic neuromuscular disease

General principles

Good management of patients with chronic neuromuscular disease typically involves regular multidisciplinary follow-up to reduce unplanned hospital admissions and emergency critical care treatment. Critical care involvement may nevertheless become necessary, not only through primary disease progression, but also through complications that the neuromuscular disorder causes during unrelated problems (e.g. lack of mobility causing complications during recovery from trauma, or postoperative respiratory depression). It is essential for the neurologist to communicate effectively with the other treating teams, and also to be aware of the patient's wishes regarding invasive treatments, of the longer-term survival and quality of life expectancy, and of the potential benefits from the various treatment options before entering into discussion with the critical care team. Too often, neurologists are involved late when significant options have already been missed, and decisions on ICU admission are based on inadequate information on both sides.

Critical care and emergency management in Duchenne muscular dystrophy and other muscular dystrophies

The potential life expectancy for patients with Duchenne muscular dystrophy (DMD) has almost doubled through today's multidisciplinary approach to care with carefully planned protocols and well-defined interventions such as NIV. Patients with DMD are now more likely to be considered for critical care treatment in the event of intervening complications, and it is essential that the critical care team understand current life expectancy and quality-of-life potential. Patients with borderline respiratory function are more likely to develop respiratory failure through intercurrent infections, and are more difficult to wean successfully. Good long-term management includes discussion of issues such as ventilation and tracheostomy with the patient before an emergency situation occurs. Many features that influence the chance of recovery after ICU treatment, such as the baseline respiratory or nutritional status, are determined by the quality of long-term care and whether NIV and cough-enhancement techniques have been instituted in a timely fashion. The option of long-term home ventilation has made the question of whether weaning from a ventilator is going to be possible a less central concern before starting ICU treatment, but has made appropriate discussions with the patient earlier in the course of management even more important.

Cardiac involvement in DMD adds to the complexity of ICU treatment for respiratory complications. The risk of dysrhythmia and cardiac failure is increased. Further anesthetic complications in patients with DMD include intraoperative heart failure, inhaled anesthetic-related rhabdomyolysis, and a malignant hyperthermia-like syndrome, and succinylcholine-induced rhabdomyolysis and hyperkalemia, for which reason depolarizing muscle relaxants are contraindicated.

Cardiac disease and transplantation in muscle disease

Cardiac involvement may be severe in muscle disease. Some myopathies (e.g. Becker muscular dystrophy or some myofibrillar myopathies) typically develop cardiomyopathy and may require

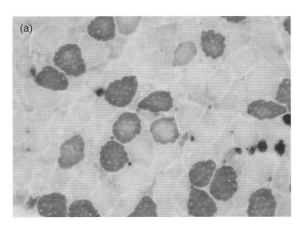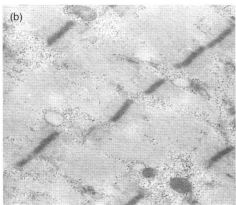

Figure 32.1. Acute myosin-loss myopathy (acute quadriplegic myopathy). (a) Light microscopy shows areas of myofibrillar loss – hematoxylin and eosin; (b) complete loss of thick (myosin) filaments – the dense Z discs can be seen, with the thin (actin) filaments radiating from them. In the midzone between Z discs there is a complete lack of thick (myosin) filaments. (Courtesy of Dr W Squier, Department of Neuropathology, John Radcliffe Hospital, Oxford, UK.)

transplantation, whereas in others dysrhythmia is more common and the need for pacemakers or implanted defibrillator–cardioverters may arise acutely (e.g. laminopathy or myotonic dystrophy). Patients with Becker-type dystrophinopathy constitute approximately half of muscular dystrophy patients who undergo cardiac transplantation.

ICU-acquired weakness and critical illness neuromyopathy

Patients receiving long-term ventilation commonly develop neuromuscular weakness, which delays weaning from the ventilator and the start of rehabilitation, and in some cases results in long-term disability. A careful search to exclude metabolic, acute cerebral, and spinal disorders is often necessary as the mode of onset is frequently unclear. Patients on ICU often receive multiple treatments or interventions that may cause acute neuropathy (i.e. drugs ranging from amiodarone to metronidazole) or rhabdomyolysis (propofol). Toxicity may occur through multidrug combinations, e.g. statin-induced rhabdomyolysis when cyclosporine is added.

Patients who develop symmetric flaccid paralysis of the limbs, often sparing facial muscles, in the absence of a clear metabolic cause often have a combination of critical illness polyneuropathy (CIP) and critical illness myopathy (CIM). These may be impossible to differentiate clinically. Abnormal sensory nerve action potentials are typical for CIP, and reduced response to direct muscle stimulation is typical for CIM, but the two entities are often difficult to separate by routine electrophysiological examination, and there is considerable overlap, so that today the term "ICU-acquired weakness" is often preferred. Muscle biopsies have shown significant muscle cell necrosis in 58%, loss of myosin in 36%, and mitochondrial abnormalities in 52%. Previous muscle biopsy reports indicated three major subtypes of CIM: a diffuse non-necrotizing myopathy affecting type 2 fibers predominantly; acute myosin-loss myopathy; and acute necrotizing myopathy. Neuropathy used to be considered more common, but today myopathic abnormalities are recognized as predominating. The importance of separating CIP and CIM is unclear, because there is no conclusive evidence that the outcome of CIM is better than CIP as has been postulated. Both CIP and CIM appear to be associated with the same risk factors: about a third of patients who are ventilated for over 7 days have some degree of neuromuscular disturbance, rising to 60–70% in those with sepsis/systemic inflammatory response syndrome (SIRS) or acute respiratory distress syndrome (ARDS), and up to

100% in those with multiple organ failure. Acute myosin-loss myopathy (clinically referred to as acute quadriplegic myopathy) has a more specific association, being most frequently described in patients receiving steroids and neuromuscular-blocking agents combined, typically for asthma. It can be seen when steroids are used without neuromuscular-blocking drugs. As the name implies, there is selective loss of the thick (myosin) filaments. Recovery is normally good, but takes several months (Figure 32.1 and Plate 32.1).

Currently, bedrest and prolonged immobility, sepsis, and corticosteroid exposure are recognized risk factors. There is no known specific treatment. Approximately half of patients with CIP/CIM recover fully, but half of the rest may retain significant long-term disability. Long-term follow-up studies with rigorous diagnostic classification are not available yet.

Bibliography

Barohn RJ, Mcintire D, Herbelin L, Wolfe GI, Nations S, Bryan W. Reliability testing of the quantitative myasthenia gravis score. *Ann NY Acad Sci* 1998;**841**:769–72.

Bleck TP. *Clostridium botulinum* (botulism). In: Mandell GL, Bennett JE, Dolin R (eds), *Principles and Practice of Infectious Diseases*, 5th edn. Philadelphia: Churchill Livingstone, 2000: pp 2543–8.

Bushby K, Finkel R, Birnkrant DJ, et al. Diagnosis and management of Duchenne muscular dystrophy, part 2: implementation of multidisciplinary care. *Lancet Neurol* 2010;**9**:177–89.

Fernández-Lorente J, Esteban A, Salinero E, et al. Critical illness myopathy. Neurophysiological and muscular biopsy assessment in 33 patients. *Rev Neurol* 2010;**50**:718–26.

Flachenecker P, Toyka KV, Reiners K. Cardiac arrhythmias in Guillain–Barré syndrome. An overview of the diagnosis of a rare but potentially life-threatening complication. *Nervenarzt* 2001;**72**:610–17.

Fletcher DD, Lawn ND, Wolter TD, Wijdicks EF. Long-term outcome in patients with Guillain–Barré syndrome requiring mechanical ventilation. *Neurology* 2000;**54**:2311–15.

Griffiths RD, Hall JB. Intensive care unit-acquired weakness. *Crit Care Med* 2010;**38**:779–87.

Gurnaney H, Brown A, Litman RS. Malignant hyperthermia and muscular dystrophies. *Anesth Analg* 2009;**109**:1043–8.

Hatheway CL. Botulism: the present status of the disease. *Curr Top Microbiol Immunol* 1995;**195**:55–75.

Hermans G, De Jonghe B, Bruyninckx F, et al. Clinical review: critical illness polyneuropathy and myopathy. *Crit Care* 2008;**12**:238.

Hermans G, Wilmer A, Meersseman W, et al. Impact of intensive insulin therapy on neuromuscular complications and ventilator dependency in the medical intensive care unit. *Am J Respir Crit Care Med* 2007;**175**:480–9.

Hill NS. Neuromuscular disease in respiratory and critical care medicine. *Respir Care* 2006;**51**:1065–71.

Plasma Exchange/Sandoglobulin Guillain–Barré Syndrome Trial Group. Randomised trial of plasma exchange, intravenous immunoglobulin, and combined treatments in Guillain–Barré syndrome. *Lancet* 1997;**349**:225–30.

Seneviratne J, Mandrekar J, Wijdicks EF, Rabinstein AA. Noninvasive ventilation in myasthenic crisis. *Arch Neurol* 2008;**65**:54–8.

Tong J, Laport G, Lowsky R. Rhabdomyolysis after concomitant use of cyclosporine and simvastatin in a patient transplanted for multiple myeloma. *Bone Marrow Transplant* 2005;**36**:739–40.

Wijdicks EF, Roy TK. BiPAP in early Guillain–Barré syndrome may fail. *Can J Neurol Sci* 2006;**33**:105–6.

Wu RS, Gupta S, Brown RN, et al. Clinical outcomes after cardiac transplantation in muscular dystrophy patients. *J Heart Lung Transplant* 2010;**29**:432–8.

Index

Neuromuscular Disorders, First Edition. Edited by Rabi N. Tawil, Shannon Venance.
© 2011 John Wiley & Sons, Ltd. Published 2011 by John Wiley & Sons, Ltd.